Psychiatry and the Humanities, Volume 5

Kierkegaard's Truth:
The Disclosure of the Self

Associate Editor
Harold A. Durfee, Ph.D.

Assistant Editor
Gloria H. Parloff

Editorial Aide
Katherine S. Henry

Published under the auspices of the
Forum on Psychiatry and the Humanities
The Washington School of Psychiatry

Psychiatry and the Humanities

VOLUME 5

Kierkegaard's Truth:
The Disclosure of the Self

Editor
Joseph H. Smith, M.D.

New Haven and London   Yale University Press

Published with assistance from the foundation established in memory of Philip Hamilton McMillan of the Class of 1894, Yale College.

Set in VIP Baskerville type.
Printed in the United States of America by Vail-Ballou Press, Binghamton, N.Y.

Library of Congress Cataloging in Publication Data

Main entry under title:

Kierkegaard's truth.

(Psychiatry and the humanities; v. 5)
"Published under the auspices of the Forum on Psychiatry and the Humanities, the Washington School of Psychiatry."
Includes bibliographical references and index.
1. Kierkegaard, Søren Aabye, 1813–1855—Addresses, essays, lectures. 2. Self (Philosophy)—Addresses, essays, lectures. 3. Personality—Addresses, essays, lectures. I. Smith, Joseph H., 1927– II. Forum on Psychiatry and the Humanities. III. Series.
[DNLM: 1. Ego. 2. Self concept. W1 PS354T v. 5 / WM 460.5.E3 K47]
RC321.P943 vol.5 [B4378.S4] 616.89s [126]
ISBN 0-300-02621-8 80-26983

10 9 8 7 6 5 4 3 2 1

Contributors

Paul B. Armstrong, Ph.D. Assistant Professor, Department of English, University of Virginia

James Collins, Ph.D. Professor of Philosophy, Saint Louis University

Harold A. Durfee, Ph.D. William Frazer McDowell Professor of Philosophy, American University

Paul L. Holmer, Ph.D. Professor of Philosophy and Theology, Yale Divinity School, Yale University

William Kerrigan, Ph.D. Associate Professor of English, University of Virginia

Bruce H. Kirmmse, Ph.D. Assistant Professor of History, Connecticut College, New London

Louis H. Mackey, Ph.D. Professor of Philosophy, University of Texas, Austin

Vincent A. McCarthy, Ph.D. Humboldt Fellow, University of Tübingen, West Germany; Assistant Professor of Philosophy, Central Connecticut State College

W. W. Meissner, S.J., M.D. Associate Clinical Professor of Psychiatry, Harvard Medical School; Faculty, Boston Psychoanalytic Institute; Staff Psychiatrist, Massachusetts Mental Health Center

Paul Ricoeur, Ph.D. Professor, Divinity School, University of Chicago; Professor, Université de Nanterre (Paris)

Mark C. Taylor, Ph.D. Associate Professor, Department of Religion, Williams College, Williamstown, Massachusetts

Michael Theunissen, Dr. phil. Professor of Philosophy, Freie Universität Berlin, West Germany

Contents

When the question of truth is raised in an objective manner, reflection is directed objectively to the truth, as an object to which the knower is related. Reflection is not focussed upon the relationship, however, but upon the question of whether it is the truth to which the knower is related. If only the object to which he is related is the truth, the subject is accounted to be in the truth. When the question of the truth is raised subjectively, reflection is directed subjectively to the nature of the individual's relationship; if only the mode of this relationship is in the truth, the individual is in the truth even if he should happen to be thus related to what is not true.

An objective uncertainty held fast in an appropriation-process of the most passionate inwardness is the truth, the highest truth attainable for an *existing* individual. At the point where the way swings off (and where this is cannot be specified objectively, since it is a matter of subjectivity), there objective knowledge is placed in abeyance. Thus the subject merely has, objectively, the uncertainty; but it is this which precisely increases the tension of that infinite passion which constitutes his inwardness. The truth is precisely the venture which chooses an objective uncertainty with the passion of the infinite.

—Søren Kierkegaard, *Concluding Unscientific Postscript* (pp. 178, 182)

Introduction

Joseph H. Smith

The truth for Kierkegaard is the truth of the self—the truth of what it is to become a self. To become such, for him, is a passionate venture in which the self achieves freedom from despair and its fundamental grounding "by relating itself to its own self and by willing to be itself . . ." (*The Sickness unto Death,* p. 147).

Subjectivity, truth, and selfhood and their connections with each other are the themes and relations upon which the psychoanalytic, literary, and philosophical contributions in this volume converge. Holmer, for example, speaks of a grammar or logic of the self. Kerrigan refers to Kierkegaard as "the prophet of the self." Collins writes on Kierkegaard's imagery of the self, Kirmmse on the social falsification of the self, Mackey on the self and the other, and Meissner reviews the place of the self as agent in the history of psychoanalysis. The importance of the issue is this: the self has assumed so central a place in the psychoanalytic thought of the recent past that to have a superficial understanding of the self is to have a superficial understanding, in general, of what it is to become a person. Our concept of the self can, I believe, be brought to both greater clarity and a more proper complexity in the light of Kierkegaard's contribution. Specifically, the current tendency to equate the self with self-representation or to consider it the integrate of conscious and unconscious self-representations will be found to fall decisively short of Kierkegaard's concept of the self as presented herein.

Of course, many of these issues regarding selfhood were raised for English readers at the time of the first Kierkegaard translations. But the renewed relevance of Kierkegaard's work arises in connection with newly gained understanding of primitive development and especially in connection with the understanding of the place of trust, on the one hand, and of guilt and precursors of guilt, on the other, in the genealogy of the self.

Good and evil are ineradicably rooted in what it is to become a person. Psychoanalytic and theological explication would both endorse that ineradicability. Each would explain it in a different though not necessarily incompatible way. Both would agree that the achieved capacities to do or be good or evil, to make the choice between good and evil, are prefigured in early forms of trust, guilt, and reparation.

Kierkegaard, in order to reach people where they were, wrote under various pseudonyms of forms of despair and stages of development that he had come to recognize as universal. The question he poses for us now is whether or to what extent we can follow his judgment of the universal significance of the stages in adult development he outlined. The aesthetic, ethical, and religious stages—are these indeed hierarchically related such that successive stages can transcend and yet include the prior stage in a higher form? Is the human situation such that every person is called upon to traverse this path? Or was Kierkegaard's journey one for him alone, the extreme solution to the extreme situation of an eccentric genius of a prior century?

These are questions variously addressed by contributors to this volume. But to the last question let me here give Kierkegaard's own answer. With absolutely no doubt of his own genius he nevertheless wrote:

> *Why did Socrates compare himself to a gad-fly?*
> Because he only wished to have ethical significance. He did not wish to be admired as a genius standing apart from others, and fundamentally, therefore, make the lives of others easy, because they could then say, "it is all very fine for him, he is a genius." No, he only did what every man can do, he only understood what every man can understand. Therein lies the epigram. He bit hard into the individual man, continually forcing him and irritating him with this 'universal.' He was a gad-fly who provoked people by means of the individual's passion, not allowing him to admire indolently and

effeminately, but demanding his self of him. If a man has ethical power people like to make him into a genius, simply to be rid of him; because his life expresses a demand. [*Journals,* pp. 97-98]

Paul Holmer, whose Weigert Lecture introduces this volume, has often reminded us of C. S. Lewis' statement that you can't study human beings but you can get to know them. That the diagnostic procedure coincides with the therapeutic one in the psychoanalytic situation also points away from the idea of purely objective study and toward a Socratic stance. The question, then, is how to evoke the individual's own conscious and unconscious knowledge of the meaning of a particular mood, thought, symptom, or any manifestation whatever that appears in the transference repetition of important life events. This is how we get to know the person and how the person comes better to know himself.

But we always also get to know ourselves better in such an encounter, and also change. I believe an interpersonal universal is involved, but one only more clearly and explicitly formulated in the work of the therapist. It is not just the therapist who "hears" what the patient is saying by also attending to his own responses, silently reviewing his own history and noting the associated mood, thought, and motive; the parent, too, in interacting with the child, similarly learns about his own parenting, both that which he gives and that which he earlier received. The parent can change on the basis of that enlarged understanding or, if too threatened, turn a deaf ear and resist change. So also with all human relationships and endeavors. We are always, more or less knowingly, concerned with the defense and/or development of ourselves. The ideal outcome of good enough mother-child, father-child, and teacher-child relationships is an individual capable of devoting himself to the relationships and work that promise the chance of further development.

In many ways, Søren Kierkegaard was an exception to the ideal development. He wrestled with the question of whether his destiny would lie in overcoming being the exception or whether, on the other hand, he was destined to devote his life to ensuring that he was a justified and not an unjustified exception. He finally accepted that his task was to be the justified exception.

To be justified, for Kierkegaard, was to become clear on that in his own life which was also a universal. To be a justified exception was to discover wherein every human is the exception. To choose being a justified exception is a choice every human is called upon to make and is to achieve being an individual, a self, a single one. Thus his outward, his conventional, exceptionality—that he could not marry Regine, that he did not take a job (for instance, the country parish he so often thought of), the oddities of his physical appearance—all became emblems of a radically inward exceptionality that he claimed was the potentiality and the task of every person. The renunciation of Regine became a sacrifice, a mutual sacrifice, in the service of a destiny that brought Kierkegaard into communion with others by delineating that exceptionality at another level, the achievement of which is the calling of each person.

A painful and passively experienced sense of being exceptional is often the motive for entering analysis. However, even though a person might think so initially, he does not undertake analysis to become normal, if normal means being like other people. The process reveals that the task is to become who he is—to actively achieve his own exceptionality. He can attempt to forsake that task in superficial adaptation to the norms of a culture or those of his analyst, as the French think Americans do, or he can assert a not-yet-gained individuality by accentuating his overt exceptionality, as Americans think the French do. But both would be forms of despair, at best, stages on the way toward a more genuine individuation.

In the mode of defensively accentuating difference, for instance, one can lay claim to acceptability either in spite of or because of his exceptionality, and Kierkegaard thought at that stage a person, like Job, should have the trust and courage to contend with God, to insist that He speak, and not just give in to misfortune with "then I must be guilty." That would be to close one's eyes and despressively insist on a childishly understood rule of retributive justice. However, when the heavens finally declare, then the contender knows that he made neither himself nor the world—that, essentially, his place in the world is not of his own doing and at that point, in the religious person, contending can give way to praise and thanksgiving.

However, Kierkegaard believed that it is only by virtue of a great struggle that a person can come to know that the struggle was not necessary. He also believed that his era was one that believed it had been granted the latter insight without struggle. He therefore took it upon himself, like Socrates, to be a gadfly, a disturber of the peace. Like other men who have achieved and become appalled by an overall view of mankind's status, he felt more hope for the common people than for the intelligentsia. At least they were not complacent, they had passion, and often misfortune, the latter perennially understood as spiritually a more advantageous position than that of being well off. The "patients" in his books, like the nameless young man of *Repetition*, are going to go further than their "doctors."

As a poet-philosopher Kierkegaard addressed himself to the intelligentsia of Denmark and the world, but his intent was to show that the task of becoming a self belongs to each person and each is equal in his potentiality to undertake it—that every person must be assumed to be in possession of what it is essentially to be a person. It is not that differences don't make a difference—they do. But what matters most is that being different from all others each person has in common with all others. The question is what each is to do about being the person he or she is.

Regarding differences of both endowment and development, Kierkegaard wrote: "The difference between the plain man's knowledge of the simple, and the simple wise man's knowledge of the same . . . . consists in the insignificant trifle that the wise man knows that he knows, or knows that he does not know, what the plain man knows" (*Postscript,* p. 204). He pictures the wise man saying to the plain man:

> My advantage is something both to laugh at and to weep over, considered as the fruit of a period of study. And yet,

> you must not hold this study in contempt, just as I do not
> myself regret it; on the contrary, it pleases me most of all
> when I smile at it, and then again enthusiastically take hold of
> the strenuous labor of thought. [*Postscript,* p. 204]

And further on he wrote:

> To be moved to reflect that before God all men are essentially
> equal, is not in truth to understand the equality, especially if
> one's daily work and striving tends in more than one way to
> bring it into forgetfulness. But precisely when most strongly
> entrenched in one's difference, then strongly to apprehend
> the equality, that is the simple wise man's noble piety. [p. 205;
> see also p. 316]

Such passages might lead us to rethink the usual differences we
attach to psychoanalysis as compared with other, sometimes
briefer, and more superficial kinds of psychotherapy. Might they
be, at their best, "superficial" only in the sense of the knowledge
here attributed to the simple wise man and at the same time be the
means of that essential knowing which, according to Kierkegaard,
both the plain and the wise man can achieve?

But strictly in Kierkegaard's terms the passages point toward
understanding his stages not in the sense that the highest endowment for and development of the aesthetic is a prerequisite
for entering into the ethical, nor, similarly, the ethical for entering into the religious. He assumed instead that all men have the
potentiality for the essentially religious. His meaning is not that
only if there is the highest development in the aesthetic or ethical
spheres is further development possible but that *even* in the case
of the highest in aesthetic or ethical development a core despair is
still enclosed. He believed that man's quest for happiness—or,
rather, man's quest for that state of being that is marked by
happiness—falls short of fulfillment whenever it falls short of the
religious.

As for the assertion that Kierkegaard wrote only as a Christian,
leaving the way of all others unmarked, there is this to be said. He
was a Christian—a believer—and he thought it as absurd to say of

Christianity "that it is to a certain degree true" as it would be to say of love that it is "to a certain degree" (*Postscript*, p. 205). However, for Kierkegaard, the "what" of belief is decisively less critical than the "how" of believing, a distinction he held even in the realm of the aesthetic (see *Postscript*, pp. 179–81).

The emphasis given here to the religious is not just an effort to understand Kierkegaard as he wanted to be understood. It has also to do with the renewed relevance of his thought. The first wave of psychological interest in Kierkegaard some thirty years ago focused on aspects of individuation, largely as typified in the adolescent era. At that time certain elements of his thought were lifted from their ultimate religious context and made the fundament of existential psychiatry and humanistic psychologies. At this time our attention is focused more on an effort to understand primitive trust—the trust of the predifferentiated state—and its relationship to adult love and adult faith, the latter still a gift but a gift to be claimed by active suspension of reason or of achieved secondary-process thought, which may be one aspect or one way of phrasing what Kierkegaard meant by a spiritual leap and what psychotherapists mean by inner change that surpasses mere intellectual insight. The current thinking, I believe, constitutes both a more essential and potentially a more fruitful confrontation between the thought of the Christian Kierkegaard and the atheist Freud.

References

Kierkegaard, S.
  The Journals of Kierkegaard [1834–55]. Edited and with introduction by
    A. Dru. New York: Harper Torchbook, 1959.
  Concluding Unscientific Postscript [1846]. Translated by D. F. Swenson
    with notes by W. Lowrie. Princeton, N.J.: Princeton University
    Press, 1968.
  The Sickness unto Death [1849] (published with *Fear and Trembling*).
    Translated by W. Lowrie. Princeton, N.J.: Princeton University
    Press, 1954.

Psychiatry and the Humanities, Volume 5

1

Post-Kierkegaard: Remarks about Being a Person

PAUL L. HOLMER

I

Just as he himself predicted with scorn and derision, Kierkegaard has been taken over by the academics. This was to him no trivial matter. He knew the academic world that surrounded him in Copenhagen and, to a lesser extent, that of Berlin. But it was not the immediate acquaintance that fed his misgivings, or the idiosyncrasies of individuals and the oddness of this or that school of thought. And it is not, surely, that he was protesting only philosophical idealism in the mode of Hegel, or historical scholarship in contrast to existential concern, or objectivity in lieu of romantic subjectivity, or, for that matter, the nihilism of the contemporary intellectuals in antithesis to the ages of faith. Anyone who believes that what he said about the academics was peculiarly engendered by the "sitz-im-leben" surely must have misread him.

So Kierkegaard notes a difference between himself and the rich men referred to in the Psalms. The latter collected wealth with great forethought and yet do not know "who shall inherit it," whereas Kierkegaard accumulated a considerable intellectual capital and knows exactly who is going to get it—the professional intellectuals, the academics. The professor or dean, the experts

The Edith Weigert Lecture, sponsored by the Forum on Psychiatry and the Humanities, Washington School of Psychiatry, Oct. 19, 1979.

on Kierkegaard, the one who makes it a job to know everything—he or she will pounce upon that literature. Kierkegaard will become what the academics can make of him, just as Shakespeare is what professors of English can make of him and Molière is what the historians of French culture say he is. It is not that the professors are less intelligent, but it is rather that there are modes of understanding, categories, and methods, easy to come by, to which they almost uniformly and thoughtlessly subscribe. The academic, we read, "is longer than the tapeworm (which a woman lately got rid of and which measured, according to her husband, who gave thanks in the paper, 200 feet), longer even than that is the 'don': and no man in whom there is the 'don' can be freed by another man from that tapeworm, only God can do that, if the man is willing."[1]

But this, obviously, poses an issue. Why, again, the scorn toward the intellectuals? Is Kierkegaard one more misologist, someone who hates or distrusts reasoning? Does he prefer passion to thought, expression to reflection, assertion to evidence, faith to reason? It is tempting to place his numerous diatribes, his remarks on absurdity, his notion that reality cannot be a system, his stress upon subjectivity, into familiar categories and thereby lump him with other anti-intellectualists, sophisticated and vulgar. But this will not finally be a successful way to understand Kierkegaard. Besides, it will only illustrate the point he is making, that the tapeworm in the professor has another way of assimilating (supposedly understanding but also dismissing) his literature than that proposed by the literature.

It might be tempting to think his scorn and sarcasm is a symptom of pride or defeated wish; but this notion, too, he predicts among the intellectuals. They will, he insists, do almost anything but engage his literature and its respective demands and will, instead, look for clues elsewhere, particularly in his life and particularly in his journal. But Kierkegaard anticipates them and promises that his journal will reveal very little of that "lowdown"

1. *The Journals of Søren Kierkegaard*, selected and trans. Alexander Dru (London: Oxford University Press, 1938), pp. 471–72.

the academics revel in. And anyone who takes the trouble to read his pages will soon enough discover that Kierkegaard has very little to hide. His works intended for publication—thirty-odd books, written mostly in an eight-year period (1842–50)—and his journals and letters, over twenty volumes, written in a twenty-year period (1835–55), are his life. This may smack of another theory, the kind he did not like, but nothing esoteric is intended. For that literature includes both objective and sheer aesthetic creations and intimate self-expression; it is both argument and logically precise polemic and passional effusion; it is in both the first-person singular and the third-person singular modes; it is both analytic description of forms of life and an unashamed avowal of Christian faith. The very multiplicity of the literature and of the kinds of responses it requires is how it tests the reader, especially the academic reader, so severely.

His notion is that his literature is primarily a way of tearing away the illusions and defenses, the silly methodologies and funded cultural responses that keep us from responding in a primitive and clear way to actual existence. His point is not to erect one more theory, one more artifice, one more permutation of reflection, by which we all are supposed to come to grips with reality. What he is about is an attack upon these and related notions. Now we come, again, to the academics. They have set forth a few notions and created some stock responses, appropriate perhaps to a wide range of topics about which we are curious. They are always after the facts; they propose hypotheses; they invent theories. This is what most of us are trained to do; and despite the vaunted difficulties and the supposed talents that are required, it cannot be too difficult to do, otherwise we could not explain how a brief period of university training succeeds so well and why there are so many who do it.

Kierkegaard is not saying what so many self-critical academics now say, almost in chorus—that the academics are positivists, or that they apply the methods of the hard sciences to all other subject matter. There are some resemblances in the criticism, but they are minor. Instead, his criticism is to the effect that the intellectuals typically fall into the pattern of thinking that forms of living, ways of being persons, ways of being aesthetic (even in the artistic sense), moral, and religious, are somehow a matter of cognitive and intellectual problems and dependent on their resolutions. His repeated remark is that we forget what it means to exist. We insist that the intellectual inquiries are the mediators, the "necessary" mediators, also, to becoming persons. We try to think existence, our personal existence, in the same way that we think everything else. He shows a radical difference.

Wittgenstein noted something similar when he pointed out that some things that people do, such as hope and grieve, fear, and even "understand," are modes or modifications in a form of life.[2] And forms of life are not so much a subject matter to be inquired into as they are a foundation beneath speaking and kinds of inquiry. Language and inquiry are more like activities engendered by a form of life than they are means of producing it. However, where Wittgenstein speaks obliquely, albeit suggestively (and this because his interest was so different), Kierkegaard speaks more fully. He draws our attention to the fact that certain forms of life, or stages, are actually like self-projections, like organized ways of responding to existence itself. Our subjectivity is in fact formed, molded, adapted, to both the way the world obtrudes upon us and the managerial pressures that each of us brings to bear upon our activities. Thus, we can be like the amoeba, without much of any form and definition. Then our responses are like tropisms. But we can also begin to adapt in conscious ways and to constitute ourselves, by choice, decisions, purposing, plans, wishes, and more. Kierkegaard's point is, however, that becoming aesthetes, or moral or religious persons, is a more primitive and more fundamental matter than is being a knower. The reason is that asking questions, becoming objective, posing problems, is something that subjects do. These activities and the relevant language-games are properly generated by the way we have responded to the need to be persons, to constitute ourselves, to effect our relations to the world around us.

2. Note particularly his *Philosophical Investigations*, 3d ed., trans. G. E. M. Anscombe (New York: Macmillan, 1970), p. 174.

The serious charge is that the reason the intellectual life produces so much confusion and so much nonsense on matters of morals and religion, such a welter of contrasting views, dozens of theologies, countless metaphysical schemes, a cacophony of "isms" on issues thought to be of the greatest moment, is that we have forgotten what it means to exist. It is not as if we lack the conclusive word and the bang-up system; our orientation is wrong. And that will not be corrected by one more theory and another conceptual system. So Kierkegaard does not provide one. But what he was sure of was that the professors would now read him as if there were a lurking scheme there nonetheless— misread his work and force it to testify to an alien scheme of reflection.

Therefore we can say with some confidence that Kierkegaard is providing a kind of diagnosis for an intellectual sickness of his time and ours. Wittgenstein noted that a certain array of philosophical issues were seemingly irresolvable, such that once one started on them one could never stop. They were not, in the form in which they occurred to one, answerable problems; instead, one's reflection would deepen the morass and the skepticism, and uncertainty would grow rather than cease. Rightly, Wittgenstein saw that language itself was the source of these problems, but this was not a trivial comment for him. He thought that the forms of language, not readily apparent to us, cause certain expectations, certain hopes, and also force questions upon us. A deep disquietude can then grip us, and we become prone to feeling that something profound is missing. We do not seem to know what time is, what length (just by itself) really means, what the good is, whether God is objective, and so forth. All of these issues we find very demanding, important, and confoundedly puzzling.[3] Wittgenstein tried with extraordinary patience and almost tireless ingenuity to show his students and readers, not a general theory about all philosophical difficulties, but, rather, the range of linguistic and other facts that were already around. For very obscure reasons, it was, he thought, very hard to get at these facts for

3. *Philosophical Investigations,* pp. 47 and 42.

oneself. Some of the problems, then, typically philosophical problems, were not genuine. One could, after a while, see that for oneself.

To say the following is not to denigrate Wittgenstein's thought. But Kierkegaard, independent of some of the currents of thought later imbibed by Wittgenstein, suggested that the confusions on moral and religious matters in particular could not be dispelled by attention only to language. It is not that there is disagreement, for their issues were not quite the same. Kierkegaard thought in addition that there was an odd reluctance, perhaps almost an aversion, to becoming clear about what it meant to be an existing human subject. Once one saw it, and then remembered it always, a kind of clarification could ensue. But as with Wittgenstein, so Kierkegaard also sees that this cannot be done for anyone else.

The tapeworm in all of us with academic proclivities begins to rebel. We insist that Wittgenstein is a linguistic analyst, and we formulate a theory about what philosophy is and does and allow the understanding of Wittgenstein's work to be consummated in our theory and his. No wonder, he, too, felt repelled by the prospect of all those intellectual hangers-on, trying to determine what he was up to. His pages are a discipline and a way, not another theory. In Kierkegaard's case, the academic world has had to invent another category, namely, existentialism. Here he becomes an advocate by induction, a progenitor by anticipation, of a school of thought, a metaphysician and a system-builder despite himself. All the while, he had predicted this and took it as one more instance of the malady of popular thought and pedagogical devices.

I have said that the chief task cannot be done for another person. Certainly a theory or a summary will not be the means. And this is where the way swings off from the typical academic pattern. Kierkegaard's entire literature, including his *Journal,* is calculated not to give theories, nor quite to provide a therapy, but is designed to be something radically different from the traditional literature on morals and matters of faith. One can scarcely exaggerate the importance of his pseudonyms, of the oddness of his writings, of the entire shape of his work. It is as if a radical reordering of thought and discourse was necessary. He had to invent a genre and, in so doing, he stands outside the mainstream of thought and language of the Western philosophical and theological tradition.

His literature is not calculated to say all the important things, for they cannot be said. For example, the reality and requirement for the individual, he notes, is to develop self-concern and an avidity for being a person. Therefore, he shows us individuals, a rich variety of them, with all kinds of self-interest, enthusiasm, despair, and the rest. The literature, then, is not a theory so much as it is a locus for forms of life and kinds of subjectivity. But it is more than a spectacle, too, more than merely word-pictures and a display of personae. It is calculated both to show something (show it, not say it) and also to create unrest and an activity in the reader. It tries to communicate so that we become something different, realize new capacities, and activate our own personality.

But we need to pause here. The literature is two things. The kinds of subjectivity, the forms of life, are there. It might well be that the reader might want to become a dashing Don Juan, an ethically modulated judge, a vagrant dreamy lover of womankind, or what-have-you. That is certainly likely given a variety of readers. But the literature also provides a comment upon itself, a kind of intellectual shaping that pulls the miscellany together and abridges in a set of rules and themes what is otherwise shown us. Kinds of pathos, indeed, but they are not random. They have conditions, causes, antecedents, relations, effects; and the commentary-literature is perpetrated chiefly by Johannes Climacus, Kierkegaard's pseudonymous-philosopher. So there is some philosophy, after all, but still not a theory.

For Kierkegaard is doing both a poetical job, sketching the differing kinds of subjectivity, and also providing what he calls a dialectical component. The latter has a genuinely philosophical ring to it. But while Hegel and Marx used "dialectic" to describe an interpretative method by which both entities and thoughts could arise, oppose one another, and be synthesized, Kierkegaard means something far plainer. For him, dialectic is simply a name for the conceptual scheme, the algebraic rubrics, that will hang matters together. It is as if there is a logic, a grammar, a catena of concepts, that rules human subjectivity too. There is a grammar of the self—some rules for human subjectivity. And the conceptual scheme describes and projects that grammar. The human self is actually the synthesizing agent, where differences are put together. But his philosophy, insofar as he can be said to have one at all, is not the truth one needs; rather, it is like an account of the relations between pathos and thought, emotion and belief, that make up the way in which we do form our lives.

Opposed to the logic of the attempt to explain human persons, even the self, by general laws and theories, Kierkegaard's writing will loom up, suggesting another logic, which involves a rethinking of the notions of subjectivity, objectivity, and the self. In all, then, I am here proposing that the logic of the self is within reach, in fact, in the Kierkegaard literature. But the self is even closer to all of us than that. If Kierkegaard's logic is right, then we have the means both to become genuinely transparent persons, defensible and justified, and to steer away from the jungle of thought that makes personality theory so bizarre and moral and religious questions so stupefyingly confusing. A big order? Of course. But Kierkegaard never said it could be done on paper or in a theory. His point was that such problems would lose their hold on us, not by being answered, but by being made pointless.

II

Kierkegaard's work, sprawling as it first seems, is closely governed by some very demanding conceptions and rules. He wrote a spate of fifteen books from 1842 to 1846, eight of them pseudonymous, another seven short ones rather mildly religious. From 1846 through 1850 came another fifteen or so, these were strenuous and more definitively Christian. Most of these fit together and articulate a plan, even a kind of logic, that is morphological and also the means of effecting a teaching aim. But this takes a little explaining.

Most readers find his pseudonymous works difficult to cite if they take Søren Kierkegaard's admonition seriously. He warns his reader not to quote them as if the opinions in them were Kierkegaard's; instead, they are the pseudonym's. Obviously, these subauthors are Kierkegaard's creation and, almost like characters in a novel, are variously related to their author. But there is a difference. Kierkegaard's pseudonymous works do play a role in the literature as a whole, and that has a purpose, a "telos," not identical with what is stated in any single book. The whole literature "shows," after a while, by its very shape and the uses that are appropriate, what cannot be said without falsifying that purpose. That purpose is a realization in the life of a reader and not one more theory about human lives.

Thinking about this from another angle, we can see that the opinions, views, and evaluations of the pseudonyms—embedded in their language about the world, themselves, and their goals— are both "about" this or that (i.e., their words typically refer) and also "of" (i.e., in part, an expression of) a "form of life," or "stage." Therefore, to cite them as if they were of Kierkegaard's point of view would mean that one could see in all of this what stage or form of life Kierkegaard himself occupied. But this is absurd, for the stages are multiple. And Kierkegaard was not concealing himself by the pseudonymous authorship. Rather, he thought it preposterous to invoke his own authority for something like a fundamental mode of living and erected ideal "personae" really to divert attention from himself and to maximize the activation of the capabilities and power of each of his readers. The intrusion of the author's authority would vitiate the creation and sustaining of an authorizing activity on the part of the reader. By the same token, Kierkegaard's point of view cannot be easily surmised from the literature.

But there is something else. The literature *says* a variety, a plurality, but it *shows* a unity. And that unifying force and movement, everything working together, is not only the anticipation of a telos but hangs together in other ways as well. There are rules embedded, a morphology that takes shape, a logic that is disclosed. Furthermore, all of that can be articulated linguistically. Perhaps this sounds like more academic shenanigans, but that depends upon whether one realizes that "how" in a way that is consonant with what is shown. For if a rule becomes clear, then a rule is a rule. But the point being made here is that a certain kind of realization, a certain kind of understanding, can also dawn in the appropriate reader. Kierkegaard begins to describe that understanding as the pseudonymous literature unwinds. But he is not providing it in his philosophical-like remarks. Such an understanding does allow a linguistic expression of it, but the linguistic expression, in turn, is not the understanding but is "of" it. Thus, "truth is subjectivity" is a piece of philosophy. It is not a super theory. It is more like what Wittgenstein would have called a "grammatical remark." Therefore, its use is, again, to call attention to the way to think about moral religious matters—not the least of which is how to use the word "truth" in these special areas of concern.

Hence, throughout Kierkegaard's work, even the pseudonymous literature, something firm, nonconjectural, and deep is being articulated. Part of that is a radically different grammar of human life that begins to show itself as his literature flows forth. But it has to be carefully described. It is not as though Kierkegaard were a philosophical innovator. Nor is this grammar and logic of the self quite a novelty and what he jokingly called another "matchless discovery." Rather, it is the very grammar of the way we must live if we are to become true persons.

So another comment about his literature as a totality is in order. Kierkegaard thought it something like a literary abridgement of human existence itself. That is why, again, it is not a theory of human existence. For the correct mood for a theory is a disinterested mood, one of detachment and even curiosity. But this is no way to respond to existence itself. Our daily life requires commitment, long-term wants, even passions and deep feelings. It is Kierkegaard's notion that understanding ourselves and our tasks already supposes highly qualified interests. Hence, he attacks the academic convention that most of us illustrate, that first we must have the understanding (the theory) and this disinterestedly; and secondly, and subsequently, that the emotions and pathos will then follow as a matter of course. Instead, he designs his literature to accord with actual existence. We are in an examination where we cannot cheat, and existence examines us and demands a response, not the other way around.

Actuality affords everywhere around us all kinds of examples. We are, as Aristotle noted centuries ago, numerically distinct, and in this sense we are individuated. And we can add details nowadays about the extent and degree of individual differences. Thus far, most would probably admit, there is nothing very interesting about the "differentia." Another task confronts each of us. We have to become persons. Kierkegaard thought there was only a limited variety of ways of being a person and this despite the radical character of individuality itself. So he sketches some idealized characterizations in the aesthetic, ethical, ethico-religious, and Christian modes. He does it with a variety of pseudonyms, most of which are variants of these "stadie." The "stages on life's way" are not strictly chronological nor are they life-phases. They are more like ways that lives get formed, when choice is exercised, when decisions are made, when ideas are taken seriously, when pathos is educated. Each of them is a synthesis of emotion, idea, disposition, will, and plan. Kierkegaard's point is that our life in the world both elicits and permits a rich variety of character and thought, of pathos and ideas of ourselves.

If this were all that his literature set forth, it might seem as chaotic as our physical and social life itself—relative, absurd, radically contingent, and almost without available criteria. But Kierkegaard's literature does not just represent or reproduce. It is designed to be an occasion for bringing the person and the self to birth. In contradistinction to existence itself, it does so by presenting idealized persons, the pseudonyms, who are more distinct than historical personages; and their oppositions, polemical postures, and criteria are thereby brought into sharper focus and a tighter compass. His literature both compresses human circumstances and distills the consequences of the forms of life we all choose, so that we can get a more acute picture of what is involved. Therefore, the literature clarifies both by its idealizations and by shortening the period between antecedent choices and their kinds of consequents. Thereupon two kinds of critieria begin to emerge. On the one hand, we begin to see that we all are made for an enduring happiness. Then the anxiety, restlessness, and other kinds of pathos, even dread and despair, do not loom up as odd and casual effects, but instead can be discerned as symptoms of the ineffectual and hapless kinds of selves we have brought to birth. Then the achievement of happiness is not only a goal but also a part of the very logic of human living.

But another kind of criterion is also made manifest. We shall note more of this matter later, but suffice it here to point out that achieving selfhood is not a biological and/or simply a sociological attainment. Kierkegaard causes us to see in the manifold of his literature that being a human individual requires us also to become agents on behalf of our own selfhood. We have to learn to think our own existence. We have to become conscious of ourselves and to develop a passionate concern about the quality of our lives. But Kierkegaard's point is, in addition, that forms of life differ in the degree that they require and sustain such self-reflection, self-concern, and self-intending. Thus, we see via his pseudonyms that an aesthete may be constituted by accident, by idiosyncrasies, by "raw material," by chance, and by the fortuitous concatenation of circumstances that a family or an environment provides. Kierkegaard contends that such a form of life breeds its own dissatisfaction, eventually a kind of despair at not thinking and willing one's own selfhood.

The ethical mode of life, by contrast, does make the individual's selfhood a topic of thought, and a genuine pursuit too. Then passion can be organized upon a major task. And Kierkegaard's reflection is to the effect that a kind of propriety and intellectual transparency then confirms the individual. We seem never to regret reflection that helps organize and constitute ourselves. Thoughtfulness that focuses upon such a conquest finds its own reward. More than this, Kierkegaard has one of his later pseudonyms summarize the grammar of this religio-moral outlook by saying that "The self is a relation which relates itself to itself. . . ."[4] To say the self is a "relation" implies that it is not a

4. This is presented in *The Sickness unto Death,* trans. Walter Lowrie (Princeton, N.J.: Princeton University Press, 1941), p. 17. But an idea like this is also marked

substance nor a material thing, neither the body nor the mind. To be a self is to be a relating agency, putting together mind and body, future and present, impulses and duties. Our thinking demands an identity between thinking and its object, and there is no identity until the self as a perduring relation comes into view. This is why we can say that all of us keep pursuing another form of the self either until happiness is achieved or until we have chosen and achieved by thought that object, that selfhood, that turns out to be satisfying. Both passion and thought, then, find their resolution and satisfaction in a form of selfhood.

The self as a relation is never done, once and for all. It is also a kind of activity, nurtured by choosing, willing, judging, and thinking. But this is thinking one's own quality of existence and hence is passionate thinking, not disinterested, not theoretical, and not objective (in the customary uses of that term). Neither is it simply wishful thinking or projection. It is about something, hence it is objective after all, meaning then that it "refers" and is not idle; but this use of "objective" does not exclude interest and concern. Kierkegaard would have it that people are people precisely because they must think about their own existence. Like Samuel Johnson, who said that we are geometers by chance, moralists by necessity, Kierkegaard knew that without moral concern and passion we would never be selves at all. The "self" is a "how," not a "what"; and the burden of Kierkegaard's literature is to activate the reader's concern about what he himself is and to provide the reader that foreshortened range of possibilities which will show them to be available under a variety of conditions.

III

It is in a context like that already noted, then, that Kierkegaard begins to clarify the reader's thought—not the least, one might easily suppose, with respect also to what being an existing person requires. But all of that is done polemically too. Much of that

---

by Judge Wilhelm, *Either/Or*, trans. Walter Lowrie (Princeton, N.J.: Princeton University Press, 1944), pp. 180 ff.

polemic is set up by what he calls "the errors of a scientific-scholarly outlook." To make his point even more decisively, he says that there has been in his day a "scientific-scholarly abrogation of the dialectical element."[5] A rephrasing of the latter might allow us to say that the concepts describing persons are now displaced: they are invariably put into a doctrinal and theoretical context. So, too, Christianity is not totally abolished, he says, but the fate of a person, as citizen, aesthete, ethicist, even as a Christian, is now couched as theory or as doctrine. Then the logic becomes wrong, even though the right components are present. The result is fantastic mistakes on several counts. We forget, but, of course, very learnedly, what it means to exist; we mis-describe the self; and we transfer our passion from the effort to become true persons to the effort of searching out the right theory or objective truth about persons.

But here we will take another hint from Kierkegaard's writings. He spoke about the abolition of the "navigation guides," about a confusion being introduced by thinking, not just by the absence of thinking. Therefore, we will turn to a difficult range of contemporary thought, where we find a kind of understanding of man, modernized by reference to the current ethos and, if Kierkegaard is right, made almost intractable by scholarly-scientific attitudes. All of these tend to cluster for us and could be given all kinds of documentation. Some of them are found among followers of Freud, but they are typically endemic to any of those who also want to be objective and scientific about persons.

In the flurry of enthusiasm for resolving typically human difficulties—wretchedness, depression, crime, antisocial behavior, and a host more—most of us are prone to think that persons are infinitely complex, that the variables are hence too many at present for our schemes of knowing. "The confusion and barrenness of psychology is not to be explained," said Wittgenstein,

5. *Armed Neutrality and An Open Letter,* trans. Howard V. Hong and Edna H. Hong (Bloomington: Indiana University Press, 1968), pp. 6 and 7. Other remarks about thinking in the wrong manner about the right matters are to be found in the *Postscript*.

"by calling it a 'young science'. . . ."[6] But most of us are not so bold. We lament the failure to produce a science of human nature, but then we excuse the present state by saying that psychology is too new a discipline and that the subject matter—namely, persons—is infinitely variegated. Wittgenstein thought that psychology was beset by "conceptual confusion," hence its barrenness. Kierkegaard would surely agree, but he also would be quick to deny the idea that the failure of the objective theory is due to the complexity of people.

This state of intellectual affairs, if not people themselves, is a confusion. Most of us have come to believe that we need to explain human behavior in order to help persons be themselves and even find themselves. Almost without thinking about it, we accede to the conviction that if we are going to explain, we must also find some general laws. But there seem to be so few, and those we have either are banalities that cover human behavior far too generally or are so specific that they address issues not germane to the problems that truly bother us. Hence, the domain called psychology has to include those who complain about the irrelevance of psychology made exact, and, on the other hand, those who insist that if it becomes humane and immediately relevant, then it becomes literature, speculation, and certainly not an exact science. It is easy to say, then, that psychology has as yet no general laws, that we still wait for a Galileo on human nature who could provide us with a powerful "field-theory." Besides, where there are still competing theories that make up schools of thought and "isms," there does seem to be something deeply awry. For Kierkegaard it was more than conceptual confusion.

Of course, we can always insist upon the subtlety of persons. That idea has a gratifying kind of flattery about it, and, besides, it keeps the idea alive that we can still have our science in the future, if not quite right now. For if persons are so subtle, it might be that we need, above all, a more refined conceptual system. The possibility that human behavior is so subtle that it slips through our

6. *Philosophical Investigations*, p. 232.

rough conceptual nets of thought has not gone unnoticed. Once more, we do have all kinds of examples, and most of them generate a need for a more detailed kind of behavior analysis and a correspondingly more precise set of hypotheses and language tools.

But this scholarly-scientific method, if Kierkegaard is right, tends after a while to generate difficulties and to maximize all sorts of uncertainties. To keep alive this mode of understanding—namely, that we cannot really know ourselves and others until we do it objectively (and by theory)—we do have to explain our failures. So, we begin to say that persons are mysterious, that they are deep, that they are private, that motives for many actions are unconscious, that they are mythic-oriented, that structures are embedded in our life-histories; some would even say that every person is radically idiosyncratic and defies anything beyond enumeration.

All of this may only seem like more philosophy of science. What I am saying here, however, has two loci in Kierkegaard's thought and hence weighty consequences. There is, first, the conviction that a fundamental mistake about persons is being made. But this is not a case of one theory versus another, Kierkegaard's versus Freud's several, or versus behaviorism or neobehaviorism. If that obtained, then we would still have to pursue the right theory or theories, in preference to the wrong ones. Kierkegaard is not suggesting even the corrigibility of a theory. His point is rather that the logic of theories is altogether faulty, that in principle theories cannot be right because people are not subtle, obtuse to our schemes, and infinitely variable. Just why and how this can be said, we will subsequently assay. The logic of this argument—again, if not people themselves—is probably subtle and certainly unfamiliar. His philosophical-like remark is not speculation or wild metaphysics; it is a kind of rulelike piece of grammar about the way people are. So he is saying that theories, indeed multiple about human persons, do not make real sense. They create dogmatism and schools simply because they are nonempirical and in consequence of the lack of another kind of self-knowledge.

There is, secondly, another issue. The attempt to generate objective knowledge about the self in order to explain and to understand human nature engenders its own cacaphony of views. There is no way out of this intellectual impasse through more research, better evidence, closer observation, and more detailed theories. And this is only, then, the other locus that his literature is. It speaks to this matter not so much directly as indirectly. For science here becomes a costly diversion. In the name of seriousness and of understanding, it distracts us even more. Kierkegaard's literature, therefore, is an attempt not to do more general philosophy except inadvertently: that grammar obtrudes itself upon us when we submit to his literature. But his literature itself does something quite different. It attacks our feelings, our pathos, our indifference, by stimulating self-concern and magnifying our anxiety, our despair, and our guilt. For these, rather than being only problems to be resolved, also have to become the very means and motives for seeking a new form of life. What science and scholarship ask us to bracket for the sake of understanding, Kierkegaard asks us to augment for the sake of bringing the self to birth.

In a journal entry for 1849, Kierkegaard notes: "In relation to good as well as evil, to the demonic as well as to the religious, it requires that we be an Ego—a well-developed ego, a subjectivity. Most men do not have sufficient subjectivity even to let Divine Governance get a grip on them, and therefore, in the deepest sense, they become neither good nor evil, only a mélange."[7] In another book, *Concluding Unscientific Postscript,* Kierkegaard's pseudonymic philosopher Johannes Climacus plots much of that extraordinary work around the issue of how the subjectivity of the individual must be qualified in order that certain issues come to exist for him.

In brief, it is the case that Kierkegaard's literature rephrases the issue of psychology and the nature of man, and this in a radical manner. The failure to achieve self-knowledge lies neither with faulty intellectual tools nor with the infinite complexity or the

7. *Papirer,* 2d ed. (Copenhagen: Gyldendal, 1968), vol. X, pt. I, pp. 50–51 (my translation). (The Danish manner of noting this entry is X' A 65, 1849.)

inherent privacy of persons. Everything here, Kierkegaard notes in a journal entry, "depends upon being well constructed."[8]

IV

One would be unfair to Kierkegaard if one left matters in this generalized psychological mode. For he is, first and last, a religious and Christian writer. But this did not keep him from noting the logic and rhythm of the subjective life and from seeing the oddness of human psychology. Still, he adds another note. This is, plainly, that Christianity provides through the Bible a kind of self-knowledge that one gets nowhere else. It is as though the Bible also educates us, not by providing the truths and the right doctrine, but by being a mirror in which we see ourselves. Then, the religious life becomes an adventure in self-knowledge and not just a matter of believing. God in Christ even supplies a new capacity in people.

This self-knowledge, too, manifests a duality, held together by the relation that is the self. So one again has a powerful passion that is born in the person. This is a love for God in virtue of which one will also love all others. Faith in God creates a happy passion, as Kierkegaard calls it, that one can never regret nor disparage. This love, of course, is not just eroticism brought to a wide compass. Kierkegaard shows us how that love is brought to our attention, not as a natural development, but from the outside, by the life and teaching of Jesus Christ. As the Apostle Paul said in introducing the hymn to love in the *Epistle to the Corinthians,* Kierkegaard too thinks that we are here shown "a better way." Some kinds of love are natural capacities and are implicit in the person and only need manifestation in our lives; but the Christian kind of love is acquired from the outside, from the story of Jesus Christ and His love for the world. Even Christianity must be chosen. An activity, a decision, a passionate preoccupation, is requisite. This is why Kierkegaard insists that human life is itself a form of "becoming," not a state of "being." Once that "becoming," that process of concern and pathos, is terminated, the self becomes

8. *Papirer,* IV A 166, 1843–44 (my translation).

obscured and character is dissipated. The point is, initially, not the truth or falsity of views of life. Respecting such an issue, Kierkegaard is convinced that there is a large measure of objective uncertainty. If one raises the question in the disinterested mode, one sees nothing but relativities and alternatives, each responsible to the facts; but one's choice is never determinable by anything like evidence, probabilities, or even authority. To ask a question in that disinterested manner is to forget the logic of existence and the fundamental grammar of life. The fact that the learned people so frequently have their passion skewed in this way, actually diverted from what they, in principle, can do something about and must do something about, to something that looks intellectual and respectable—namely, the objective truth—but which finally cannot be ascertained, is all the more a reason for Kierkegaard's work—which aims to make one's personal existence the major concern. His work does this by making the case for the objective uncertainty glaringly, by stirring self-consciousness, by clarifying despair so that it at least is acknowledged, by proposing anew the idealities, like happiness, forgiveness, peace of mind, hope, so that they will indeed attract one to a high calling.

This, then, is also how Christianity becomes amenable and commensurate with persons. For only when one is desperate, even broken-hearted about oneself, does faith begin to cohere with one's life. Only when we are sick and need the physician will the life of faith acquire any plausibility. Otherwise it is only one more cultural accretion and by and large a superstition, a bit of poetry, or a kind of speculative metaphysics. Logically it will all look like paradox, which says little that is cogent or pertinent. But once the pathos of the individual is developed, a rich subjectivity cultivated, then and then only will any kind of relation between the finite and the infinite, between God and man, even become likely. In Christian terms, man's need for God is his highest perfection. That need for God will not occur unless there are crises in the subjective life. Until pathos has been made deeply unhappy by the consciousness of what we have made of ourselves there will be no need for a savior. Then a new pathos can ensue as we dare to let go and allow God to make of us what we could not. Here is where a new subjectivity and the true self emerges.

Is it any wonder then that Kierkegaard could say:

> What the age needs is true pathos (in the same way that scurvey requires vegetables); for not even the work of drilling an artesian well is any more subtle than the calculated dialectics of humor, emotion, and passion, with which I have sought to establish a provident flush of feeling. The misfortune of our age is reflection and understanding. . . .[9]

The grammar of human life suggests that sense has to be made out of ordinary lives. This is the grammar, the logic, that Kierkegaard has stated algebraically and formally with his theme of "stages on life's way." But the grammar is only useful if it is a rule for how we conduct ourselves. Kierkegaard obeyed that grammar himself by so poetizing the aesthetic, the ethical, and even the Christian forms of life that they would incite, not just inform; that they could stimulate an activity, not just titillate curiosity. Almost incidentally but with a firm hold upon both the details and the morphological issue, it becomes clear both that a science of selfhood is a chimera and that knowledge of oneself and others as selves is dependent upon moral development, not cognitive skill.

9. *Papirer*, VIII A 92.

2

Reading Kierkegaard—Disorientation and Reorientation

PAUL B. ARMSTRONG

I

Reading Kierkegaard is a bewildering experience. The dialectical verbal pyrotechnics, the paradoxical turns in the argument, the pseudonyms that mask an author who refuses to make his point straightforwardly—all of these and other characteristic features of Kierkegaard's strategy of indirect communication disorient even the most sophisticated reader. Kierkegaard disorients readers in order to expose and criticize their habits of construing the world—habits that would not be questioned if the expectations they project were confirmed. Since the reader's habits of understanding reflect his presuppositions, a challenge to those habits is also a challenge to his beliefs. Shaking him loose from his customary bearings, Kierkegaard disorients the reader in order to reorient him.[1] The bewilderment he experiences paves the way for an introduction to new ways of understanding and for a reorientation of his beliefs.

Most of Kierkegaard's best students agree that he attempts to educate his audience through the very activity of reading.[2] But it

1. I borrow the notion of "reorientation by disorientation" from Paul Ricoeur, "Listening to the Parables of Jesus," in *The Philosophy of Paul Ricoeur,* eds. Charles E. Reagan and David Stewart (Boston: Beacon, 1978), p. 244.

2. Mark C. Taylor summarizes the consensus when he argues that "Kierkegaard becomes a Socratic midwife" through his pseudonyms: "the reader becomes a participant" in a "dialogue" where "the midwife seeks to bring to birth

is rare for them to examine in detail the experience of reading that his indirect works propose. This may reflect the fact that literary theorists have only recently developed ways of studying the experience of reading without lapsing into the vague impressionism that Wimsatt and Beardsley warn against when they denounce the "affective fallacy."[3] Every reader experiences a work differently in some respects, but we can still identify and describe the role a work assigns to readers as the condition of a legitimate response. Since each of Kierkegaard's works sets somewhat different tasks for his readers, we must single out one text for detailed study. Kierkegaard's *Fear and Trembling* has been called "the work that most perfectly expresses his special genius" in the art of indirect communication.[4] A close examination of *Fear and Trembling* may reveal in heightened form the kind of education that the strategy of indirect communication offers.

Before we begin our analysis, two frequently cited obstacles to the study of the reader's role deserve brief consideration: the changing situations of readers throughout history and the difficulty of validating a description of an experience that seems essentially private. Reading is unquestionably a historically situated activity. Kierkegaard's contemporaries and modern readers necessarily approach his works from different vantage points. His contemporaries would be in a better position to understand Kierkegaard's attacks against Hegelianism, for example, and his ref-

---

truth in the reader" (*Kierkegaard's Pseudonymous Authorship: A Study of Time and the Self* [Princeton, N.J.: Princeton University Press, 1975], p. 60). For an analysis of the experience of the reader in the Socratic dialogues, see Stanley E. Fish, *Self-Consuming Artifacts* (Berkeley: University of California Press, 1972), pp. 5–21.

3. See William K. Wimsatt, Jr., and Monroe C. Beardsley, *The Verbal Icon* (Lexington: University of Kentucky Press, 1954), pp. 21–39. The most persuasive program for studying the reader's experience is Wolfgang Iser's "The Reading Process: A Phenomenological Approach," in *The Implied Reader* (Baltimore: Johns Hopkins University Press, 1974), pp. 274–94. Also see Iser, *The Act of Reading* (Baltimore: Johns Hopkins University Press, 1978).

4. Stephen Crites, "Pseudonymous Authorship as Art and as Act," in *Kierkegaard: A Collection of Critical Essays,* ed. Josiah Thompson (Garden City, N.Y.: Doubleday, Anchor, 1972), p. 219. Also see Edith Kern, *Existential Thought and Fictional Technique* (New Haven: Yale University Press, 1970), p. 17.

erences to persons and events in Copenhagen. But particularly innovative texts such as his pseudonymous works may require interpretive abilities that only develop in future generations of readers.[5] It is wrong to attempt to turn back the clock by pretending that we can reconstruct the experience of the contemporaneous reader. What matters is how the horizons of past and present meet in the process of engaging a text. My analysis focuses on aspects of reading Kierkegaard that a modern audience might experience.

The problem of validity is responsible for charges that analyses of reading may fall into the trap of relativism, even solipsism. These charges are misguided, since interpretations of the reading experience raise no difficulties of validation that are not shared by all methods of literary analysis. Any interpretation, whatever the method behind it, can claim validity only to the extent that it persuades other readers that what it discloses is confirmed by their own experience with the text. The charge of subjectivism often reflects a reification of the literary work into a "formal structure"—a reification which ignores that the literary "object" exists only as a construction abstracted from concrete experiences of reading. Like all other kinds of interpretation, my analysis seeks to claim validity by persuading readers either that they have experienced what I describe or, if they haven't, that they would become more adequate readers by attuning themselves to the process I outline.

The process of reorientation by disorientation in *Fear and Trembling* is geared toward two issues central to Kierkegaard's thought: the status of "truth" and the problematic, paradoxical relation between the finite and the infinite. According to one of Kierkegaard's pseudonyms, "truth exists for the particular individual only as he himself produces it in action."[6] As part of its program of disorientation, *Fear and Trembling* seeks to upset the

5. For a further exploration of this issue, see Hans Robert Jauss, "Literary History as a Challenge to Literary Theory," in *New Directions in Literary History*, ed. Ralph Cohen (Baltimore: Johns Hopkins University Press, 1974), pp. 11–41.

6. Søren Kierkegaard, *The Concept of Dread*, trans. Walter Lowrie (Princeton, N.J.: Princeton University Press, 1957), p. 123.

reader's confidence that truth exists absolutely, in fixed and certain form independent of human action. What we understand as "true," Kierkegaard's readers learn, depends on how we comport ourselves, so that "truth" varies according to the position from which we act and the presuppositions that govern our practice. If truth depends so completely on man's finite practice, then the infinite is not ultimately comprehensible except as the horizon of human activity. In Kierkegaard's view, as one writer puts it, "God is revealed to man only negatively, as man's limit."[7] *Fear and Trembling* disorients the reader by dramatizing the limits that prevent religious belief from attaining the security of positive, certain knowledge. It reorients the reader by showing how, paradoxically, man can nonetheless comport himself toward what lies beyond his horizons by making "the movements of faith."[8] Kierkegaard's reader is shown that faith is a way of understanding that occupies a privileged but precarious position on the boundary between the finite and the infinite.

The movements of disorientation and reorientation in *Fear and Trembling* are inextricably intertwined. Every disorientation is also a reorientation. For the sake of clarity, however, let us split these movements apart—concentrating on the disorienting aspects first.

7. Josiah Thompson, *Kierkegaard* (New York: Knopf, 1973), p. 186.

8. Søren Kierkegaard, *Fear and Trembling* (published with *The Sickness unto Death*), trans. Walter Lowrie (Princeton, N.J.: Princeton University Press, 1954), p. 48; *Frygt og Bæven* in *Søren Kierkegaard: Samlede Værker* (Copenhagen: Glydendal, 1963), 5:36. Subsequent references will be given parenthetically in the text with the English edition cited first and then the Danish in italics, thus: p. 48/*36*.

Translations pose a particularly thorny problem for analyses of reading. Reading Kierkegaard in Danish is obviously different from reading him in an English translation. Most of these differences occur on the phonetic and syntactic levels—the levels where individual signs combine. With a good translation, the broad movements of meaning on the semantic level should closely approximate the original. I will point out important divergences between the Danish text and the English translation when they occur. For the most part, however, my analysis operates at a general semantic level where the experience of construing meaning is comparable for Danish and English readers.

II

In his prolonged meditation on the story of Abraham, the narrator of *Fear and Trembling* demonstrates a remarkably resourceful command of a variety of disorienting strategies. The policy behind Johannes de Silentio's many strategies is to frustrate his readers' expectations by making strange what they take for granted. He makes authority strange, for example, in order to show that truth may come to seem fixed and certain not because it is ultimately independent of human action but because the privilege claimed by such institutional arbiters of validity as philosophers and pastors has gone unquestioned. By frustrating their expectations, Kierkegaard's narrator also shows his readers that what they think they understand perfectly may only be something they are overly familiar with. If we are too familiar with something, he suggests, we can easily forget that our knowledge depends solely on our own actions and expectations.

Johannes de Silentio challenges authority by making it strange in the very first sentences of *Fear and Trembling:*

> Not merely in the realm of commerce but in the world of ideas as well our age is organizing a regular clearance sale. Everything is to be had at such a bargain that it is questionable whether in the end there is anybody who will want to bid. Every speculative price-fixer who conscientiously directs attention to the significant march of modern philosophy, every *Privatdocent,* tutor, and student, every crofter and cottar in philosophy, is not content with doubting everything but goes further. [p. 22/9]

Specifically targeted at the speculative Hegelian philosophers of his time, the narrator's polemic against "going further" than faith may seem somewhat outdated to modern readers. But the general thrust of his attack retains the power to reach across historical distance. Even modern readers do not expect to find philosophers compared to "price-fixers" and salesmen. The commercial metaphor makes strange the status of philosophers in order to open for question their privileged role as arbiters of truth. As an indictment against them for cheapening understanding, this metaphor attacks the "virtuosity in self-deception" (p. 130/*109*) that allows the unquestioning (and not just the philosophers) to "live secure in existence" (p. 73/*58*). The narrator's attack aims to undermine the fixity of accepted ideas that pretend to deliver certain truth but actually deceive in the very pretense that truth is fixed and certain. Although "doubting" and "going further" may seem the height of activity, the demystifying commercial metaphor indicts the philosophers for reifying truth—for treating meaning as a product rather than a process, as a commodity to be obtained rather than an activity to be pursued. Truth is not a commodity that specially trained workers produce for the reader to purchase ready-made in the market place. Thrust back on his own authority, the reader must produce truth for himself.

Johannes de Silentio also challenges authority and attacks the reification of truth by playing with different strategies of beginning. Ordinarily, readers expect meaning to disclose itself in a stable, regular fashion, as the beginning of a sentence, a text, or any intelligible state of affairs leads to the middle and then to the end.[9] But the narrator of *Fear and Trembling* complains that "people are curious about the result, as they are about the result in a book—they want to know nothing about dread, distress, the paradox" (p. 74/*59*). As part of his assault on his readers' habits of understanding, the narrator refuses their quest for "the result" by refusing to orient their expectations straightforwardly at the outset. His title page pretends to meet the reader's expectations, for example, but actually defies them. Readers expect a title to help them anticipate what will follow; but what does *Fear and Trembling* refer to? It gives little direct hint that an extended meditation on Abraham is ahead. In addition to a title, the first page of Johannes de Silentio's book gives a generic classification of the work. A

---

9. See Iser, "The Reading Process," on the reader's effort "to fit everything together in a consistent pattern" (pp. 283–90); also see Frank Kermode, *The Sense of an Ending* (Oxford: Oxford University Press, 1966).

sense of the genre to which a work belongs allows readers to gear themselves toward it according to their expectations about that genre. But what is a "Dialectical Lyric"? Aren't these two terms contradictory—the one philosophical and logical, the other poetic and personal? Like the title, this generic self-description pretends to orient the reader while refusing to do so.[10] As part of the process of disorientation, the title page leaves the reader wondering and bewildered about how to begin. Kierkegaard's text defies its readers to submit themselves to it as an authority that will hand over its "truth" in a simple report of results.

Refusing to deliver "results," *Fear and Trembling* begins not once but several times. The middle and the "result" are postponed again and again as the reader is invited to begin first with the "Preface," then with the "Prelude," then with the "Panegyric upon Abraham," and then with the "Preliminary Expectoration," which introduces the "Three Problemata." Every one of these introductory sections makes a fresh start toward understanding the paradox of faith. They do not build on each other in a logically developing sequence of argumentation, as the reader might expect. Each beginning approaches the wonder and danger of faith from its own perspective. And the paradox of faith seems to become more rather than less mysterious as each perspective proves limited in its explanatory power. By beginning so many times, *Fear and Trembling* refuses to give the reader a fixed point of departure, a single origin that could claim unequivocal authority. This strategy of multiplying beginnings should give rise to what Edward Said calls a "strong sense of doubt that the authority of any single voice, or group of voices, is sufficient unto itself."[11] A

10. I do not mean to suggest, of course, that the title and subtitle bear no meaningful relation to the work that follows them. The many interpretations that have been given of their meaning suggest that they do. My point is only that the recognition of this relation must occur retrospectively, since the title and subtitle do not adjust the reader's expectations prospectively with the same directness as, say (to choose an example from Kierkegaard's nonpseudonymous works), *The Point of View for My Work as an Author: A Report to History*.

11. Edward W. Said, *Beginnings: Intention and Method* (New York: Basic Books, 1975), p. 88; also see pp. 76–78, 85–87, 380–81.

multiplicity of competing origins suggests that to begin means to sacrifice wholeness, since every point of departure excludes many other possibilities of understanding.

   The title of one of *Fear and Trembling*'s beginnings suggests a similar point. The heading "Prelude" is a figurative translation of the Danish *Stemning,* a word that literally means "mood, feeling, tone, atmosphere." It is a close relative of the German *Stimmung,* which Heidegger employs in his argument that all understanding is directed by its "situational attunement."[12] In Heidegger's view, our situation "attunes" our understanding—that is, it sets our attention in advance according to the predisposition, presuppositions, and interests that make up our point of departure. Most literary works attempt to situate the reader at the outset by invoking the appropriate mood to gear his expectations. But the situation of the reader changes as the mood of *Fear and Trembling* shifts in its many beginnings. The most strikingly dramatic of these shifts may be the narrator's jump from the polemical tone of the "Preface" to the fairy-tale opening of the "Prelude" ("Once upon a time . . ." [p. 26/*13*]). The polemical tone understands by demystifying, while the fairy-tale mood acts in a revelatory manner to evoke the mystery and wonder of faith. Here and elsewhere, the narrator abruptly changes the mood of his exposition in order to dramatize how understanding varies according to the perspective opened by its situation.

   Johannes de Silentio is self-consciously humble about his own authority and the limits to his perspective. "The present writer is nothing of a philosopher," the narrator explains; "he is, *poetice et eleganter,* an amateur writer who neither writes the System nor *promises* of the System" (p. 24/*11*; original emphasis). In the context of his polemic against Hegelian hubris, the narrator's humility here is, of course, an assertion of authority. But it is an ironic assertion which calls authority into question in the very act of

12. See Martin Heidegger, *Being and Time,* trans. John Macquarrie and Edward Robinson (New York: Harper & Row, 1962), pp. 172–79, 182–95. Emanuel Hirsch translates *Stemning* as *Stimmung* in *Furcht und Zittern* (Düsseldorf and Cologne: Eugen Diedrichs, 1950). Also see Louis Mackey, *Kierkegaard: A Kind of Poet* (Philadelphia: University of Pennsylvania Press, 1971), pp. 206–07.

claiming it. Furthermore, at the stage of "infinite resignation," beyond the realm of ethics but at "the last stage prior to faith" (p. 57/44), Johannes de Silentio openly confesses how his situation limits him: "I can well describe the movements of faith, but I cannot make them" (p. 48/36). There are at least three ways of explaining why Kierkegaard chose Johannes de Silentio as his narrator, but all are fundamentally similar. First, Johannes de Silentio's shortcomings cast him in the role that Gregor Malantschuk describes as typical of the Kierkegaardian pseudonym—the role of "an ironist, standing . . . at the threshold between a stage already experienced and a new stage" so as "to point to a further development" that readers might undertake in their own existence.[13] We should also recall, secondly, that a knight of faith could not write *Fear and Trembling;* the inwardness of his belief and the absolute character of his relation to the infinite prevent him from communicating with others about his experience. Finally, Johannes de Silentio's ambiguous position, between the ethical community and the paradox of faith, makes him particularly well suited to provoke others to feel wonder and bewilderment toward Abraham. The narrator's at times pained ambivalence about Abraham reveals both the marvels and the risks of faith. All of these explanations have one thing in common. They all assume that Kierkegaard's use of a limited narrator draws the reader's attention to the relation between "truth" and its situation. By repeatedly reminding his audience of the limits to his perspective, Johannes de Silentio emphasizes the relation between what anyone knows and the position from which he understands.

Johannes de Silentio's insistence on his limitations also helps to make unfamiliar what is all too familiar. The narrator of *Fear and Trembling* claims that he cannot understand Abraham's faith. He contrasts himself to those "countless generations which knew by rote, word for word, the story of Abraham"; but, he asks, "how many were made sleepless by it?" (p. 39/28). He demystifies their certainty about the meaning of Abraham's story by exposing it as excessive familiarity—as "bondage to the law of indifference" (p.

13. Gregor Malantschuk, *Kierkegaard's Thought,* trans. Howard V. Hong and Edna H. Hong (Princeton, N.J.: Princeton University Press, 1971), p. 230.

38/27). He combats this indifference by making Abraham strange. He wonders, for example, about a parishoner who, after hearing a simplistic sermon about Abraham, might very well decide to murder his son in emulation of the knight of faith. And then he wonders what makes Abraham different from a potential murderer. Most Christians would not expect to hear Abraham's faith compared to a criminal act. Most would not expect to see anyone take the biblical past as a literal model for conduct in the present. But Johannes de Silentio defies the reader's expectations by wondering why what happened to Abraham "might not have taken place on a barren heath in Denmark" (p. 26/*13*). The juxtaposition of past and present, of the Holy Land and the Scandinavian countryside, does more than insist on the contemporary relevance of Abraham's trials; it also makes those trials strange by removing them from their familiar context in the pages of the Bible. Johannes de Silentio shows that certainty about Abraham's story does not come from attaining a secure hold on its "truth" but, rather, from acting toward it in a specific way that covers over the problematic paradox of faith. The disoriented readers of *Fear and Trembling* learn that they failed to understand Abraham precisely because they were so certain about their knowledge. Kierkegaard's narrator calls on the reader to exchange active indifference for active questioning and wonder toward faith.

The narrator's challenge to the reader to see Abraham's story anew is part of a call to reconsider a whole range of unquestioned categories. In the process of making Abraham unfamiliar, Johannes de Silentio also renders strange a variety of overly familiar notions like "temptation," "sin," "love," and "ethics." Consider, for example, his claim that Abraham faces "a trial, a temptation":

> A temptation—but what does that mean? What ordinarily tempts a man is that which would keep him from doing his duty, but in this case the temptation is itself the ethical ... which would keep him from doing God's will. But what then is duty? Duty is precisely the expression for God's will. [p. 70/*56*; original ellipses]

The familiar meanings of "duty" and "temptation" are reversed here. Abraham's "duty" (to sacrifice Isaac) is the opposite of ordinary, ethical duty (a father's responsibility to his son); his "temptation" (to obey ethical restrictions) is the reverse of what the term usually refers to (transgressing the law). This reversal juxtaposes what these terms mean in the context of faith and what they mean when used ethically. It suggests, consequently, that the meaning of these and other categories is not fixed and certain but, rather, varies according to their use in different contexts. Through repeated, unquestioned use, terms seem to become absolutes; this disguises that what they mean depends on their use. As categories of understanding, ethical "temptation" and religious "temptation" differ because of the conflicting presuppositions embodied in the ethical and religious positions. By making familiar categories strange, Johannes de Silentio challenges the reader to reflect about the limits of his habitual ways of understanding and about the beliefs they represent.[14]

In disorienting the reader out of his complacency about faith and understanding, the narrator of *Fear and Trembling* pays particular attention to the categories and operations of logical discourse. He questions the authority of logical language, its rhetorical claim to deliver and guarantee the "truth." The reader learns the limits of logic by experiencing them. Johannes de Silentio dramatizes the finitude of logical procedures by exploiting their possibilities in order to bring the reader up against their limits. Consider, for example, the language of the following passage:

> If there is not a concealment which has its ground in the fact that the individual as the individual is higher than the universal, then Abraham's conduct is indefensible, for he paid no heed to the intermediate ethical determinants. If on the

14. For a related argument, see Stanley Cavell, *Must We Mean What We Say?* (New York: Scribner's, 1969), pp. 165–66. After the passage I quoted from *Fear and Trembling*, Kierkegaard introduces the term *Anfægtelse* to distinguish religious temptation from ethical temptation (*Fristelse*). Lowrie is correct to translate both terms as "temptation" but to note their differences parenthetically. He thus draws attention to their similarity and difference in meaning as related but conflicting categories of understanding.

other hand there is such a concealment, we are in the presence of the paradox which cannot be mediated inasmuch as it rests upon the consideration that the individual as the individual is higher than the universal, but it is the universal precisely which is mediation. [pp. 91–92/75]

Fear and Trembling abounds in "if-then" (*er-saa*) constructions, in logical terminology like "mediation" and "intermediate determinants," and in vocabulary like "the universal" and "the individual as the individual" that the narrator defines with philosophical precision. By invoking logical discourse, Johannes de Silentio tries to prove faith; but his inability to do so demonstrates that faith is beyond proof by logical means. In this passage, the reader is invited to follow a carefully crafted sequence of premises, conclusions, and reasons that promise a rigorous inquiry into the logic behind Abraham's silence. This kind of language is difficult for the layman; but it is ultimately reassuring, since it pretends to break a problem down into its most basic elements and to solve it once and for all by rigorously disciplined reasoning about their necessary relations to each other. But if the reader accepts the invitation to follow the narrator's demonstration here, he finds himself at the end cheated of the reassurance he had expected. The paradox of faith cannot be mediated, and Abraham's silence remains unjustified. By employing the tools of logic to justify faith, Johannes de Silentio has subverted them. After undergoing a rigorous exercise in logic, the reader is left without conclusive results but with further questions about faith and the limits of logic.

A similarly disorienting strategy of subverting logic by using its tools is evident in the following assertion: "Either there is a paradox, that the individual as the individual stands in an absolute relation to the absolute/or Abraham is lost" (p. 129/*108*). Kierkegaard uses the words "either/or" often, for many different purposes. This "either/or" (*enten/eller*) construction is a logical device. It attempts a proof by reduction to the absurd. Since the narrator's readers cannot accept the absurd alternative that "Abraham is lost," they must accept the proposition that faith transcends ethical universals. But this method of proof is ludicrous if, as the narrator claims, Abraham makes the leap of faith "by virtue of the absurd" (p. 67/53). As in the passage before, the narrator invites the reader's confidence in logical tools only to disorient him by ironically undercutting them.

The three Problemata pretend to explore faith logically. In setting them up, Johannes de Silentio proposes to answer three basic questions about the paradox of faith in what seems like a conventional philosophical format—Problem I, Problem II, Problem III. The division of the paradox into three successive problems to be solved seems to promise a sequential, progressively developing argument. Actually, the three Problemata only *seem* to develop into each other with progressive logic. Despite their different emphases, they all circle around the same central mystery. They repeat each other since none of them can resolve systematically and syllogistically the problems they address. Faith is "a paradox" that is "inaccessible to thought," the narrator claims; "faith begins precisely there where thinking leaves off" (pp. 66, 64/52-53, 50). The reader may be bewildered about what lies beyond logical thinking, but that will be one of the topics of his reorientation.[15]

If logic cannot explain faith, neither can reasoning by analogy. Ordinarily, analogies seek to appropriate the unfamiliar by comparing it to the familiar. Reversing this procedure in a disorienting manner, Johannes de Silentio uses analogies to make the familiar unfamiliar. This contributes to his effort to undermine the reader's complacency about religious belief and confidence about the meaning of Abraham's story. Throughout much of *Fear and Trembling*, the narrator tells stories that seem to offer an analogy to some aspect of Abraham's case. So numerous and various are these stories, in fact, that Abraham seems at times to have disappeared from view altogether. At least it comes as a bit of

15. Kierkegaard's critique of logic is one of the major factors behind charges that his "position must be regarded as radically irrationalistic." See Henry A. Allison, "Christianity and Nonsense," in Thompson, *Kierkegaard: Critical Essays*, p. 302. The next section of my argument will suggest that it might be useful to rephrase the debate over Kierkegaard's "irrationalism" in hermeneutic terms.

a surprise and a relief when, toward the end of Problem III, Johannes de Silentio finally asks:

> But now as for Abraham—how did he act? For I have not forgotten, and the reader will perhaps be kind enough to remember, that it was with the aim of reaching this point I entered into the whole foregoing discussion [of stories about silence]—not as though Abraham would thereby become more intelligible, but in order that the unintelligibility might become more desultory. For, as I have said, Abraham I cannot understand, I can only admire him. It was also observed that the stages I have described do none of them contain an analogy to Abraham. The examples were simply educed in order that while they were shown in their own proper sphere they might at the moment of variation [from Abraham's case (translator's note)] indicate as it were the boundary of the unknown land. [p. 121/*101*]

The relief of returning to Abraham is frustrated by the narrator's insistence that the detour through other stories has not made the knight of faith "intelligible." Now the stories that illustrate why aesthetics prefers concealment and why ethics demands revelation do help to explain why the knight of faith, in the anguishing isolation of his private relation to the absolute, cannot communicate to others as the "tragic hero" can. But Johannes de Silentio refuses to let his readers rest easy, with the sense of a secure explanation. At the moment when comprehension seems in sight, his disclaimer about the value of the route he has taken undermines his explanation of Abraham's silence. He thereby prevents clarification from diminishing the reader's wonder and bewilderment about the paradox of faith.

Although Johannes de Silentio claims that none of his stories "contain an analogy to Abraham," his description of them actually offers a good definition of the process of analogizing. By their "variation" from the unknown, analogies indicate what the unknown is. All analogies are both like and unlike what they hope to clarify. And both their similarities with and their differences from their object help to make it comprehensible by indicating what it shares with the familiar and what makes it unique. Most analogies emphasize the "like" in order to stress the assimilation they offer. But Johannes de Silentio emphasizes the "unlike." Ordinarily, the "unlike" in an analogy acknowledges the crucial role of negation and differentiation in understanding; our knowledge of what something *is* depends on our sense of what it is *not*. But Johannes de Silentio plays subversively with the customary use of differentiation. His emphasis on the "unlike" makes faith strange by insisting that it defies complete explanation by ordinary methods of comprehension. Just as God is only available to humanity as its negative limit, so the disorienting strategies of *Fear and Trembling* reveal faith to the reader negatively, as the limit of what the narrator's discourse can disclose.

Let us conclude our survey of Johannes de Silentio's disorienting strategies by examining the variations on Abraham's story in the Prelude. They offer a small-scale model of the process of disorientation in *Fear and Trembling*. They also point toward the reader's reorientation. Under the guise of bringing Abraham closer to the everyday realm, short of his religious grandeur and horror, the narrator gives four versions of what the knight might have done if he had lacked faith. The Prelude is doubly interpretive. Prefaced by part of the biblical text of the story, the variations are attempts, first of all, to make Abraham comprehensible by imagining him in the more familiar realm of ethical obligation of father to son. These indirect efforts to understand the story of Abraham are followed in turn by four refrains about a mother weaning a child. The refrains offer a kind of interpretive commentary on the variations. Taking the reader further into the ethical realm of relations between parent and child, the metaphors of weaning hope to show the meaning of the variations by showing what they are not—by showing instances of separation between parent and child that are ethically good (unlike the sacrifice of a son that the variations address) and where, unlike the variations, there is no need for "dreadful expedients" (p. 28/*15*). In this way, the refrains parallel the variations, which also try to clarify Abraham by showing what he is not.

Still, although the variations interpret Abraham, just as the refrains interpret the variations, neither aspect of the Prelude fulfills the function exegetical commentary is expected to perform—namely, to make the hidden meanings of a text more intelligible by explication. Only adding to Abraham's mystery, the variations increase the narrator's sense that "no one is so great as Abraham! Who is capable of understanding him?" (p. 29/16). And if the variations ultimately fail to enlighten the biblical text, then the metaphor of weaning refuses to clarify the variations fully. As metaphorical discourse, the refrains about the mother and her child have the density of polyvocal symbols, not the transparency of univocal propositions which exegesis ordinarily employs. By raising the expectation of hermeneutic elucidation only to defy it, the variations and the refrains should set the reader's own interpretive activity to work. Disorienting the reader away from complacency about faith's mediation of the finite and the infinite, they call on him to reject the reified "truth" of standard religious dogma. What the reader then needs is a reorientation that will give him instruction about the activity of understanding appropriate to faith.

III

The reorienting movements of *Fear and Trembling* do not offer the reader a genuine "truth" to replace the inadequate "truth" he is called upon to sacrifice. Rather, they induct the reader into the implications of a world where "truth" varies according to the activity of its producer. This is a world of conflicting interpretations—a world where, as we saw in the last section, what such categories of understanding as "temptation" and "duty" disclose depends on the hermeneutic position they represent.[16] The conflict of interpretations is dramatized most vividly in the last and longest of the three Problemata as the narrator leads the reader through a series of investigations into how aesthetics and ethics understand silence. Johannes de Silentio shows that Kier-

16. My theory of hermeneutic conflict owes much to Paul Ricoeur, *The Conflict of Interpretations,* ed. Don Ihde (Evanston, Ill.: Northwestern University Press, 1974).

kegaard's much-discussed "stages" are not only possible modes of existence. The aesthetic and the ethical stages are also hermeneutic standpoints—ways of understanding which gear their attention to the object of interpretation according to the presuppositions and beliefs that define their positions.[17] Through the stories and interpretations he gives of the various meanings of silence, the narrator of *Fear and Trembling* inducts the reader into the conflict between the aesthetic and the ethical as ways of understanding. This experience should then orient the reader toward the hermeneutic standpoint of faith.

Faith is one competing mode of understanding among others, in conflict with aesthetic and ethical ways of construing states of affairs like "silence," "love," "time," and "language." But it is not simply one among equals. As we shall see, Kierkegaard asserts the superiority of faith over aesthetics and ethics by claiming that it enjoys privileged powers in relation to its rivals in the conflict of interpretations. But the reader learns as well that the superior understanding which, in Kierkegaard's view, faith makes possible also has perils that reflect the incommensurability of God to man. The reoriented reader can choose faith's privilege— but only at the cost of accepting its perils.

The conflict between the aesthetic and the ethical is well illustrated by the narrator's account of the dispute between those standpoints over how to understand the story of Agamemnon. Faced with the necessity of sacrificing Iphigenia, Agamemnon first remains silent. Then, after his secret comes out, he withstands the temptation to spare his daughter despite the tear-filled pleas that she and Clytemnestra make (see *Fear and Trembling*, pp. 96-97/79-80). From an aesthetic point of view, Agamemnon's silence makes his dilemma more interesting by heightening its dramatic tension. According to the high value it places on the "interesting," aesthetics understands the disclosure of Agamemnon's secret as a dramatic instrument that complicates his heroic

17. Cavell makes a similar point when he compares "a Kierkegaardian stage of life" to "a Wittgensteinian form of life" with a language of its own (*Must We Mean What We Say?*, p. 172).

stature by putting him through trials to test his resolve. But an aesthetic interpretation of his situation cannot reveal how, from an ethical perspective, a "tragic hero" like Agamemnon must feel trapped by the demand of silence. Interpreted ethically, his silence deprives Agamemnon of the opportunity to justify his course of action by explaining to others how it will serve the universal good of the community. The disclosure of the tragic hero's secret restores his relation to the community. It allows him to express his allegiance to the universal in open argumentation, which engages him with others in the community and which can justify his action as an individual through an appeal to the public welfare. The aesthetic category of the "interesting" cannot explain the tragic hero's responsibility to the community. On the other hand, though, ethical considerations alone cannot disclose the full dramatic interest of Agamemnon's dilemma.

The aesthetic and the ethical are pitted against each other elsewhere in Kierkegaard's work, most notably in the two volumes of *Either/Or*. In Problem III of *Fear and Trembling,* however, Kierkegaard escalates the conflict between them by taking the reader back and forth between the aesthetic and the ethical standpoints in just a few pages—or, as in the narrator's discussion of Agamemnon, in just a few paragraphs. The point of the often almost dizzying to-and-fro movement between the aesthetic and the ethical in Problem III is not only to show the reader how Abraham's silence transcends the categories of understanding that belong to them. It also gives the reader a vivid, at times bewildering, experience of how every hermeneutic standpoint reveals some aspects of a state of affairs only at the cost of disguising others.

By taking his readers back and forth between the aesthetic and the ethical, the narrator teaches them about one way of understanding—only to reveal its limits and challenge it with the interpretation suggested by the other position. At the narrator's direction, the reader assumes with him the aesthetic perspective in order to understand what it reveals about one of the stories in Problem III. But then the narrator shifts ground, and the reader moves with him to examine what the aesthetic interpretation disguised but what ethics reveals. Shortly, however, either with the introduction of a new story or sometimes in the consideration of the same tale, narrator and reader move back to the aesthetic position. This "dialectical" strategy of presentation, as the narrator calls it, takes the reader through the possibilities of comprehension opened up by a certain perspective—pursuing them so rigorously and so single-mindedly that the reader is brought up hard against the wall that marks their limits. These limits then call for a change to the field of vision available from a different position. And the process of revealing the hermeneutic possibilities of a position in order to disclose their limits begins once again.

This back-and-forth movement between the aesthetic and the ethical aims to reawaken readers to the positioned, provisional nature of understanding, which, in its unquestioning certainty about itself, everyday knowing tends to forget. But Johannes de Silentio's hermeneutic agility in shifting from position to position does not depict interpretation as relativistic in any simplistic sense. The aesthetic and ethical positions are not equal, with nothing to decide between them. To begin with, the narrator shows that the aesthetic and the ethical perspectives are privileged by what they can reveal about something, just as they are undercut by what they cannot account for. Adjudicating their conflict involves more, however, than merely deciding their relative value for any given task of interpretation. Since their field of vision reflects their underlying assumptions about the world, the reader must ultimately decide between them—or decide to transcend them—by accepting or rejecting their beliefs. This is where the role of the aesthetic and the ethical as "stages of existence" meets their role as hermeneutic positions within the field of conflicting interpretations.

Ultimately, however, *Fear and Trembling* offers faith as the only truly satisfactory solution to the problem of relativism. For Kierkegaard, faith occupies a peculiar, paradoxical position at once within and beyond the field of conflicting interpretations. Faith is privileged not only as a stage of existence superior to ethical and aesthetic ways of being but also as an attitude of understanding that transcends their conflict. According to Johannes de Silentio, "religion is the only power which can deliver the aesthetical out of its conflict with the ethical" (p. 103/85). It does so not by deciding the conflict in favor of one party over the other or by declaring the battle insignificant in light of the higher stakes involved with the problematic of faith. Rather, invoking the Hegelian process of *Aufhebung*, Johannes de Silentio argues that faith resolves the conflict between aesthetics and ethics teleologically, by suspending their positions and transcending their dispute so that "what is suspended is not forfeited but is preserved precisely in that higher thing which is its *telos*" (p. 65/51). One might suspect some dialectical sleight of hand here. After all, if interpretations necessarily conflict because their positions of observation differ, then how can one hermeneutic perspective encompass the others it disagrees with? This is not the place to enter into a discussion of the teleological relation that Kierkegaard ascribes to the aesthetic, ethical, and religious stages of existence. What matters is the rhetorical purpose his dialectical maneuver serves here. By invoking dialectics, Kierkegaard acknowledges the conflict of interpretations but at the same time asserts a privilege for faith.

Where the conflict between aesthetics and ethics made the battleground of rival interpretations seem like a horizontal field, dialectical thinking transforms it into a vertical one. The religious stands at the top rung of the ladder; it can look down at the others, although they cannot look up. Johannes de Silentio describes faith not as one position among others that deserves to be chosen on its merits. Rather, faith is a way of understanding that transcends other modes of interpretation by including them within its own compass. Faith can understand the other positions, but they cannot understand faith. The reader can finally get beyond the dizzying back-and-forth clash of relative hermeneutic position with relative hermeneutic position only by making the other positions relative to faith.

From his position of infinite resignation, just short of faith, Johannes de Silentio can move freely among subordinate positions, back and forth between the aesthetic and the ethical in their different understandings of silence. But no more than they can he interpret Abraham's silence adequately: "Here is evident the necessity of a new category if one would understand Abraham" (p. 70/56). Actually, rather than requiring a "new," all-powerful "category" of understanding, Abraham's silent faith might seem to move him altogether beyond the finite realm of understanding and interpretation in his solitary confrontation with the infinite. According to Johannes de Silentio: "By faith Abraham went out from the land of his fathers and became a sojourner in the land of promise. He left one thing behind, took one thing with him: he left his earthly understanding behind and took faith with him" (p. 31/18). He believed by virtue of the absurd, and "the absurd is not one of the factors which can be discriminated within the proper compass of the understanding" (p. 57/44). Everything depends on what "understanding" (*Forstand*) means in these passages. Abraham's faith takes him beyond such kinds of "earthly understanding" as logical reasoning, aesthetic appreciation, and ethical deliberation. But it does not take him beyond interpretation entirely—beyond the hazards and responsibility of construing signs as knowing subjects to which our finitude commits us by depriving us of infinite omniscience.[18] Although incomprehensible to any position outside it, Abraham's faith does not deliver him out of the limits of human understanding. Rather, it con-

18. The word *Forstand* would be more precisely translated as "intellect" in the sense of "logical faculties." Its meaning is more limited than *Forståelse* (understanding) or *Fortolkning* (interpretation). The debate about Kierkegaard's irrationalism risks confusion because it does not always keep this distinction in mind. Those who charge Kierkegaard with irrationalism often argue that faith defies and denies understanding. It would clarify the debate, I think, to recognize that faith does not go beyond interpretation but, rather, as a hermeneutic standpoint, challenges the limits to reason as a competing mode of understanding. Faith is unquestionably "irrational" in the sense that its position of understanding conflicts with the hermeneutic standpoint of reason. The crucial issue raised by the charge of "irrationality," however, is one of validity: can faith justify its understanding of man's relation to God? As a hermeneutic standpoint incommensurate with the position of reason, faith cannot be asked to justify its understanding with the tools of logic. But "validity" is a category that applies to all modes of understanding. And as we shall see, what many describe as the "irrationality" of faith is indeed the ultimate impossibility of validating its understanding with the certainty about itself that, within their limits, such ways of knowing as the aesthetic and the ethical can claim.

fronts those limits resolutely in a way that shows how they make faith perilous and even scandalous.

Like all finite subjects, whatever their positions and presuppositions, the knight of faith knows the object of his understanding only according to how he acts toward it. The knight must make "the movements of faith"—a phrase that emphasizes that faith is an activity, a way of comporting oneself so as to reveal certain phenomena which other attitudes of understanding would not disclose. Elsewhere, one of Kierkegaard's pseudonyms describes faith as "the inward certainty which anticipates infinity."[19] "Inwardness" is an attitude actively taken up and carried on by a subjectivity, and its "certainty" is nothing more than its expectation that what it "anticipates" will prove justified.[20]

Like all attitudes of understanding, then, faith discloses meaning according to its expectations. Abraham "expected the impossible" (p. 31/*18*), and only by projecting this kind of anticipatory understanding could he comprehend what happened to him. As the Prelude suggests, if Abraham hadn't comported himself in this way, he could not have understood his trial on Mount Moriah or the return of Isaac. The second variation in the Prelude argues that Abraham would have felt resentment toward God rather than joy in the return of his son if the appearance of the ram had fallen outside of his range of expectations. He may not have had a complete, precise prevision of how events would unfold on Mount Moriah. But the ram did not surprise and upset him because his horizon of expectations allowed for it, if only implicitly. By contrast, able in his infinite resignation to envision only the sacrifice of the finite, Johannes de Silentio declares that the return of Isaac would have embarrassed him because it would have completely contradicted his expectations (see p. 46/*34*). Only because he geared his expectations in an appropriate manner was Abraham able to understand what would simply bewilder the

19. Kierkegaard, *The Concept of Dread,* pp. 140–41. Vigilius Haufniensis acknowledges Hegel as the source for this phrase.

20. This is also one of the implications of the famous slogan "Truth is subjectivity" in Kierkegaard's *Concluding Unscientific Postscript,* trans. David F. Swenson and Walter Lowrie (Princeton, N.J.: Princeton University Press, 1968), p. 169.

narrator. The knight of faith does not transcend the hermeneutic circle whereby understanding and expectation mutually define each other.[21] Instead, through acts of belief, he makes an entry into the circle that enables him to comprehend what other ways of understanding could not account for.

Still, the hermeneutic circle runs the risk of becoming a vicious circle unless criteria of validation test the legitimacy of the beliefs according to which understanding projects its expectations. Abraham's faith seems scandalous to Johannes de Silentio because the extremity of his belief seems to outrun the demands of validation. Nothing troubles the narrator more than the question of whether Abraham was justified in his faith: "Though Abraham arouses my admiration, he at the same time appalls me" (p. 71/56). The narrator seeks to convey to the reader not only his wonder at Abraham's belief but also his bewilderment, even fear and trembling, at the great risk of error, even self-delusion, that the knight runs. Abraham is justified in several ways—most of all, perhaps, because his expectations are fulfilled. But the criterion of validation by the fulfillment of expectations is a weak test at best, since expectations can be self-fulfilling. Intersubjective agreement provides a stronger test. But because, in his silence, Abraham stands in an absolute relation to God that leaves behind all social, intersubjective mediation, the knight of faith is close to madness, in that realm of risk beyond the assurance that agreement with other knowing subjects can offer.[22] Returning again and again to the dangerous similarity between faith and madness, Johannes de Silentio repeatedly draws the reader's attention to the risk of delusion that accompanies the knight's isolation from any intersubjective confirmation.

The narrator's great worry about the scandalous perils of faith reflects his own shortcomings, since his fear of these dangers

21. On the role of anticipation and expectation in understanding and interpretation, see Heidegger, *Being and Time*, pp. 188–95.

22. This dilemma reflects Kierkegaard's much-discussed and rightly criticized "veneration of the individual's isolation from other selves" (Taylor, *Kierkegaard's Pseudonymous Authorship*, p. 355; also see Richard H. Popkin, "Kierkegaard and Scepticism," in Thompson, *Kierkegaard: Critical Essays*, p. 372).

prevents him from emulating Abraham. But his worry also shows that faith does not escape the responsibility of validating its understanding. In the isolation of his inwardness, the knight "did not then enjoy himself in the silence but suffered pain—but this precisely was to him the assurance that he was justified" (pp. 102–03/85). The knight's pain shows that the demands of validation still accompany faith. The knight suffers because he has no immediate assurance that his belief is valid. And if his pain assures him that he is justified, it is at most an unsettling assurance, since it results from his lack of certainty. Abraham's pained uncertainty should recall the oft-quoted description of faith from *Concluding Unscientific Postscript:* "*An objective uncertainty held fast in an appropriation-process of the most passionate inwardness is the truth,* the highest truth attainable for an *existing* individual."[23] The "objective uncertainty" is a sign of the peril that goes hand in hand with the privilege of faith as "the highest truth attainable" in a world of conflicting interpretations. In its borderline position, both within and beyond the conflict, faith shares the responsibility of asking about the "certainty" of its "truth"—but cannot answer with the secure assurance of validity that, within their limits, other ways of understanding can claim. The knight's silent suffering is not the same as Johannes de Silentio's outspoken fear of the risks of faith. But both suffering and fear are expressions—different according to the different standpoints of faith and infinite resignation—of the perils that come with the privilege of the religious position.

It might seem strange that a strategy of communication that aims to reawaken its readers to faith should place so much stress on the perils and uncertainties of belief. By emphasizing the perils that accompany faith's privilege, however, the narrator helps to make sure that the reoriented reader won't forget what he learned in his disorientation. Johannes de Silentio's worry about the uncertainties of faith complements the disorienting strategies in their work of undermining complacency about the ability of religious belief to mediate the finite and the infinite. His

23. *Concluding Unscientific Postscript,* p. 182; original emphases.

worry also reinforces the other major lesson of disorientation—
that "truth" exists only in the hazardous enterprise of producing
it in action, an enterprise all readers must undertake for themselves.

IV

Fear and Trembling ends with the story of Heraclitus and his
misguided disciple. The disciple "went further" than Heraclitus.
In the process of transcending the master's teachings, however,
the disciple actually went "back to the position Heraclitus had
abandoned" (p. 132/*111*). The moral of the story seems to be that
readers should go further than their teacher Johannes de Silentio
by transcending the stage of infinite resignation—but not by reverting to positions that the process of disorientation and reorientation should have led them to abandon. The narrator does not
interpret his story, however. Even to the end, he frustrates the
reader's desire for "the result," for closure that would put a false
finish to the never-ending activity of pursuing meaning through
understanding. By offering the story without interpreting it,
Johannes de Silentio closes *Fear and Trembling* by inciting his
readers to keep active, as they have been in reading. They must
ponder the story for themselves, just as they must choose for or
against faith on their own.

Fear and Trembling prepares for this choice by appealing to the
reader's freedom in the very activity of engaging the text. All texts
must solicit the cooperation of the reader's free subjectivity to
make the black marks on the page come alive with meaning and
significance. The reader must agree to lend his subjectivity to the
subjectivity lodged in the text so that it might speak with borrowed powers. Readers exercise their subjectivity and their freedom at the same time, since they must decide how to actualize
even the most univocal text by choosing from a range of different
possibilities of construing and evaluating its meaning. The process of reading is disturbed at its heart if the text cajoles the
reader—if, that is, it makes him the object of a polemic and

thereby denies the subjectivity that makes possible its own actualization.[24]

Kierkegaard's strategy of indirect communication acknowledges the reader's freedom by refusing to objectify his subjectivity through polemical instruction. Moreover, the difficulties of reading Kierkegaard seek to awaken the reader's freedom by calling for a heightened application of his subjective powers. Readers do not exercise to the fullest their possibilities of interpretation, reflection, and self-discovery with books that, in the words of Johannes de Silentio, "can easily be perused during the afternoon nap" (p. 24/11). Kierkegaard's pseudonyms see it as their "task to create difficulties everywhere"—"It is thus left to the reader himself to put two and two together, if he so desires; but nothing is done to minister to a reader's indolence."[25] An indolent reader might prefer texts that allow his subjectivity to rest easy in objectlike passivity. Still, texts less self-consciously difficult than Kierkegaard's pseudonymous works can also leave much for the reader to do. But with a readership so prone to self-deceptive, self-protective "indolence" about matters like truth and faith, Kierkegaard apparently thinks that only difficulty that calls attention to itself can awaken his audience out of its lethargy to become fully active in reading. Kierkegaard's strategy of making difficulties for his readers allows him to appeal to them to change their lives by reawakening instead of reifying the powers that make change possible.

Kierkegaard's practice of communicating indirectly, through pseudonyms, shows a liberating rather than dominating solicitude for the reader's welfare. By withdrawing behind the pseudonyms, Kierkegaard claims, "The communicator disap-

24. My analysis of the relation between reading and freedom derives from Jean-Paul Sartre, *What Is Literature?*, trans. Bernard Frechtman (New York: Harper & Row, 1965), particularly pp. 32–60. In Sartre's view, a writer appeals to the reader's freedom in order to open the possibility of his political and social rather than religious liberation. Mark Taylor offers a necessary corrective to Kierkegaard's limited understanding of the relation between individual freedom and its historical, social situation (see *Kierkegaard's Pseudonymous Authorship*, pp. 356–72).

25. Kierkegaard, *Concluding Unscientific Postscript*, pp. 166, 264–65.

pears, as it were, makes himself serve only to help the other be-come."[26] This withdrawal is necessary, he believes, because "it is impossible for me to compel a person to accept an opinion, a conviction, a belief. But one thing I can do: I can compel him to take notice. In one sense this is the first thing; for it is the condi-tion antecedent to the next thing, i.e. the acceptance of an opin-ion, a conviction, a belief. In another sense it is the last—if, that is, he will not take the next step."[27] As we have seen, the experience of reading a pseudonymous work like *Fear and Trembling* offers a challenge to unexamined ways of understanding and the "opin-ions, convictions, beliefs" they embody. But Kierkegaard com-municates his challenge indirectly rather than dogmatically be-cause he understands the limits to how much someone can help someone else. A dominating solicitude oversteps these limits by leaping in and taking over for the other. A liberating solicitude holds itself back so as to allow the other the freedom and respon-sibility of confronting his own possibilities.[28] Kierkegaard's pseudonyms challenge readers "to take notice" of the in-adequacies in their habits of understanding and behaving in order to open up the possibility of changing their existence. But they must decide to take the next step.

Actually, they must also decide to take the first step. Kier-kegaard cannot "compel" them to take notice. Since everything depends on how readers respond to Kierkegaard's challenge, they can choose to respond by ignoring or misunderstanding it. Kierkegaard often despaired at ever finding his "real reader." The great courage of Kierkegaard's strategy of indirect com-munication is also its great risk—the risk he takes by making the

26. Kierkegaard, *Journals and Papers*, trans. Howard V. Hong and Edna H. Hong (Bloomington: Indiana University Press, 1967), no. 657.

27. Kierkegaard, *The Point of View for My Work as an Author*, trans. Walter Lowrie (New York: Harper & Row, 1962), p. 35.

28. On the relation between solicitude and freedom, see Heidegger, *Being and Time*, pp. 158-59. Here and throughout this section of the essay, I am trying to explain how Kierkegaard's strategy of indirect communication enables the reader to take the step that Crites calls crucial to the pseudonymous project—the step from reading to making "an existential movement" that "can only be realized in the life of an individual" ("Pseudonymous Authorship as Art and as Act," p. 225).

possibility of misreading such an integral part of his project. He increases the risk of not finding his "real reader" because his strategy of indirect communication leaves open the possibility of inadequate readings more courageously than more direct and dogmatic modes of discourse do. Every aspect of reading *Fear and Trembling* that I have described can be ignored by the reader if he chooses to refuse Kierkegaard's challenge. If he would not deny the reader's freedom, a freedom necessary to the choice of faith, then Kierkegaard must allow the reader the freedom to misread—to refuse to hear the call the indirect works make. If readers choose to read Kierkegaard correctly, however, they will be helped toward a decision about faith by experiencing a disorienting and reorienting education.

3

Kierkegaard's Imagery of the Self

JAMES COLLINS

The Research Situation

English-language work on Kierkegaard is currently in a state of healthy ferment. A third generation of scholarship is now emerging gradually yet unmistakably. It builds upon the groundwork laid by the pioneers in this field. The task of the first generation was to get Kierkegaard translated into English and to furnish some general outlines of his thought. Through the heroic labors of Swenson, Lowrie, Dru, and a few others, the English-reading world was confronted with a vast new source literature and given some preliminary guidance on how to find one's way around in it. Here was an unusual case in culture history where large-scale translating efforts took the lead in establishing a new intellectual presence among us and provoking some introductory responses. A point was reached sometime in the 1960s, however, when introductions (even translated ones) could no longer satisfy but had to be succeeded by a second generation of Kierkegaard studies. These studies were characterized by a concentration in depth upon specific topics, by a more detailed comparison with other thinkers, and by a growing cross-disciplinary interest. Considerable progress toward understanding Kierkegaard was made by these particular approaches, but the limits reached indicated the need for still newer directions.

Third-generation activities are taking several forms. Increas-

An earlier version of this essay was delivered as the Wade Memorial Lecture, Saint Louis University, October 1979.

ingly, scholars are following the example of Unamuno by learning Danish. Kierkegaard is no exception to the rule that a thinker must eventually be studied in his own language in order to appreciate his precisions and connotations. Although Kierkegaard always felt that his mother tongue made his writings culturally provincial, scholars today feel that they are on the periphery if they cannot consult him in the original. Their efforts are greatly facilitated by McKinnon's massive *Kierkegaard Indices,* which uses computer methods to count the Danish word frequencies and contexts and also to establish line correlations with existing Western translations (except the Italian ones). But the most pressing need is for a new English version of Kierkegaard. As far as his *Journals and Papers* are concerned, a much fuller selection is now provided by Howard and Edna Hong's six volumes of text plus an index volume. And we are now at the outset of the great project of a complete new translation (under Howard Hong's general editorship), *Kierkegaard's Writings,* in twenty-five volumes and a cumulative-index volume. Both projects are careful to give the Danish source references for every translated text.[1]

What impact are these projects likely to have upon ongoing research? The most obvious effect is to induce a more careful reading and analysis of the terminology, phrasing, and argument in the Kierkegaard books that until now have been the staple fare. Yet three other tendencies in internal studies are fairly predictable. First, Kierkegaard's numerous upbuilding discourses and Christian discourses can no longer be kept uncomfortably in the

1. Alastair McKinnon, *The Kierkegaard Indices,* 4 vols. (Leiden: Brill, 1970–75). This work has now been published by Princeton University Press, 1979. *Søren Kierkegaard's Journals and Papers,* ed. and trans. Howard V. Hong and Edna H. Hong, 7 vols. (Bloomington: Indiana University Press, 1967–78). Referred to hereafter by volume and page thus: *JP* 3:146. Autobiographical materials are arranged chronologically in vols. 5 (1829–48) and 6 (1848–55). *Kierkegaard's Writings,* general ed. H. V. Hong, to be in 26 vols. (Princeton, N.J.: Princeton University Press). Issued in 1978: vol. 14, *Two Ages;* vol. 25, *Letters and Documents,* trans. Henrik Rosenmeier, referred to hereafter by page thus: *LD* 283. Research materials are gathered in the Kierkegaard Library at St. Olaf College and in the Kierkegaard-Malantschuk Library Collection at McGill University.

shadows. The religious books accompany the conventionally emphasized writings; they have both an intellectual structure of their
own and a modifying effect upon the rest; and their contribution
to Kierkegaard's total meaning is considerable for every problem
and comparison.

A second line of inquiry, not unrelated to the first, is to give due
attention to the publications of his last few years (1846–55), to
what is called "the second literature" in his authorship. This has
not been combed as thoroughly for its thought as for its biographical significance—that is, the role it played in Kierkegaard's
open conflict with the church establishment. He was conveying
much more than a passionate outburst, however, and what he
argued has a retroactive effect upon our understanding of his
earlier positions and their implications. Such reconsiderations are
affecting the comparative as well as internal interpretations, as
recently witnessed by conflicting accounts of his personality given
by two Danish psychiatrists.[2]

The third research path leads toward a more intensive scrutiny
of Kierkegaard's journals, papers, and letters. They furnish the
living context and continuity for his thought and publications.
Without them, we would be left groping about the exact prove-
nance and intent, transitions and implications, of the books he
authored by indirect and direct communication. But they possess
an integrity of their own, not just an ancillary value with respect to
his other writings. It is this intrinsic significance that is now being

2. Hjalmar Helweg, *Søren Kierkegaard, En Psykiatrisk-Psykologisk Studie* [Søren
Kierkegaard, a psychiatric-psychological study] (Copenhagen: Hagerup, 1933;
English translation forthcoming), proposes that Kierkegaard had a manic-
depressive psychosis. Ib Ostenfeld, *Søren Kierkegaard's Psychology* (Waterloo, On-
tario: Wilfrid Laurier University Press, 1978), denies that Kierkegaard has this
psychosis but emphasizes the many family and social stresses affecting his personality. This is the first volume in *The Kierkegaard Monograph Series*, general ed.
Alastair McKinnon. The problem of "Kierkegaard on the psychoanalytic couch" is
surveyed by Henning Fenger, *Kierkegaard, The Myths and Their Origins: Studies
in the Kierkegaardian Papers and Letters*, trans. George C. Schoolfield (New
Haven: Yale University Press, 1980), with an inclination to accept Helweg's
interpretation.

explored, and it is being found to be much more complex than expected.

The first four volumes of Kierkegaard's *Journals and Papers* testify to this intellectual and affective complexity, arranged as they are under 5,050 topical headings. Even then, the Hongs felt that much had eluded their sieve, and that is why they presented two more volumes as autobiographical materials. Of course, no rigid demarcation can be drawn here, since almost everything Kierkegaard records has a covert autobiographical aspect, just as the items selected as autobiographical have a larger significance in terms of the thought and argumentation in his books. Added to this fund of information is Kierkegaard's lifelong correspondence, now completely translated in Rosenmeier's edition, *Letters and Documents.* As with other noted letter writers, Kierkegaard knows how to blend the passing circumstance and the lasting reflection in a skillful way.

My own objective can now be stated. For the most part, I restrict myself to the English translation of the two autobiographical volumes of *Journals and Papers,* along with the *Letters and Documents.* Instead of attempting a global approach, I concentrate upon one theme that looms large in these sources: imagery of the self. This topic can be taken in two senses—namely, the images Kierkegaard develops about his own self, and those that contribute to his general conception of the self as presented in these sources. Such a distinction does not rest upon two neatly separated sets of images but usually represents aspects and phases in his presentation of the same imagery. My main interest here lies in Kierkegaard's self-imagery considered as a process, well grounded in his own life and yet striving toward communication with others and hence toward an interpersonal significance of selfhood.

The images of self sought here, therefore, are those that reach out from Kierkgaard's personal reflection and kindle some recognition of similarity by other people who may be touched by his thought and language. These images are presented in a roughly chronological order, to show the developmental quality of Kierkegaard's reflections on the self and to preserve their concrete context. At the end, I will consider some methodological implications of my approach to this theme and some further tasks imposed upon our research.

The Storied Self

The young Kierkegaard is no solipsist in his treatment of selfhood. He immerses himself in those cultural expressions that strike him forcefully and that hold promise of making definite contributions to his own questioning. Indeed, it would be surprising if he were to ignore the work of a generation of romantic philosophers and poets, folklore collectors and tellers of fairy tales. The ideals and personages they celebrate provide him with multiple glints of human selfhood, different ways in which to realize our potential for becoming selves. Through the mediation of these materials, Kierkegaard keeps his reflections open, sharpens his hermeneutic and analytic skills, and recognizes diverse possibilities for forming his own self. His position in relating to his precursors is not unlike the uses that might currently be made of the study of Dostoevsky and Chekhov, Camus and Joyce, Melville and Faulkner.

Two points strike him at once: figurations of self with national origins are nevertheless transposable into other cultures, and the masterly expression of some such figuration in one art form does not exclude its representation in another art form. On the first score, he muses: "It is also remarkable that Germany has its Faust, Italy and Spain their Don Juan, the Jews (??) [SK's question; Jews not then represented by a country] the Wandering Jew, Denmark and north Germany, Eulenspiegel" (*JP* 5:42). But as testified by Kierkegaard's favorite opera, *Don Giovanni,* a particular cultural genesis does not prevent the transmission of a storied person into another cultural setting and artistic medium. On this second score, Kierkegaard adduces *Faust* not only in Goethe's great poem but also in its translations, in theater directions for staging it, in chapbook collections of the legend, and in some now mercifully forgotten operas and plays. From this transcultural and pluriform artistic evidence, Kierkegaard is convinced that some broadly representative traits and options of the human self are being imaginatively treated. Little wonder that, for a while, he even thinks that his own notions of the self can be effectively organized around Faust and Don Juan, the Wandering Jew, and Til Eulenspiegel.

Actually, his use of these archetypes is uneven. The tale of Ahasuerus, the Wandering Jew, reached painfully close to home in its illumination of human character. Kierkegaard took the trouble to transcribe E. T. A. Hoffmann's question about one who discerns the secret thoughts of others: "Does not this fatal gift bring over him that frightful condition which came over the eternal Jew, who wandered through the bright tumult of the world without hope, without pain, in apathetic indifference which is the *caput mortuum* of despair, as if through an uncomfortable, comfortless wasteland?" (*JP* 5:475). This mood overcame Kierkegaard himself for a long while after he fathomed his own father's sense of being doomed because of a boyhood act of blasphemy. Such a benumbing indifference to present values and future prospects could chill the self in all its relations. Kierkegaard anticipated T. S. Eliot in regarding the wasteland outlook as one of the real shapers of modern personal and social life.

Don Juan represents another formation of human existence, one that perhaps begins in a livelier way but ultimately also locks itself into despair. There is a strong aesthetic quality in this image: "The Don Juanian life is really musical" (*JP* 5:100). We feel irresistibly drawn toward Mozart's opera, not only as a supreme work of art but also as a powerful embodiment of the aesthetic mode of existence, as one compelling image of the self.[3] Especially under the actual conditions of attending an opera or play on this theme, we are enthusiastic about intense love given for the moment, along with an eventual search for yet another and another conquest. Kierkegaard attributes the attraction of this idea not only to the context of a musical performance but also to

3. For some Kierkegaard texts on "self," see *JP* 4:36–41. For a helpful working list of passages on the self in Kierkegaard's books, as well as of secondary studies on this topic, consult *JP* 4:634–37. The specific connection between musicality and aesthetic existence is analyzed by T. H. Croxall, *Kierkegaard Commentary* (New York: Harper, 1956), pp. 47–59.

its articulation of an age-old image of self-comportment and aspiration. "The great poetic power of folk literature is expressed in various ways, also in the intensity of its craving and coveting. . . . It inevitably must at least shake people up, and in its descriptions it does not allow anything to be scaled down by the cold calculation of probability and pedestrian understanding. D. Juan still glides across the stage with his 1,003 mistresses and no one smiles at it" (*JP* 5:139). Leporello's catalogue arouses a thousand desires of one's own.

But a further maturing of selfhood comes with the realization that life includes its offstage, after-performance conditions. Practical considerations do not just *intrude* upon the storied self but *educate* it regarding the problems of existence. If he were writing a reminiscence of childhood (his own early dreams and those of the human race), Kierkegaard mused, he would use as a motto this line from Kruse's account of Don Juan's fantasies: "But they wither and soon fade away" (*JP* 5:114). The withering process is inherent in the aesthete's dedication to momentary pleasures, his incapacity for enduring attachments and continuities, his low satiety threshold, and his boredom with other people and exploitation of them. By way of contrast, Kierkegaard valued the fidelity and mutual integrity that we are also capable of cultivating.

During his early years, he himself found more significance in the legends about Til Eulenspiegel and Peer Mikkelsen than was usually spelled out. Kierkegaard concretized this added meaning in his theme of the master-thief, who exemplifies the noble outsider. This figure combines kindness toward others with ingenuity and extraordinary bearing. Despite some ambiguity, he recognizes the reality (although not the fully humane actuality) of the state, even though he attacks its abuses and remains apart from the established order. Yet his is not a simpleminded antiestablishment attitude, since he distances himself from other thieves, endures punishment "as a man who is conscious of having lived for an idea" (*JP* 5:7), and retains a sense of humor about life's discrepancies. He maintains also an affectionate relationship with his mother (who is, however, critical of his deeds) and with his beloved, who perceives his humane geniality.

Nevertheless, Kierkegaard discovered a twofold defect in his image of the self as master-thief. First, although not a misanthrope, the master-thief cannot overcome "a touch of melancholy, an encapsulation within himself, a dim view of life-relationships, an inner dissatisfaction" (*JP* 5:13). A self thus patterned is unable to break through its inner confinement, even at those points where it would like to experience joyful mutual relations and not just dream about them. This pent-up reserve can be traced to a second and more basic defect: the idea for which the master-thief lives and from which he draws his sense of self-worth is too indefinite. He cannot specify it sufficiently so that it can serve as a pattern for his own striving and for communicating with others. Eventually, these shortcomings led Kierkegaard to deemphasize the master-thief motif and incorporate its viable portions into his image of God's spy.

Before doing so, however, Kierkegaard used the occasion of his 1835 trip to the rough sea-country around Gilleleje to reduce somewhat the indefiniteness in his own life plan. His famous journal pages for this journey are filled with self-imagery that can have an attraction for other people as well. The following are three examples of such imagery.

1. It is good to withdraw sometimes from the consuming busyness of the world. One seeks an Archimedean point, an anchor, an inner poise, a sense of selfhood apart from this deceptively solid and engrossing world. Thoreau's withdrawal (a decade later) to the heart of nature is of longer duration than Kierkegaard's but is not more intensely reflective. "Here the soul opens willingly to every noble impression. Here one comes out as nature's master, but he also feels that something higher is manifested in nature, something he must bow down before. . . . Here he feels himself great and small at one and the same time" (*JP* 5:33-34). Realism about the self consists in that Pascalian sense of man's grandeur and misery alike, or in Kant's feel for the dignity of the perceiver's own worth when he grasps the moral symbolism of sublimity in natural forces.

2. Kierkegaard also advances a linguistic image of self-growth. One tries to improve upon the child's object-oriented

expression—"me hit the horse"—by gaining an interior understanding of one's free initiation of action. "For only thus will I be
able, like a child calling itself 'I' in its first consciously undertaken
act, be able to call myself 'I' in a profounder sense" (*JP* 5:38–39).
This profounder sense consists in recognizing that even in wor-
shiping the unknown God, one cannot dissolve one's selfhood but
must accentuate one's own individuality and responsibility. To
emasculate the individual would thwart our vocation of engaging
in an always uphill struggle. The name of Sisyphus comes as
readily to Kierkegaard as to Camus, with the difference that for
Kierkegaard it stands for man's alliance with God and not for a
godforsaken absurd situation.

3. A further way of clarifying the master-thief's principle of
living for an idea is to make a twofold distinction regarding imperatives directed at the self. The first is a contrast between an
external and an *internal* imperative. A person who relies upon
some fortunate set of circumstances is an other-directed self: his
rule of acting is set by these external conditions, which ultimately
fail to bring satisfaction. Internal imperativity is the law of the
inner-directed self, looking to one's own understanding and
abilities in relation to life's burdens and opportunities. But Kierkegaard is unwilling to concede that realization of the deepest
roots of one's own existence comes simply from the shift from
outer to inner directedness.

Thus, his second distinction is between the inner-directed attitudes of the *spectator* and the *agent*.[4] These images of self correspond to internal imperatives of two kinds: that of knowledge and
that of living and acting in accord with one's knowledge. The
spectator feels obliged only to improve his knowledge, whereas
the agent seeks to incorporate that knowledge into a line of action.
Kierkegaard does not go so far as to turn this distinction into an
antithesis, since human action springs from knowledge that is
rendered practical. But the Socratic maxim to know oneself can
never be fully realized by the spectator attitude if it is regarded as

4. A congenial Kantian analysis of this distinction is made by Lewis W. Beck,
The Actor and the Spectator (Cambridge, Mass.: Harvard University Press, 1975).

a sufficient interior imperative. "The crucial thing is to find a truth which is truth *for me,* to find *the idea for which I am willing to live and die.* . . . I certainly do not deny that I still accept an *imperative of knowledge* and that through it men may be influenced, but *then it must come alive in me,* and *this* is what I now recognize as the most important of all" (*JP* 5:34, 35). In the most pregnant sense, to live for an idea is to appropriate personally a knowledge that yields an actional imperative. The agent self is the young Kierkegaard's deepest penetration into the meaning of selfhood and foreshadows his theory of truth as subjective and intersubjective.

In sharp contrast to this intersubjective and implicitly theistic image stands that of Faust, who turns the imperative for knowledge into an absolute that excludes the influence of the God-man interpersonal relationship. Like everyone else who tries to interpret Faust, Kierkegaard is never fully satisfied and done with his rendition. On the negative side he rejects part two of Goethe's portrait, since the Kierkegaardian Faust remains unrepentant and unconvinced by any divine plan of redemption through work (which would be synonymous with accepting Kierkegaard's actional imperative of an idea to live and die for). The positive drive is toward identifying Faust as essentially a spectator and incorporating that attitude into the range of permanent attitudes that can characterize a human self. It is the Faust of part one of Goethe's masterpiece that dominates the Faustian imagery used by Kierkegaard.

In a letter to the biologist P. W. Lund, who was doing fieldwork in Brazil, Kierkegaard discussed the doubting moment, or negativity, involved in a search for knowledge. He then personified this phase of self-growth when it is rendered absolute.

> For many, it is this Faustian element that makes itself more or less applicable to every intellectual development, which is why it has always seemed to me that we should concede cosmic significance to the *Faust* concept. Just as our ancestors worshipped a goddess of yearning, so I think that Faust represents doubt personified. . . . He surrendered himself to the

Devil for the express purpose of attaining enlightenment, and it follows that he was not in possession of it prior to this; and precisely because he surrendered himself to the Devil, his doubt increased (just as a sick person who falls into the hands of a medical quack usually gets sicker). For although Mephistopheles permitted him to look through his spectacles into man and into the secret places of the earth, Faust must forever doubt him because of his inability to provide enlightenment about the most profound intellectual matters. In accordance with his own idea he could never turn to God because in the very instant he did so he would have to admit to himself that here in truth lay enlightenment; but in that same instant he would, in fact, have denied his character as one who doubts. [*LD* 43]

This passage succinctly expresses the main traits of a self that seeks to confine its life-ideal to the skeptical attitude and a search for knowledge alone, separated from actional moral responsibilities toward the human community.

For several years, Kierkegaard toyed with the plan of delivering a series of lectures on the Faust theme. They would inspect this image of self internally, point out its attractiveness, and show its ultimate frustration and failure to reach human fulfillment. But although the project generated some interesting notations, it was abandoned as a primary vehicle of expression. The Faust-figure was kept as one manifestation of the aesthetic sphere of existence, but it had to be adjusted to two other lines of inquiry. What happens to a self that subordinates the drive for knowledge to the further internal imperative of moral action? And what consequences for self-development are adumbrated in the above-quoted phrase: "turn to God"? In a word, the aesthetic stage of a Faustian doubting of all things belonged within Kierkegaard's more ample context of the moral and religious modes of existential selfhood.

The theme of the storied self would remain incomplete without including the fairy tale among its sources. Not unexpectedly in the age of the Grimm brothers and of his own compatriot H. C.

Andersen, Kierkegaard takes special relish in reading fairy stories.

Just as perceptively as any psychiatrist writing today, he analyzes their workings upon himself and hence their contribution to his view of selfhood. Interrogating his own experience, Kierkegaard asks:

> Why does the reading of fairy tales provide such fortifying relaxation for the soul? When I am weary of everything and "full of days," fairy tales are always a refreshing, renewing bath for me. *There* all earthly, finite cares vanish, joy, yes, even sorrow, are infinite (and for this reason are so enlarging and beneficial). One sets out to find the blue bird, just like the Crown Princess who lets someone else take over the care of the kingdom while she goes to look for her unhappy lover.... One completely forgets the particular private sorrows which every man can have, in order to plunge into the deep-seated sorrow common to all. [*JP* 5:112]

Through the fairy tale, one can tap the mother lode of our common human experience. Here, the storied selves enlarge our empathy, invite us to fellowship in life's joys and woes, and thus provide a hopeful perspective within which to interpret our personal predicaments after a time of imaginative release.

Finally, the theme of the storied self evokes its counterpart in the *storying self*. Kierkegaard is himself a good storyteller. His imagination takes active hold upon the archetypal figures and fairy-tale characters, elaborates upon them in reference to his own searching for self-realization, and moves his hearers and readers through the retelling. Communication through a story in another key enriches both the teller and the listener in coming to self-understanding. Despite his worries about the role of the imagination in the religious self, Kierkegaard develops this talent into the parable form.[5] In and through the numerous parables studding his works, he offers us the opportunity to share in the

---

5. Examples of his storytelling art are gathered in *Parables of Kierkegaard*, ed. Thomas C. Oden (Princeton, N.J.: Princeton University Press, 1978).

enlargement of the storying self as well as in the educative potential of the storied self.

The Socratic Self

The portrayals of Socrates by Plato and Xenophon have led to centuries of meditation on and rethinking of the character and significance of Socrates.[6] This theme received a powerful impetus in Germany and Scandinavia from J. G. Hamann's *Socratic Memorabilia* (1759) and from Schleiermacher's translation of Plato's dialogues (1807-28). Even before reading Plato, Kierkegaard was strongly attracted to the figure of Socrates, an attraction he felt very early in life and upon which he continued to reflect until the end. Like Nietzsche after him, Kierkegaard offered several interpretations of Socrates, correlated with different situations in his own life. He used these thoughts to clarify his self-understanding and to propose certain possibilities to other human selves. Thus the theme of the Socratic self constituted both a path of personal exploration and a concrete ideal for anyone else seeking a demanding ideal of self-imagery.

The references to Socrates in Kierkegaard's correspondence are few but revealing. They show a spread of responses to life that range from the playful to the stinging, from a perception of everyday incongruities to a sense of the divine. During his stay in Berlin as a student, Kierkegaard sandwiched in between his ironical reports on Schelling's lectures a remark that he never sends postage-due letters. "I always pay the postage, and in this I not only attempt to model myself after but even to outdo that great sage Socrates, who never accepted a fee for his tutorials. I say that I outdo him, although this is really incorrect, for I [outdo] his ideality merely by putting out money; . . . but this outdoing is really only an expression of my attempt to imitate" (*LD* 117). A Socratic person does not live grandiosely off his ideas but always

6. An excellent anthology of interpretations of Socrates through the centuries is edited by Herbert Spiegelberg, *The Socratic Enigma* (Indianapolis: Bobbs-Merrill, 1964). Kierkegaard's own dissertation is *The Concept of Irony, with Constant Reference to Socrates,* trans. Lee M. Capel (New York: Harper & Row, 1965).

pays his own freight in life. He regards himself (in Locke's famous image) as a humble under-laborer clearing away, with his own hands, the rotten twigs of illusion about himself and the world. Into such a self goes the readiness to remove clutter and confusion and to do so by personal example that arouses imitation existentially.

Another component in a Socratically modeled personality is set forth in an 1848 letter sent by Kierkegaard to a law-professor friend. This letter takes as point of departure two items in the newspaper. One is a report that railroad trains were being equipped with brakes. Since the Danish word *bremse* means both a "brake" and a "gadfly," Kierkegaard makes a pun by remarking how crazy it is to use a gadfly to make a train stop. Then he uses the second circumstance—newspaper reports on the revolutions of 1848 and plans to halt them—to draw an analogy. It is even crazier to try to use the gadfly of a counterrevolution to brake a revolution, which itself constitutes a social gadfly.

Kierkegaard moves beyond the word game by asking what a personal or a social vortex needs, and by supplying as an answer: a fixed point. More specifically, he notes that his own fixed point is expressed in the technical term "that single individual" (*LD* 261). These three words connote an existing concrete self who is lucid about his or her own reality, who grounds it in some relation to the divine, and who freely criticizes social movements rather than silently conforms to them as primary shapers of selfhood.

In this sense, Socrates is preeminently a single individual and hence identifies himself as a gadfly, not in order to halt life but to set men searching for a fixed point of reference. Whereas politicians and sophists ask *where* they are going, the Kierkegaardian Socrates asks *whence* one begins, what one's point of departure and foundation are, what lies behind one's strivings. "His point of departure lay in himself and in the god. That is to say, he knew himself, he possessed himself. . . . The living Socrates understood intellectually that only a dead man could conquer, as a sacrifice—and he understood ethically how to direct his whole life to becoming just that" (*LD* 263). Kierkegaard does not agree with the Platonic Socrates that knowledge is an act of reminiscence and that there is a timeless back-door entrance into eternity.[7] But he does recommend the Socratic precepts of becoming a distinctive individual through cognitive and affective acts of self-comprehension, through careful attendance to one's unique call from the divine source of existence, and through living one's personal ideal to the point of a costing sacrifice.

From beginning to end of his unpublished autobiographical materials, Kierkegaard keeps developing his portrait of Socrates as a model for attaining human selfhood. Here, I will concentrate upon four aspects of this theme of Socratic guidance in becoming a self or single individual: affinity, ignorance, education, and liberation. My choice is guided by those traits that are both important to Kierkegaard and capable of having wider application to others.

Affinity. Sometimes interpreters take Kierkegaard's stress on the authentic individual's singularity to mean that the self is unique to the point of being completely isolated and unrelatable to the rest of humanity. One piece of evidence against this inference is Kierkegaard's own sense of affinity with the Greeks, especially Socrates. He expresses this bond in frequent phrases and sentences. During the heat of the attack upon him in the public press, Kierkegaard describes himself in third-person terms as "an author essentially educated by Socrates and the Greeks." Hence, "it is not at all surprising that Socrates made such a deep impression upon me. It may be said that there is something Socratic in me" (*JP* 5:343, 6:251). Before considering what that something is, we should recognize that a self is essentially educable and open to the impressions of others, whether they be historical sources or contemporaries. One does not remain passive but admits of being influenced by the best personal examples and thoughts of other people. A growing self will have to criticize, to appropriate individually, and to transform the human heritage, but it does not remain aloof and unaffected by the values expressed in other lives.

7. From a theological viewpoint, Socrates is presented by Robert L. Perkins as a humanistic temptation and alternative to Christian historicity, in *Søren Kierkegaard* (Richmond, Va.: John Knox Press, 1969), pp. 9–13.

Kierkegaard has a special reason for emphasizing his debt to Socrates and Shakespeare, Hamann and Lessing. If the self were impermeably shut off from such human influences, it might also remain unreachable by God's power and grace. Perhaps this is why Kierkegaard speaks with such respect of Socrates and applies to him some terms otherwise reserved for Christ (without ever fusing the two). This connection is explicitly made when Kierkegaard speaks about tracing Christianity "back to the simplicity of faith, about which I have learned inexpressibly much, formally, from that noble 'simple' wise man of old" (*JP* 6:279), which is Kierkegaard's customary way of referring to Socrates. This text contains two qualifying words: the quotation marks around the word "simple" are a reminder that the ignorance of Socrates is wiser than the complicated talk of the sophists, and the word "formally" is included lest anyone confuse the Socratic faith in the divine with the distinctive structure of one's faith in Christ. That Kierkegaard learns so much about the religious attitude from Socrates indicates that even the most self-possessed person can be instructed and enriched by human and divine teachers.

The other index of the self's essential openness is found in the application of the distinctive terms "prototype" and "governance" to Socrates' life, although always within human limits. One's representation of Socrates is not only historically descriptive but also morally normative. The image not only is informative but also conveys an imperative: Do something similar with your own existence and power of expression. In this way, the human self recognizes that it is not the absolute measure of being and that it has need for imitable ideals. To experience Socrates in his prototypal relation to us is thus to clear up any confusion between God and the human self, between the creative source of moral law and its free acceptance and reaffirmation by us.

Yet there should be no misunderstanding about Socrates or anyone else accorded a humanly prototypal relation to the developing self. Socrates remains that sort of pattern who is himself patterned. His responsiveness to the daimon symbolizes his distinctness from divinity and his attentiveness to its inner check. In taking Socrates as prototype, then, we also accept his attention and response to the divine. Kierkegaard refers to God's active and individually directed providence as governance. The existing human self should become aware of governance, open his individual being to it, and thus shape his singularity by confident following of its promptings (which are more active than the check or reining-in of behavior, as reported by Socrates himself). Without being granted any special visions, Kierkegaard is sure that he is at least *on the right road* in his fidelity to governance. Something like this modest yet firm assurance characterizes every well-grounded self, whatever the obstacles, opposition, and disappointment encountered in life.

Ignorance. Although Socratic ignorance has become proverbial, it is invested with special significance by Kierkegaard. It serves two polemical purposes that are defined by corresponding aspects of his selfhood and his personal relationship to religious existence in his own time.

The first use of the Socratic analogue is to aid us in understanding how agreement is often reached by people who were initially far apart on religious issues. Kierkegaard gives a phenomenological description of the technique of religious reductionism. Sharply defined meanings are whittled down so that the body of beliefs dies a slow death, under a thousand qualifications and accommodations.

> In order to get men along, one may (out of consideration for what men are like these days and what one is himself) reduce the Christian requirements, reduce Christianity, make concessions in that direction. This way one gets to be the most earnest Christian himself and wins many such people over to Christianity. This does irreparable harm, and it is inconceivable that anyone has dared to take this responsibility upon himself, for it is winning men over to Christianity by doing away with Christianity. One may, however, do the reverse and present Christianity without such deference, and then, lest one seem to be judging others, judge oneself as being so far behind that one can scarcely claim the name of Christian, yet deeply desires to become a Christian and strives to be that.

> This is the right way. In due time it may have a resemblance
> to the relation of Socratic ignorance to the glut of human
> knowledge. [*JP* 6:45-46]

A Socratically patterned self raises questions about truth and
faith, justice and human dignity, in order to remove the misap-
prehension that we all understand and accept these values. Such a
self proclaims its ignorance about them, as a way of dissipating the
illusion that they are obvious and that a whole society gives them
thoughtful allegiance.

The Socratically ignorant self maintains only a relation of *striving to become* a person whose life may eventually incorporate such
values. One moves back a step from the knowledge explosion so
that everyone may see the necessity of reflecting upon this glut
rather than just riding on the assumption that its outcome will
obviously be to humankind's benefit.

Kierkegaard's second gloss upon Socratic ignorance takes a
similarly ironical twist. Here the question concerns the uncon-
scionable use of authority on the part of specialists, be they operat-
ing in scientific or governmental, ethical or religious fields. The
human temptation is to glide imperceptibly from modest, limited
competence to very broad claims of authority as though one were
the originator of, and embodied warrant for, the whole field.

How can this attractive delusion (affecting both the claimant to
authority and those who accept him in the attitude of accepting
his words as authoritative) be contravened? Since his own interests are ultimately ethical and religious, Kierkegaard answers in
very personal terms, but his response carries implications for
other affirmations of selfhood.

> *The category* for my undertaking is: to *make men aware* of the
> essentially Christian, but this accounts for the repeated
> statement: I am not that, for otherwise there is confusion. My
> task is to get men deceived—within the meaning of truth—
> into religious commitment, which they have cast off, but I do
> not have authority; instead of authority I use the very oppo-
> site, I say: the whole undertaking is for my own discipline and
> education. This again is a genuinely Socratic approach. Just

as he was the ignorant one, so here: instead of being the teacher, I am the one who is being educated. [*JP* 6:252]

Self-actualization includes a dimension of putting oneself at the service of others. If that service consists solely in consciousness-raising, however, it entails the danger of stimulating others only to one's own conclusions and words, accepted extrinsically in mindless slogans that carry the weight of authority.

Drastic measures are required to enkindle personal searching and free acts of becoming aware. Hence a Socratically minded self will deliberately *de-authoritize* its discourse at some strategic point where the other persons must carry on their own inquiry and form their own convictions. Both Socrates and Kierkegaard find that this point can be reached most readily by declaring their own ignorance, by including themselves among those being taught, in the relationship of dialogue rather than in that of magisterial discourse to others. To arouse personal search, one must shun being an "authoritative somebody."

Education. One self may influence another across the ages, through comportment and practical consequences that carry a message. In this sense, Socrates the educator taught Kierkegaard some somber lessons about what is likely to happen to anyone engaging in the radical pursuit of self-being and interpersonal relations, within the rigidity of a social structure.[8] Three points of instruction were highlighted in Kierkegaard's journals, because they aided in clarifying his own existence and might serve a similar function in other lives.

Kierkegaard confessed, first of all, that he puzzled for years over the paradoxical difference between Socrates' relation with his contemporaries and his relation with later generations. Whereas the former group gave him the cup of hemlock, the latter held him in the highest esteem. This was no accident but expressed the fate of anyone living for his ideals and achieving a unity of those ideals with his very selfhood. "All those who truly

---

8. On the ways in which Kierkegaard uses the model of Socrates for communication, see Ronald J. Manheimer, *Kierkegaard as Educator* (Berkeley: University of California Press, 1977), pp. 3–58.

have served the truth get into trouble with their contemporaries
while they are alive and no sooner are they dead than they are
idolized. . . . This, then, is the law: the person who does not want
to operate with illusions will unconditionally get into trouble during his lifetime, will be trampled down, sacrificed. On the other
hand, as soon as such a person is dead, the deceivers (orators,
poets, professors, etc.) promptly take him over and exploit him—
and he is idolized by the next generation" (*JP* 6:473). Kierkegaard
traced this alienational law to the antipathy that people feel toward unadorned accounts of actuality and hence to the need for
an imaginative distance from honest reports before acknowledging their truth and honoring their existential bearers.

A second consideration was aimed against any special condemnation of the time of Socrates or of Kierkegaard's own generation. "Far be it from me to indict the present age as if the world
had been so wonderful before. No, as far as I am concerned, I
would have a bad time of it in any age. Socrates was right in saying
that banishment would have helped him very little, since it would
have gone badly for him in every country. The root of the matter
was that Socrates was the inciter" (*JP* 5:407). For his own sanity
and balance, it was essential also for Kierkegaard to avoid a con-
spiratorial view of his day and age, an exaggerated pessimism
about it that would trace his troubles back to others taken separately from his own incitive self. Whenever and wherever he
might have lived, he would have had to endure the opposition his
inherently polemical self would have stirred up. And his implicit
suggestion was that anyone else bearing strong witness to personally held ideas could expect the same strife to develop and ought
not to bemoan the parlous times as a peculiar burden.

Thirdly, Kierkegaard's interpretation of Socrates educated
him to criticize the elitism apparently entailed by opposition to the
masses. A major entry on this issue is tart and precise.

> "The crowd" is really what I have aimed at polemically, and
> that I have learned from Socrates. I want to make men aware
> so that they do not waste and squander their lives. The aristo-
> crats take for granted that there is always a whole mass of

men who go to waste. But they remain silent about it, live secluded, and act as if these many, many human beings did not exist at all. . . . Men are not so corrupt that they actually desire evil, but they are blind and really do not know what they are doing. Everything centers on drawing them out into the arena of decision. [*JP* 5:368]

Written in 1847, when everything was pointing toward the social upheavals of the following year, this passage conveys the sort of revolution sought by Kierkegaard.

For him, the terms "crowd" and "masses" are not completely rigid, objective classifications of groups of people. Rather, they are modal qualifiers applicable to a particular way of living *into which anyone* can fit, and also *from which anyone* can get free. These terms characterize an unaware, unreflective manner of being and acting, one that thrives upon a thoughtless conformity and evasion of personal deliberation. Kierkegaard's project of making men aware sets him on an inevitable course of conflict with this attitude but does so in such fashion that it keeps him related energetically with the people in whom this attitude is found. He does not withdraw aristocratically from them and write them off as a necessary but unimportant condition of civilized living. Instead, "to make aware" is to aim at kindling a self-recognition on the part of all people as human beings and at encouraging them to make free decisions for themselves. This is the radically humane equality in which a Socrates and a Kierkegaard locate the reality of the self, the transformational quality that enables all persons to break out of caste and class categories.

Liberation. Occasionally, Kierkegaard speaks admiringly about Socrates' laughter and dance of life. These are celebratory expressions by a reflective self who also affirms the peaks of joy that an entire society can share. But while Kierkegaard commends the Socratic acts of celebration consecrated to the divine, he does not let laughter have the final say, lest it turn into a comic act. His own highest joy lies in the thought that "my life is a service in the royal court" (*JP* 6:540), which is a way of stating his own manner of remaining faithful to God's call to himself.

Thus in the end Socrates set Kierkegaard free to actualize his own self-being freely and within his distinctive mode of existing. In turn, Kierkegaard regarded it as a duty to invite others to liberate themselves from him. As a remarkable series of letters testitifes, he had toyed for some time with the idea that Professor Rasmus Nielsen might be his own disciple and academic spokesman.[9] But eventually he cut the umbilical cord so that their relation could be less formally structured and intellectually one-sided. For the larger theme of selfhood, then, Kierkegaard held that interrelations among persons should involve a link with the community along with liberation from all obstacles to maturity and reciprocity.

Friendly Selves

Much about Kierkegaard's life and thought suggests that the relation among selves is bound to be painfully alienating or even hostile, rather than friendly. His melancholy father not only sharpened his dialectical wit and imagination but also left him "a primitive depression . . ., a huge dowry of distress" (*JP* 6:12-13). At least part of Kierkegaard's break with Regine Olsen was due to his reluctance to make her a partner in this inheritance, which had shadowed his childhood and left him unable to break out of his chamber of melancholy. As for the rest of the world—the public attitude represented by the press and the church establishment—he set his face against it, declaring that he delighted in war and laughed at mankind. The metaphors coming most readily to describe his condition were those of the stormy petral and the Eskimo in a kayak, metaphors of strife and social loneliness made bearable only by trust in God's providence.[10]

If we turn to the entries in the *Journals and Papers* gathered topically under the heading of "Friendship," we find scant com-

9. Cf. *LD* vii, "Correspondence Register," Letters from Søren Kierkegaard to R. Nielsen. Until his early death, P. M. Møller was Kierkegaard's teacher and friend.

10. Kierkegaard's masterly use of metaphors provides concrete instantiation of the psycholinguistic and analogical theory of meaning developed by Paul Ricoeur in *The Rule of Metaphor* (Toronto: University of Toronto Press, 1977).

fort on this theme. Yet they do yield some of Kierkegaard's intellectual grounds of criticism, directed not at the value of friendship itself but at certain notions about it that aroused his opposition and irony. His objections crystallized around four misconceptions.

First, some people identify friendship with hearty fun and games, from which all thoughtful interchange is excluded as a spoiler. But Kierkegaard asks: "What is friendship without intellectual interaction, a refuge for weak souls who are not able to breathe in the atmosphere of intelligence but only in the atmosphere of animal exhalations?" (*JP* 2:78). Conviviality without some thoughtful interchange is a surcease from life rather than its intensification. Such a relationship is a form of mutual insurance against arousing the critical mind, leading at most to business arrangements from which the free giving of selves has fled.

Secondly, and at the opposite extreme, there is an extravagant overestimating of the scope of understanding generated by friendship. "Certainly understanding is part of friendship, but not the kind which makes the one continually aware of what the other is going to say" (*JP* 2:78). This is Kierkegaard's way of requiring friendship to respect the spontaneity and individual differences proper to the persons involved. One party cannot claim to know everything about the other's experiences and conversational initiatives, on pain of reducing that other person to a marionette and thus destroying the relation of friendship. Into the relation of friendship must be incorporated the factors of freedom, surprise, and distinct manners of existing.

Precisely out of this distinctiveness arises the third, or teleological, problem. It is amazing to hear someone speak about his great number of friends. Their bond in this case is generated by what Kierkegaard calls their finite aims and interest, their agreement in devoting themselves to the pursuit of some tangible useful goods attainable in the short run. This basis does not differ greatly from the mutual insurance mentioned above, except that people may plan together and thus share in a pragmatic interaction of intelligence. But what if a person seeks the highest, a union with God that entails sacrifice and suffering? There is then a sloughing off of interests, replaced by the same sort of discouraging counsel offered to Job by those who called themselves his friends. As the telic split grows wider, the possibility of friendship diminishes. What prevents it from vanishing entirely is, in Kierkegaard's estimation, only that honesty about the connection between sacrifice and the search after God which upbuilding conversations between friends are intended to evoke.

The tendency of church leaders to muddy this connection constitutes the fourth obstacle to genuine friendship. Kierkegaard is specially distressed by Bishop Mynster's sermons on our friendship with God, on our having a friend in heaven. "This business of a friend in heaven is a sentimentality which has made a thorough mess of Christianity. Yes we may call Christ the Friend of sinners, for this is the same as Savior and Redeemer. But simply to call Christ a friend in heaven, this does away with God the Father and makes Christ into something altogether wrong" (*JP* 2:80). We never grow so old and technologically powerful as to take over our own providence, thus ceasing to need the Father-child relation. And we never simply relate ourselves to Christ as colleague, but must qualify our relation to him as redeeming us from sin and suffering. The unrealistic sentimentalizing of man's friendship with God manifests itself also in Mynster's all-too-easy gilding over of Christ's choice of disciples as friends. It would be as if one were to scrutinize polemically the whole contemporary age and then settle upon an apprentice tailor and shoemaker as friends—a friendship at which Mynster would laugh.

Given these many considerations, it was not easy for Kierkegaard to develop positive imagery of friendly selves. Yet he did do so, aided by some other aspects of his life and reflection.

Within his extended family, he helped to develop a friendly climate.[11] Kierkegaard was a favorite of his nephews and nieces. He entered into their games, told them fairy stories and challenged them with riddles, gave out flowers and toys at appro-

11. This aspect of friendly selfhood is studied by J. R. Scudder, Jr., "Kierkegaard and the Responsible Enjoyment of Children," in *Kierkegaard's Presence in Contemporary American Life*, ed. Lewis A. Lawson (Metuchen, N.J.: Scarecrow Press, 1970), pp. 240–49.

priate times, and lightened their households with laughter and open affection. When he went abroad, he kept in contact with them through letters filled with droll descriptions and drawings. Yet his Berlin letters to the youngsters conveyed no traces of his anguish about Regine Olsen, who liked the children's company and might thereby have learned indirectly about his concern for her. When he became a controversial public figure, he seldom visited with them lest the storm engulf them along with himself. Only after he had spent himself and entered the hospital to die, did he receive frequent visits from his niece Henriette Lund. Her letters and recollections are a primary source on his familial relationships.

Kierkegaard's steadfast friend from childhood until death was Emil Boesen, who took the same theological studies and became a pastor. It was he who went to the theater with Kierkegaard just after the latter broke his engagement to Regine. And it was to Boesen that Kierkegaard sent from Berlin a series of letters conveying his intimate thoughts and motivations concerning Regine, as well as describing his disappointment with Schelling's lectures. But the correspondence between them also recorded their own friendship, the chief experiential basis for the Kierkegaardian meaning of "friendly selves."

In his first extant letter to Boesen (written a few weeks before the death of Kierkegaard's father, and hence before his meeting Regine Olsen and going to Berlin), Kierkegaard hails him thus: "You, my friend, *the only one,* through whose intercession I endured the world that in so many ways seemed unbearable, the only one left when I let doubt and suspicion like a violent storm wash away and destroy all else—*my Mount Ararat,* where is it?" (*LD* 51). Although this may seem to be an extravagant mode of address, on closer inspection it proves to convey an accurate metaphor. A friend is a Mount Ararat, a supportive presence that gives hope and fidelity even when one's own suspicious and combative nature turns other people away. Yet this Ararat is a friendly peak within the human world, not the Archimedean point outside the world that Kierkegaard also mentions in the same letter and that he finds in the love of God. Boesen is never turned into a

minor deity, and hence their relationship is able to include some
sharp mutual criticisms across the ensuing years.

Kierkegaard calls Boesen his stablemate and comrade, with
whom he can share the ups and downs of life and the ideals that
make existence bearable. In a solemn journal entry written
shortly after his father's death, Kierkegaard not only speaks of a
transfigured filial image but also of a need to develop it through
conversation. "Right now I feel there *is* only *one* person (E.
Boesen) with whom I can really talk about him" (*JP* 5:122). In the
crisis following his break with Regine Olsen, Kierkegaard again
registers his strong need to talk freely with his friend and confid-
ant, Boesen.

> How good it was to talk myself out once in a while, but, as you
> know, I need a rather long time for that even though I talk
> fast. . . . You know how I am, how in conversation with you I
> jump about stark naked, whereas I am always enormously
> calculating with other people. . . . I confide only in you. I am
> used to doing that and I depend on your silence. [*LD* 102,
> 115, 140]

Conversational openness, mutual trust, and discretion comprise
the marrow of friendship among colleagues. Even in such intimate matters as his relationship with his father, his concern about
his former fiancée, and his ideal of a religious community, Kierkegaard finds healing and growth in spoken and written communication with Boesen.

Yet two further points cannot evade Kierkegaard's reflection
and explicit statement. One is the painful contrast between this
collegial bond and his wary, many-guised modes of relating to
others. Although Kierkegaard does not expect to achieve friend-
ships on all sides, he does want to reach out (if only polemically
and through upbuilding discourses) to other people in ways that
will alter their existence. There is authorial intent as well as emo-
tive force in this optative declaration to Boesen: "I need a voice as
piercing as the glance of *Lynceus,* as terrifying as the groan of the
giants, as sustained as a sound of nature, extending in range from
the deepest bass to the most melting high notes, and modulated

from the most solemn-silent whisper to the fire-spouting energy of rage" (*LD* 54).[12] This romantically tinged wish is also a good forecast of the spectrum of communicative means he was to employ in his authorship, which was to become his closest analogue of friendship with his contemporaries.

The second point is a certain reservation that Kierkegaard is always careful to include in his remarks to Boesen about their friendship. He values Boesen not despite but precisely because of the restricted areas where Boesen's opinions carry weight.

> I shall certainly not readily forget that you have been decent enough to remain steadfast, to believe even though you could not understand [Kierkegaard's behavior in breaking off his engagement]. . . . You are and always will remain the only person who has a seat and a vote in the council of my many and various thoughts. . . . When I assured you in my first letter that you held a seat in the council of my thoughts, that was true enough, but that means primarily that I often include you in my thoughts, that you really do have a seat and a vote in many aspects of my life, but especially with respect to all of my modest production. [*LD* 114, 116, 133]

These reservations conform with Kierkegaard's attack upon the sentimental notion that a friend experiences everything one does, knows all of one's motivations, and joins in all of one's decision-making. Through his remarks to Boesen, Kierkegaard concretely dissociates himself from requiring omniscience about oneself and total involvement in all one's decisions as the criteria of genuine human friendship. As in our relations with God, so also in the human sphere, friends must often believe without understanding and accept each other's course of action without being completely privy to its every aspect.

Within the limits of human finitude, however, the individual self benefits greatly from admitting a friend to one's own voting

12. Since this sentence is used again, five years later, in *Either/Or*, trans. David F. Swenson, Lillian M. Swenson, and Walter Lowrie, rev. Howard A. Johnson, 2 vols. (New York: Doubleday, Anchor, 1959), 1:23, it illustrates the intimate relationship between all modes of writing in Kierkegaard.

council. To take into account what a friend would think of one's imaginative designs and practical deliberations, even within a restricted range of concerns, is a major step toward breaking out of isolation and entering into human unions. Kierkegaard testifies that he is enormously cheered by the awareness that Boesen cares about him and seeks his well-being for its own sake. This sense of a friend's caring helps Kierkegaard to clarify his own selfhood by a good presence, to determine the course of his authorship or relation to the wider community, and thus to achieve portions of his own identity through living up to some shared ideals. Even the gradualness of self-formation as a temporal process is brought home strongly when Kierkegaard looks forward to talking again with Boesen and feeling a deeper harmony between them, in consequence of confidences interchanged and storms weathered together.[13] These are signs of jointly maturing comrades.

In Kierkegaard's journals, there is another set of considerations affecting his view of friendship, namely, its relationship with love. Drawing upon Plato and Aristotle, the Bible, and extracts from medieval theologians and mystics, he recognizes three modes of love. They are *eros* or erotic love, *philia* or friendship, and *agape* or religious love of God and neighbor.[14] Hence Kierkegaard proposes giving "twelve lectures on erotic love, friendship, and love" (*JP* 5:374, a plan realized in his book *Works of Love*). Although capable of being combined in several ways, they remain distinct and capable of distinctive realization. Kierkegaard's imagery of the self as fulfilled by friendship is always complicated by images of the other two sorts of self-realization through love.

Problems arise concerning the different ways in which the indi-

13. The conceptual issues raised by a temporally developing selfhood are explored by Mark Taylor, *Kierkegaard's Pseudonymous Authorship: A Study of Time and the Self* (Princeton, N.J.: Princeton University Press, 1975).

14. Two basic studies on these forms of love are Anders Nygren's *Agape and Eros* (New York: Harper Torchbooks, 1969), and Martin D'Arcy's *The Mind and Heart of Love* (New York: Holt, 1947). Kierkegaard's sustained contribution is *Works of Love*, trans. Howard V. Hong and Edna H. Hong (New York: Harper Torchbooks, 1964).

vidual self relates and orders these modes of love. Kierkegaard's engagement and break with Regine posed the issue of whether or not erotic love is to be integrated with friendship. Even after he revoked their engagement, Kierkegaard retained friendship for her as a permanent shaping of his self-reality. This is manifest in the letter addressed to Regine after her marriage to J. F. Schlegel. "I offer you for the second time what I can and dare and ought to offer you: reconciliation [*in earler drafts, first:* my love, that is to say my friendship; *later:* friendship; *and finally:* reconciliation]" (*JP* 6:255). We can be grateful to the editor for recording the stricken phrases, since they show vividly how difficult it was for Kierkegaard to adapt ordinary usage to his purpose. His precise intent was to affirm that *philia, amor amicitiae,* that sort of love which holds among friends, had become an indelible strand in his selfhood as related to Regine, but one calling for a response in kind. As for his relation with Boesen, it did not involve erotic love. In this case, Kierkegaard's repeated use of the term "comrade" was sufficient to indicate they were bound together by *philia,* by the nonerotic love among friendly selves.

But what about *agape*? This is a question concerning the ordering of relational strands in the realization of self-being through the modes of love. Kierkegaard regards it as part of his vocation of living and writing "as if we were God's spies" (*JP* 5:140, 499; his favorite quotation from *King Lear*) to assert the primacy of love-of-God-and-neighbor over the other two kinds of love. Agapic love is not set off at a distance eminently above other expressions of love but suffuses and transforms them, at least among persons of religious faith. Faith-ful friends are united by their dedication to a jointly affirmed religious ideal. That is why Kierkegaard's letters to Boesen often mention their mutual adherence to "our motto: '*A church stands in the distance*'" (*LD* 54; the italicized line is from the Danish poet A. Oehlenschläger). Since Kierkegaard's later attack on the established church is a deepening of his search after a Christianity not deformed by official Christendom, he regards his friendship with Boesen as being deepened. These friendly selves hold tenaciously to each other, even when there is no full understanding between them about the particulars of

Kierkegaard's call for simple ethical honesty about the social expression of agapic love.

There is another facet in his insistence upon the intervention of the agape-factor in the social growth of friendly selves. Without such a presence, the individual self may never communicate effectively with others in terms of either erotic love or friendship or both. "Even in David's psalms there are examples of the kind of self-encapsulation or closed-upness which seeks to avoid every human relationship in order to remain *Du und Du* with God" (*JP* 5:280). To maintain a Thou-speaking relation of personal intimacy with God, right away and without any redirecting of the heart, is both fraudulent and impoverishing. It is fraudulent insofar as it ignores the need for man to declare his sins, and for God to come as a forgiving, loving savior. And it is impoverishing insofar as it also ignores and conceals the difficulties attendant upon one's efforts to achieve erotic love and friendship with others in the human community. Kierkegaard satirizes all dimensions of the easy thou-and-thou relationships, since they conceal the struggles needed for overcoming what he recognizes as the human self's condition of "self-encapsulation or closed-upness."

Thus his theme of the ordering and relating among the modes of love contributes to Kierkegaard's reflections on the human self and its ways to fulfillment. But perhaps the last word should be reserved for the person with whom he became friends for life. Reporting on Kierkegaard's frame of mind during his final stay in the hospital, Emil Boesen records the concern Kierkegaard felt for any troubles brought on by their friendship. "I am so glad you [Boesen] are here. Thank you, thank you. . . . Good-bye, thank you, forgive me for having been the cause of your having difficulties which you would not otherwise have had."[15] Kierkegaard's

15. *The Journals of Søren Kierkegaard,* trans. Alexander Dru (New York: Oxford University Press, 1938), pp. 551, 552. Boesen's report is given here on pp. 548–53; sections on Kierkegaard in the memoir of his niece Henriette Lund are found on pp. 555–61. Kierkegaard's visual mode of communication is described here by his philosopher friend Hans Brøchner: "His smile and his look was indescribably expressive. He had a particular way of greeting one at a distance with a look. It was

final words of gladness, gratitude, and solicitude aptly express the fruit of a lifelong solidarity between friendly selves.

Conclusion

Having concentrated until now upon specific content, I have an inductive basis for making a few methodological remarks on how to study Kierkegaard's view of the self.

Often there is a concentration upon certain books in which he expresses his position most formally and at great length. Major treatments of the self are made in *The Concept of Anxiety* [Dread] and *The Sickness unto Death*.[16] These and his other books supply plentiful materials, but they also often lead scholars into a purely conceptual and analytic approach. Kierkegaard does indeed use many concepts drawn from his philosophical and theological readings, and uses them constructively as well as polemically. But his conceptual schemata are always contexted and modified by vivid imagery and concrete descriptions of states of the soul. The imaginal and concrete elements are not a decorative fringework but an essential part of his thinking on the self.

My emphasis upon imagery of the self is intended to take into account his actual practice and the intent behind it. Kierkegaard deliberately establishes a tension between formal *concepts* and *images*, so that his meaning of the self will grow out of their polar

---

just a little movement of the eyes, and yet it expressed so much. He could put something infinitely gentle and loving into his gaze, but he could also goad and tease people to a frenzy by a look. With a single look at a passer-by he could as he expressed it 'put himself in touch with him'" (p. 563).

16. These sources are penetratingly examined by John Elrod in *Being and Existence in Kierkegaard's Pseudonymous Works* (Princeton, N.J.: Princeton University Press, 1975), pp. 29–113; by George Stack in *Kierkegaard's Existential Ethics* (University, Ala.: University of Alabama Press, 1977), pp. 138–78; and by Kresten Nordentoft in *Kierkegaard's Psychology* (Pittsburgh: Duquesne University Press, 1978), pp. 81–89, 187–99. In his forthcoming work, *Kierkegaard: An Ethicist in 'Christendom'* (Princeton University Press), Elrod distinguishes between the naturally selfish and the neighbor-loving or ethical self, as treated in Kierkegaard's later writings.

relations.[17] The intention governing his procedure is twofold. First, he seeks to correct the claims of the Danish Hegelians that truth comes only with pure concepts. On the contrary, human true reflection on the self consists in the maximal interplay between image and concept, without the latter ever properly surmounting the former. Secondly, Kierkegaard does not think about the self in splendidly pure speculation but constantly relies upon his actual experience for problems and confirmations. Both these intentions become very evident when one observes his free development in journals, papers, and letters.

Another way of organizing the Kierkegaardian account of selfhood is to build an exposition around his doctrine on the stages and spheres of existence. This approach is especially effective in bringing out the developmental aspect of self-realization and the plural choices that present themselves in this free process of shaping individual and social selfhood.

My exposition here does not rigidly follow this guiding theme of the stages on life's way. But there is a rough analogy between aesthetic existence and the present account of storied and storying selves; between ethical existence and the figure of Socrates; and between religiousness (as distinguished by Kierkegaard into forms A and B) and the motif of friendly selves. Perhaps the chief advantage here of staying close to the journals and letters is the opening up of every existential realm more diversely and experientially than a restriction to Kierkegaard's published books would permit.

I have refrained, however, from explicitly broaching the related problem of the pseudonyms. It is implied, indeed, in Kierkegaard's call for a many-toned voice, as well as in his transcription of many autobiographical statements (sometimes in a transformed shape) into his pseudonymous writings. This complex double expression of reflections on the self indicates a need for cautious qualification of such reflections, as well as for further

17. Nietzsche does much the same thing, as brought out by contributors to *Nietzsche: Imagery and Thought,* ed. Malcolm Pasley (Berkeley: University of California Press, 1978).

research on the gnarled issue of Kierkegaard's uses of pseudonyms and "editors." Precisely on the matter of understanding his own self, the following testimony by Kierkegaard should give pause to an interpreter. "For many years my depression has prevented me from saying '*Du*' to myself in the profoundest sense. Between my '*Du*' and my depression lay a whole world of imagination. This is what I partially discharged in the pseudonyms" (*JP* 5:369). The pseudonyms are cathartic expressions that both reveal and help to remove Kierkegaard's alienation from himself. This function furnishes yet another reason for his criticism of thou-speaking, in this case because such language underestimates the difficulty of coming to understand the speaker's own self-reality as obscured by states of depression.

Many of the texts I have used also get a public lease on life by inclusion, in one form or another, in Kierkegaard's upbuilding and religious discourses. There is no good textual ground, either in the books or the papers, for stopping short of his discourses, meditations, and final polemics. They continue to develop his own self-being and his understanding of human selfhood in the single individual and in society. Whatever Kierkegaard's later vicissitudes, he holds firmly to two beacon lights. "You must want only the truth, neither vainly wish to be flattered nor self-tormentingly want to be made a pure devil. . . . No true self-knowledge without God-knowledge or [without standing] before God" (*JP* 4:40). The absolute requirements that Kierkegaard demands of himself and others are an undeviating honesty and thirst for truth about oneself, and a sufficient amount of courage to stand before God and look at oneself in the mirror provided by God's presence and word.

It is appropriate to conclude by asking the story-telling Kierkegaard how long this process of searching, measuring, and becoming a human self should go on.

> Suppose a man were assigned the task of entertaining himself for an entire day, and he finishes this task of self-entertainment as early as noon: then his celerity would not be meritorious. So also when life constitutes the task. To be

finished with life before life has finished with one, is precisely not to have finished the task.[18]

An early finish to the task of self-understanding and self-upbuilding is no finish at all.

18. Oden, *Parables of Kierkegaard,* p. 85; a remark assigned to the pseudonym Johannes Climacus in Kierkegaard's *Concluding Unscientific Postscript,* trans. David Swenson and Walter Lowrie (Princeton, N.J.: Princeton University Press, 1941), p. 147.

4

Metaphilosophy in the Shadow of Kierkegaard

Harold A. Durfee

This essay intends to suggest that the metaphilosophical implications of Søren Kierkegaard's philosophical and theological
reflections point to the radical deconstruction of the classical
foundations of Western man's metaphysical adventure and to
reconstruction on new foundations at the very ground of the
philosophical enterprise itself. I would not claim that what follows
is derivable directly from the Kierkegaardian corpus, hence the
word "shadow" in the title; but just as Karl Jaspers suggested that
we must philosophize now "in the light of the exception,"[1] so
likewise I will argue that Kierkegaard's work cut the roots of
classical philosophical endeavor and both implies and demands
its reconstitution on a fundamentally new basis. I would also
suggest that the seriousness of this transformation has hardly
been recognized within the discipline, for such recognition would
significantly transform its self-understanding. Consequently, I
invite the reader to reflect upon the initiation of philosophy
within Kierkegaard's shadow.

The Foundations of Philosophical Reflection

The relationship of human reflective activity and accomplishments to the real that such reflection intends to capture,

1. See K. Jaspers, *Reason and Existenz* (Noonday, 1955), Lecture 1. Each section
of my essay could be expanded into another essay. I hope to supply those expan-
sions in future publications, but at this time I have chosen to offer a more synoptic
vision of these metaphilosophical considerations.

resemble, and understand is the occasion for three thousand years of intense debate. While such reflection can express itself in everyday talk, scientific conclusions, poetry, myth, religious affirmations, mathematical systems, or even in nonverbal codes such as dance or musical composition, one constant elaboration of its findings lies in philosophical, theological, or scientific theories. Immediately the question arises as to the ultimate foundations of such theoretical activity. In the history of Western philosophical reflection a very strange tension has developed, however, concerning the ultimate foundations of philosophical life itself. This tension not only continues in twentieth-century theory, pervading nearly every philosophical position, but has become more intense as philosophy has become increasingly self-reflexive, attempting to understand itself. To the question concerning foundations, a somewhat common answer has suggested reliance upon what reason is able to discern and justify regarding the nature of the real and, further, has suggested that the reason, when so engaged, can be considered self-authenticating. So it is assumed, with little explicit discussion or explanation, that philosophy is the rational self-inspection of human rationality, combined with empirical evidence, to establish the appropriate conclusions regarding being. But with this kind of "answer," one is impressed by how constantly the question of philosophical foundations has been avoided. Reflective humanity waited 2,500 years for Descartes's *Meditations* upon philosophical methodology, and one looks in vain, even today, for serious studies as to how one begins the philosophical undertaking or how one enters a particular philosophical orientation. Handbooks for philosophy students are almost devoid of intelligible suggestions as to how one enters any of the theoretical positions elaborated. The tension between the assumed self-authenticating self-reflexivity of reason as the gateway to the land of sophisticated theory and the tendency to avoid the problem of clarification of the appropriate entrance to a philosophical position remains an odd ambiguity in the very center of Western theorizing.

This ambiguity leads to my thesis, which is that Kierkegaard offered debatable but penetrating suggestions, both implicitly and explicitly, as to the entré to theoretical structures. Furthermore, Kierkegaard's proposals stand in profound opposition to, and raise most serious questions concerning, the classical self-reflexive foundations assumed in the history of Western thought and thereby make obvious the serious tension within major twentieth-century theoretical alternatives. This tension, though pervasive, is regularly neglected, thus leaving the basic ground of theoretical life ambiguous and seriously in need of exploration. Philosophy still does not understand its own foundations. This essay will not overcome that obscurity but does intend to isolate the ambiguity foundational to philosophical and psychological theory, to heighten our consciousness of the tension and of Kierkegaard's shadow, and thereby to offer the theoretician opportunity to address the matter directly. Although I shall concentrate upon philosophical theory, I am assuming that consideration of the foundations of psychological theory is implicit.

The Tradition upon Which the Shadow Falls

As background for the appreciation of Kierkegaard's contribution, one should have in mind the theme of the authority of reason as it developed in Greek philosophy. Everything was made subservient to the rational authority, so that even Greek philosophy itself was a rationalized explication of Homeric and Hesiodic religious insight and a philosophical rationalizing of the Greek gods. Let us note also that this development of Greek philosophical rationalism eventually confronted a quite different elaboration of man's central concerns when it encountered the Hebrew-Christian tradition. For Western civilization this was a confrontation at the very foundation of our culture from which we have not yet recovered. While the Greeks had elaborated variations on philosophical reflection, they had not developed man's religious insight as had the early Hebrew and Christian sages. While the Hebrews and early Christians, and other Middle Eastern peoples, had concentrated upon the centrality of God, the loyalty of the person and the people, and the disloyalty of all, as well as the final hope of all, they had never developed the rational philosophical and metaphysical speculation that had characterized the Greek mind. Once Athens and Jerusalem confronted each other, Western man devoted his attention to the new problem of relating these two great cultural achievements. Although all of us may be too secularized to recognize the momentous character of this confrontation, we should not forget that a major and underlying theme in the history of Western thought, ever since Saint Paul spoke on Mar's Hill, has concerned the proper relationships of these two traditions. Even serious atheistic proponents (Camus, Nietzsche, Russell, Sartre) develop their analysis relative to the Athens-Jerusalem confrontation and the Hebrew-Christian affirmations. Contemporary philosophy is the locus for the destruction of the attempted ontotheological synthesis that has been the genius and burden of two thousand years of Western philosophy.

It should be obvious that Kierkegaard participates vigorously in this debate—in his *Philosophical Fragments,* for example, wherein he inquires as to the essential distinction between Christianity and Socrates. Let it also be noted that Paul Holmer plays an equally explicit role in this debate, constantly functioning as iconoclast, destroying the gods of theoretical systems, either philosophical or theological, and recalling modern man to the profound simplicity of biblical affirmations of loyalty, repentance, and truth. Holmer's destruction of philosophical and theological idols stands in deep continuity with the Kierkegaardian spirit.[2]

The rationalism of Greek philosophy, appearing well before Socrates, assumed a profound intimacy between the realm of human reason and the realm of reality. Only because there was some basic continuity or connection between reason and the real could one expect philosophical reflection to discern the nature of the real. The character of this intimacy, of course, was analyzed in various ways, but regardless of the descriptive details, in one manner or another thought was believed to be in sufficient intimacy with the real to be able to discover the nature of being itself.

2. P. Holmer, "Post-Kierkegaard: Remarks About Being a Person," this volume, chap. 1.

As early as Parmenides it was suggested that "it is the same thing that can be thought and can be." I am not concerned with analysis of what this might have meant for Parmenides, nor with assessment of its validity; I want only to point out the early appearance of the proposed intimacy of thought and the real and to suggest that in a variety of modes this Parmenidean theme has dominated the history of Western philosophical reflection. It was because thought seemed to have an intimate connection with being that it was appropriate to offer philosophical analysis in the first place, to build systems of thought, and to follow rules of logical validity; such analysis aimed not only at understanding thought but also at understanding the real.

Does not the same theme lie at the foundation of Saint Anselm's famous ontological argument for the existence of God? It was because thought and reality were so intertwined that Anselm could move from the idea of God to the existence of God. To deny the argument would be to contradict oneself, and contradiction could not reflect the real. Once it was determined that "that than which no greater can be conceived can not be conceived not to exist," then one could move from what was necessary in thought to what was necessary in reality, and so it was concluded that that being "than which no greater can be conceived" must in fact exist. Once again I am not concerned with debating the validity of the argumentation but only with noting the underlying assumption regarding the intimacy of reason and the real.

Consider further the attempted proofs for the existence of God in modern Thomism. Garrigou-Lagrange, professor in the Collegio Angelico in Rome and a recent leading spokesman for the position, has elaborated this concern most distinctly. In initiating the discussion of the Thomistic proofs for the existence of God he writes:

> It will be seen that the proofs for God's existence rest ultimately upon the principle of identity or of non-contradiction, their proximate basis being the principle of sufficient reason, and their immediate basis the principle of causality. Each of the proofs will establish clearly the fact that

> the principle of identity, which is the supreme law of thought, must be at the same time the supreme law of reality.

He continues later:

> The intelligible world is the sole object of true science.... In fact, the certitude properly called scientific grows in proportion as what one affirms approaches nearer to those first principles which are, as it were, the very structure of reason—the principle of identity implied in the idea of being, that most simple and universal of all ideas, the principles of contradiction, causality, and finality. If the principle of identity and non-contradiction is not only a law of thought, but also of being, if the other principles (in order to escape the charge of absurdity) must necessarily be referred to it, then every assertion necessarily connected with such principles will have metaphysical or absolute certainty, and its negation implies a contradiction.[3]

Here again I wish simply to call attention to the assumed intimacy of the first principles of thought with the first principles of being.

Consider also the famous Cartesian methodology of doubt used as a proof for the inevitability of the ego. One is to doubt until one discovers something indubitable, and what is found indubitable in thought then must be so in reality as well. In a recent reinterpretation of Lessing, quite conscious of the relationships between Lessing and Kierkegaard, Leonard P. Wessel writes of Descartes:

> The Cartesian self that has *thinkingly* isolated itself from all objective being and become aware of itself as an isolated *cogito* becomes aware in the very same reflective act of itself as existing, as a *sum*. The self as an object of cognition is identical with itself as the subject of cognition and, therefore, there

---

3. R. Garrigou-Lagrange, *God: His Existence And His Nature* (St. Louis: Herder, 1939), pp. v, 63–64. For further discussion of this Thomistic thesis see E. Gilson, *The Spirit of Medieval Philosophy* (New York: Scribner's, 1936), pp. 236–37.

is no division between subject and object, between thinking and being, between seeming and reality. . . .

The "I" as a process of rational thinking posits a host of ontological principles in the very same act of positing and cognitively grasping its own reality. In other words, that which is entailed as a necessary ingredient making possible the very act of self-cognition must be granted real ontological reference since the being of the self manifests reality. That which holds formally for the reality of the self's being must by extension hold for the being of reality *per se*. Since the reality of the self's being is only revealed in and through the rationality of thinking, the principles underlying rational thinking must of necessity reveal the ontic structure of being *per se*. In short, the *cognitionis humanae principia* must contain within themselves the essential outline of the being of all possible things. . . .[4]

The theme of the intimacy of thought and being, so pervasive of Western philosophy in a wide variety of positions, reaches its culmination in the great Hegelian system of the nineteenth century. Hegel understood this underlying logos of intellectual history and brought it to fulfillment in his central thesis of the identity of thought and being. "The real is the rational and the rational is the real." It is irrelevant for our purposes that Hegel analyzed this intimacy in a uniquely dialectical manner, although this has been traditionally the character of German reflection, at least since Jacob Boehme and Nicolas of Cusa. Neither is it of central concern to us that Hegel elaborated the intimacy of thought and the real in a uniquely idealistic way, although perhaps it may be difficult to maintain such a position and do otherwise. The Parmenidean thesis itself finds in Hegel a modern fulfillment, and has always lent itself rather readily to an idealistic interpretation, but the Thomistic and Cartesian references above at least show that such an idealistic twist was not the only form that the thesis could take.

4. L. P. Wessel, *G. E. Lessing's Theology: A Reinterpretation* (The Hague: Mouton, 1977), p. 54.

It is crucial that we concentrate upon the curious proposal that what satisfies the basic reflection of humankind defines the nature of what is—the real; that if you penetrate the stronghold of the rational you discover being itself. No more precise statement of this abiding thesis could be offered than that presented by J. N. Findlay in his 1975 presidential address to The Metaphysical Society of America.

> And if anything is to be learnt from the history of philosophy it is that one only achieves nonsense if one imagines that the conditions of intelligibility fail to march with the conditions of Being and *vice versa,* so that the same principles which order the mind also order what is.[5]

One may be philosophically unhappy with the content and structure of the Hegelian system and attempt to replace it with a more valid orientation, as did Marx and many others. But it should be carefully noted that any revision, or replacement, of the Hegelian system with a more adequate orientation is probably going to be founded upon the very same fundamental Hegelian thesis of the identity of thought and being. The intimacy of the real and the rational is apt to pervade the substitute system as well, and thus it is not so easy to overcome the Hegelian thesis, even when developing an alternative system. Hegel thought that he had captured and brought to fulfillment an underlying logical structure of Western philosophy, and the proposed alternatives to the Hegelian system may well concede, and in fact evidence, that this is the case. Consequently, any attack upon Hegelianism will, of necessity, need to take a most radical form and obviously will have the weight of the history of Western reflection standing against it. The fortress will be difficult to penetrate at best, for it is built upon the rational authority initiated by the Greeks and defended by the charge of self-contradiction leveled at all serious critics.

It is not surprising, but also worthy of note, that the elabora-

5. J. N. Findlay, "The Three Hypostases of Platonism," published in *Review of Metaphysics* 28 (1975), p. 677.

tions of insights of reflection, which also become descriptions of the real, resulted in theoretical (for our purposes either philosophical, psychological, or theological) systems. The systems intended to grasp the unity of the real, inclusive of its diversity, and thus to master reality by thought. Such was the culmination of the insight that philosophical reflection was grounded in the rational authority, and any attack upon this edifice—any attack upon the identity of thought and being, or upon the systematic character of reality reflected in our philosophical systems— quickly receives Findlay's charge of "nonsense." It is, however, just such an attack that Kierkegaard launched; it is on this very strong and heavily defended theme that his shadow falls.

Rational Authority and the Problematic of the Self

Western culture has now entered a period in which an attack upon rationalism—the rationalism that has extended from the Greeks, through the Enlightenment, to the modern scientific world view—has been seriously initiated. The nature of the critique is sometimes ambiguous, the adjustment to and compromise with rationalism often tenuous, the development of the newer orientation far from clear, and its eventual culmination obscure. But the critique has been initiated, and modern philosophical and psychological theory participate, however unwillingly, in this dialectic. Freud's introduction of the unconscious may be a part of this development, regardless of the scientific rationalism that pervaded his analysis of psychological structures. The voluntarism of Schopenhauer, extended even further by Nietzsche, developed an important existential departure from the authority of reason. Nietzsche poses the problematic of rationalism in an extreme form in contemporary culture. Consider the following excerpts from a recent study on the philosophical import of Nietzsche.

> God is dead—specifically the God of monotheism, the monotonotheistic God. The gods have died, Nietzsche writes, but they have died of laughter upon hearing the Jewish God claim to be the sole God.

The Will to Power is an abyss (*Abgrund*), the groundless chaos beneath all the grounds, all the foundations, and it leaves the whole order of essences groundless.[6]

The implications of this Dionysianism and critique of rationalism are here indicated by the Sorbonne philosopher Michel Haar:

But by devaluing contradiction, we bring into evidence a moral prejudice at the very basis of knowledge.

Values that advise being prudent—or taking risks—are dictated by a particular type of force. In exactly the same way, the supposedly immutable principles of logic, as well as the discoveries of science, serve as a support, as a basis of operation for a determinate type of humanity.... Thus Nietzsche strives to demonstrate, by the genealogical method, that science (and knowledge in general), contrary to its own pretensions, is not at all disinterested, but rather is supremely "interested."[7]

Consider finally Haar's deathblow for rationalism in Nietzsche's behalf.

With God there disappears the guarantee for an intelligible world, and therewith the guarantee for all stable identities, including that of the ego. Everything returns to chaos.[8]

6. A. Lingis, "The Will to Power," in D. B. Allison, *The New Nietzsche* (New York: Dell, 1977), pp. 40, 38.

7. M. Haar, "Nietzsche and Metaphysical Language," in Allison, *The New Nietzsche*, pp. 18, 16. For a useful analysis of the relationship between Nietzsche and Kant see G. DeLeuze, "Active and Reactive," in Allison, p. 89.

8. Haar, "Nietzsche and Metaphysical Language," p. 14. In this same voluntaristic connection it is appropriate to call attention to the association Harold Bloom proposed between Schopenhauer and Freud in his 1978 Weigert Lecture, "Freud's Concepts of Defense and the Poetic Will," in J. H. Smith, ed., *The Literary Freud: Mechanisms of Defense and the Poetic Will, Psychiatry and the Humanities*, vol. 4 (New Haven: Yale, 1980). It is also appropriate to call attention to Wolfgang Loch's attempt at an elaboration of a theory of truth for psychoanalysis, drawing heavily upon Nietzsche, as evidence of the intimate connection between such

Another major expression of the critique appears in the analysis of Spinoza's God, the geometrician, by Shestov, himself a serious student of and commentator upon Kierkegaard.[9] Even in philosophy of science one sees evidence of this tension, as in the work of Feyerabend, with his opposition to prescribed methodologies. Still another major critic is Rorty, who proclaims the end of the epistemological era in philosophy, the end of an era of man as the mirror of nature. Rorty interprets philosophy as edification and hermeneutic, and sympathizes with Derrida's thesis of the deconstruction of the philosophical tradition.[10] The philosophical establishment, with but a few exceptions, does not know what to make of these exercises, and often resolves the difficulty by ignoring them. In doing so it continues to fail to recognize its neglect of the questions concerning the foundations of the philosophical enterprise.

Kierkegaard, as I have indicated, does not avoid this question. His contribution concerns the intimacy of the self with the philosophical position that it develops and includes the problematic of the identity of thought and being. The relationship of the self to the theoretical elaborations of Western philosophy has remained virtually unexplored. While in some sense Socrates' dedication to truth was relevant to his philosophical proposals, this is not the feature of Socrates or Platonism that has occupied the center of attention. The Augustinian theme that faith pre-

---

philosophical criticism of rationalism and the elaboration of psychoanalytic theory. Has any serious psychoanalytic theory been elaborated as yet on Nietzschean foundations? See W. Loch, "Some Comments on the Subject of Psychoanalysis and Truth," in J. H. Smith, ed., *Thought, Consciousness, and Reality, Psychiatry and the Humanities,* vol. 2 (New Haven: Yale, 1977).

9. See L. Shestov, *Potestas Clavium* (Athens: Ohio University Press, 1968), and *Kierkegaard and the Existential Philosophy* (Athens: Ohio University Press, 1969). As is well known, Spinoza is a major exponent of the rationalism that I have discussed. "We may add that our mind, in so far as it perceives things truly, is part of the infinite intellect of God; therefore, the clear and distinct ideas of the mind are as necessarily true as the ideas of God." B. Spinoza, *The Ethics* (New York: Tudor, 1941), note to proposition 41, p. 114.

10. See R. Rorty, "Derrida on Language, Being, and Abnormal Philosophy," *Journal of Philosophy* 74 (1977): 673–81.

ceded reflection has hardly been studied, let alone accepted, by modern man. Although Fichte proclaimed that the kind of philosophy a man held depended upon the kind of a man he was, the validity, profundity, and implications of this theme for philosophy have not been seriously developed.[11] The tendency, rather, has been to neglect the relationship between the self holding a certain view of the universe and the view that is held, as if the self had nothing to do with the interpretation of the position.[12] Philosophical positions have been elaborated as if they were rationally established conclusions to which any mind would be driven if only it thought with clarity. The self proposing the position has been neglected as irrelevant to the position and the reason offering the proposal considered autonomous with no other function than to reason with clarity, perhaps stimulated by empirical data, or perhaps serving as an avenue enabling objective structures to make themselves known.

It is well known that Kierkegaard offered serious criticism of Hegelian rationalism and of the attempted systematic capturing of reality, and thereby of philosophy itself. The implications of this for the foundations of philosophy, for the nature of the faith-reason controversy, for the relationship of the self and its philosophical orientation, and for the relationship of passion and reason, have been little clarified and mainly unacknowledged. I shall now concentrate upon what I take to be the fundamental contemporary metaphilosophical implications of Kierkegaard's contribution.

Philosophical Immediacy and Decision

Kierkegaard is well aware of the Hegelian thesis of the identity of thought and being and attacks it directly. With the acknowl-

11. The import of Fichte's position for philosophy as a science in the context of modern philosophy, especially phenomenology, is to be found in a highly relevant recent essay by T. Rockmore, "Fichte, Husserl, and Philosophical Science," *International Philosophical Quarterly* 19 (1979): 15-27.

12. A significant and much too neglected exception to this general tendency can be found in H. W. Johnstone, Jr., *Philosphy and Argument* (State College, Pa.: Pennsylvania State University Press, 1959), especially chap. 9.

edgment of the gap between man and the transcendent introduced by sin, and with the recognition of what it means to exist,
Kierkegaard sees little reason to propose such continuity between
man's reflection and the structure of being.[13] Immediacy would
only be possible on Socratic-Hegelian grounds of continuity. He
writes:

> The systematic Idea is the identity of subject and object,
> the unity of thought and being. Existence, on the other hand,
> is their separation. It does not by any means follow that exis-
> tence is thoughtless; but it has brought about, and brings
> about, a separation between subject and object, thought and
> being. In the objective sense, thought is understood as being
> pure thought; this corresponds in an equally abstract-
> objective sense to its object, which object is therefore the
> thought itself, and the truth becomes the correspondence of
> thought with itself. This objective thought has no relation to
> the existing subject; and while we are always confronted with
> the difficult question of how the existing subject slips into this
> objectivity, where subjectivity is merely pure abstract subjec-
> tivity (which again is an objective determination, not signify-
> ing any existing human being), it is certain that the existing
> subjectivity tends more and more to evaporate. And finally, if
> it is possible for a human being to become anything of the
> sort, and it is merely something of which at most he becomes
> aware through the imagination, he becomes the pure
> abstract conscious participation in and knowledge of this
> pure relationship between thought and being, this pure iden-
> tity; aye, this tautology, because this being which is ascribed
> to the thinker does not signify that he is, but only that he is
> engaged in thinking.[14]

13. The issue of God and the concept of sin are very questionable concepts for
the modern mind. I make no apologies, however, for introducing them here
without entering that debate, as they are the basic conceptual structures with
which Kierkegaard is prepared to work. My concern is to analyze something of the
metaphilosophical import of his suggestions, which assume such categories as
meaningful.

14. S. Kierkegaard, *Concluding Unscientific Postscript*, trans. D. Swenson and W.
Lowrie (Princeton, N.J.: Princeton University Press, 1941), p. 112.

Not for a single moment is it forgotten that the subject is an existing individual, and that existence is a process of becoming, and that therefore the notion of the truth as identity of thought and being is a chimera of abstraction, in its truth only an expectation of the creature; not because the truth is not such an identity, but because the knower is an existing individual for whom the truth cannot be such an identity as long as he lives in time. Unless we hold fast to this, speculative philosophy will immediately transport us into the fantastic realism of the I-am-I, which modern speculative thought has not hesitated to use without explaining how a particular individual is related to it; and God knows, no human being is more than such a particular individual.[15]

One may not be able to establish rationally that this continuity does not exist, for to propose that reason can establish that would be to concede too much to the very identity of thought and being that is in question. It seems clear, however, that those who understand what it is to exist, recognizing the discontinuity, will not be so optimistic concerning what reason can do. Such hesitancy is intimately related to the recognition of the serious depth of sin's infection, including the impact upon the reason. Consequently, sin has separated man from God and thereby disrupted the independence of and ability of the reason even more than Thomists such as Garrigou-Lagrange and Gilson have acknowledged, and surely more than the Socratic-Hegelian rationalists have recognized.

We are confronted, therefore, with the question of the impact of the fall upon human rationality and our rational philosophical capacities; we are confronted with the question of the fall of reason itself. We are also asked to consider the extent to which philosophical reflection, which frequently has asserted the identity of thought and being, would thereby offer Western man a doctrine of salvation by works, and a saving of ourselves by our own rational efforts. In such a context we are likewise faced with

15. Ibid., p. 176; subsequent references to this work are given parenthetically in the text.

the question of what it might mean, especially in philosophical reflection, if one were to be serious about the doctrine of *sola fide*. What would it mean for reason to participate in the fall and to need salvation by faith? To the best of my knowledge the implications of the doctrine of man's fall and salvation by faith have never been carefully developed regarding reason and the philosophical enterprise itself.[16]

Kierkegaard's attack is also launched upon the initiation, or the beginning, of the Hegelian system. He requests that we become clear about how one enters that system and asks if entrance is purely by reflection, as it proposed. This inquiry is the source of Kierkegaard's metaphilosophical suggestions. The proposal is that Hegel does not enter his orientation as a pure mind, nor do any of us enter our particular orientations as pure intellects, even if we have deceived ourselves into thinking that we do.

> The System begins with the immediate, and hence without any presuppositions, and hence absolutely; the beginning of the System is an absolute beginning. This is quite correct, and has also been sufficiently admired. But before making a beginning with the System, why is it that the second, equally, aye, precisely equally important question has not been raised, taken understandingly to heart, and had its clear implications respected: *How does the System begin with the immediate? That is to say, does it begin with it immediately?* The answer to this question must be an unconditional negative. If the System is presumed to come after existence, by which a confusion with an existential system may be occasioned, then the System is of course *ex post facto,* and does not begin immediately with the immediacy with which experience began; although in

16. This deficiency is but a part of the philosophical neglect of reformation concepts and the failure by philosophers to recognize that such conceptualization may have implications for their own philosophical tools and activity. We still lack a reformation doctrine of reason and of philosophical reflection. It may be too late culturally for such an elaboration ever to be offered, but it is that context out of which Kierkegaard reflects, and it is reformation categories of understanding and interpretation of existence that make him wary of Hegel's identity of thought and being.

another sense it may be said that existence did not begin with the immediate, since the immediate never is as such, but is transcended as soon as it is. The beginning which begins with the immediate *is thus itself reached by means of a process of reflection....*

and that no logical system may boast of an absolute beginning, since such a beginning, like pure being, is a pure chimera. [*Postscript,* pp. 101–02]

Hegelian logicians have quite rightly perceived this, and they therefore define this "immediate," with which logic begins, as the most abstract content remaining after an exhaustive reflection. To this definition there can be no objection, but it is certainly objectionable not to respect the implications of what is thus asserted; for this definition says indirectly that there is no absolute beginning. "How so," I think I hear someone say, "when we have abstracted from everything, is there not, etc., etc.?" Aye, to be sure—*when* we have abstracted from everything. Why can we not remember to be human beings? This act of abstraction, like the preceding act of refelction, is infinite. How then does it come to an end—and it is only when . . . that . . . Let us try an experiment in thought. Suppose the infinite act of abstraction to be *in actu.* However, the beginning is not identical with the act of abstraction, but comes afterwards. With what do I begin, now that I have abstracted from everything? Ah, here an Hegelian will perhaps fall on my breast, overcome by deep emotion, blissfully stammering the answer: with nothing. Very well, but now I must offer my second question: *How* do I begin with nothing? Unless in fact the infinite act of abstraction is one of those tricks of legerdemain which may readily be performed two at a time; if, on the contrary, it is the most strenuous of all acts of thought, what then? Why then, of course, all my strength is required to hold it fast. If I let slip any part of my strength, I no longer abstract from everything. And if under such circumstances I make a beginning, I do not begin with nothing; precisely because I did not abstract from everything when I began. That is to say, if it is at all possible for a human being to abstract from everything in his thinking, it is at any rate impossible for him to do more, since if this act does not transcend human power, it absolutely exhausts it. To grow weary of the act of abstracting, and thus to arrive at a beginning, is an explanation of the sort valid only for costermongers, who do not take a little discrepancy so seriously. [*Postscript,* pp. 103–04; original ellipses]

Rather than enter a world view by such abstraction, Kierkegaard proposes that we enter by existential and decisional voluntaristic affirmations. This is surely not the way that philosophers traditionally have talked about themselves and the entrance to their orientations, for entrance usually has been proposed as much more objective and rationalistic. But Kierkegaard seems convinced that the perspective one holds upon the world was entered by a leap of faith, a decisional commitment and that Hegel entered his world that way as well.

How do I put an end to the reflection which was set up in order to reach the beginning here in question? Reflection has the remarkable property of being infinite. But to say that it is infinite is equivalent, in any case, to saying that it cannot be stopped by itself; because in attempting to stop itself it must use itself, and is thus stopped in the same way that a disease is cured when it is allowed to choose its own treatment, which is to say that it waxes and thrives. [*Postscript,* p. 102]

And what is it that I require of him? I ask him for a resolve. And in so doing, I do well, for in no other way can the process of reflection be halted. But a philosopher is never justified, on the other hand, in playing tricks on people, asserting one moment that the reflective process halts itself and comes to an end in an absolute beginning; and the next moment proceeding to mock a man whose only fault is that he is stupid enough to believe the first assertion, mocking him, so as to help him to arrive in this manner at an absolute beginning, which hence seems to be achieved in two different ways. But if a resolution of the will is required to end the preliminary process of reflection, the presuppositionless character of the System is renounced. Only when reflection comes to a halt can a beginning be made, and reflection can be halted only by something else, and this something else is something quite different from the logical, being a resolution of the will. Only when the beginning, which puts an end to the process of reflection, is a radical breach of such a nature that the absolute beginning breaks through the continued infinite reflection, then only is the beginning without presuppositions. [*Postscript*, p. 103]

Whenever a beginning is *made,* on the other hand, unless through being unaware of this the procedure stamps itself as arbitrary, such a beginning is not the consequence of an immanent movement of thought, but is effected through a resolution of the will, essentially in the strength of faith. [*Postscript*, p. 169]

While this objection is directed toward Hegel it should be clear that it is implicitly directed at all modern philosophy, whether rationalistic, empirical, phenomenological, or linguistic, that would attempt to begin with the immediate, without presuppositions, with the intimacy of thought and being, and resolve the philosophical problems by objective reflection. Thereby a major issue is posed for the disciplines of theory. Are philosophical theories constructions that are not only elaborated by reflection but initiated by objective reflection and grounded upon the self-authentication of reflection, or are they elaborations of decisional stances in the world? We shall return to this matter momentarily.

Kierkegaard's criticism does not suggest that world views are useless, although there may be those who carry on this venture in a minimum way, nor does it suggest that they cannot be elaborated. Rather, we are to understand that they offer the mind and life of man a set of possibilities, possible interpretations of the universe and one's place within it. A logical system is possible. Between such alternative systems reason cannot arrive at objective conclusions but man must choose.

Furthermore, this criticism does not mean that there is no world system, or no correct system of reality. It does not even mean that ultimate reason and ultimate reality are not compatible. "Does this mean that no such system exists? By no means; nor is it implied in our assertion. Reality itself is a system—for God; but it cannot be a system for any existing spirit" (*Postscript,* p. 107). We are not God, and consequently the divine system is not ours; nor should we maintain the imperialism of human rationality, claiming that our little systems are God's. To do so would simply evidence the pride of reason gone insane. Our little systems, doing the best that they can, are but the history of our failures to get it right and capture the world as it is. The high tides of reality eventually always seem to do them in. The French structuralist and literary critic Roland Barthes has captured this point with precision, "Is it not the characteristic of reality to be unmasterable? And is it not the characteristic of any system to master it?"[17]

The criticism suggests that because of our deficiencies and the limitations of existence, there is no identity of thought and being allowing us reflectively to establish the accurate interpretation of the universe. Theoretical systems will propose possible worlds entered by decisional appropriation and not established by the self-authentication of reason. Those plural systems offer us logical possibilities, but no assurances, so that the selection between them must be by decisional and not rational criteria. Furthermore, while there may well be a system for God, our little systems, in Jaspersian terms, always "suffer shipwreck." Consequently, an existential system is impossible, for one cannot arrive at a system that somehow adequately grasps what it is like to exist. No system appropriately captures the very self that holds it.

In order to focus upon the metaphilosophical implications of the foregoing, let us return to the decisional foundations of philosophical orientations. This is hardly the interpretation philosophy has offered of its own activity. Contemporary philosophy has elaborated serious metaphilosophy, but where has it been proposed that the root or entrance to a philosophical position is a

17. R. Barthes, *Roland Barthes* (New York: Hill & Wang, 1977), p. 172.

convictional decision or a "leap of faith"? The Parmenidean-Findlay axis of rational authority has been developed in the history of Western thought to grand proportions. Reason with the aid of experience—although just how reason was to aid became a serious matter of dispute—assumed authority in the realm of theory and intended to master the real. Seldom does one hear even a hint that something less rational—such as conviction, decision, will, trusting, and stances to live by—plays any role at all in the development of theoretical orientations. Greek and Enlightenment and scientific rationalism, in spite of their deep differences, have each quite neglected to take into account any of the Hebrew-Christian features of trust, loyalty, decision, and convictions to live by at the point of initiation of theoretical orientations, although at times they will concede, without elaboration, that one needs to "trust reason." Theoretical life has presented itself as the attainment of objectivity, and crucial aspects of betting one's life and taking a chance on the world and on a certain orientation are lost in assurances of what reason can clearly discern, reflecting the intimacy of thought and being.

This intended objectivity of reflection is challenged by the Kierkegaardian suggestion that even such rationalistic theory is not as objective as intended and pretended, that it contains seldom recognized and explicated features of decision, will, conviction, and faith at its initiation, and that to understand even such proposals of objectivity Western thought must concentrate much more attention on the relationship of the self who develops the theory, and whose convictional dispositions are foundational, to the theory itself. Only then will we clarify what otherwise remains ambiguous, namely, how one enters the structure with which one views the world. If there are existential decisional foundations here, as Kierkegaard is convinced there are, then it is appropriate that modern philosophers offer some concentrated attention on the way this matter works. Kierkegaard has only opened the door, but if a decisional feature plays as crucial a role in the disciplines of theory, and especially philosophy, as I have suggested, then proper analysis of the initiation of a theoretical position would change our entire perspective on just what it is that philosophy is to do, the way it functions as a mode of human existence and a form of life, and would seriously transform the current proposals of metaphilosophy. What a radically different view of the philosophical adventure one would have if it were understood as the elaboration of possibilities between which one may select—possibilities that can only be appropriated by selection—and if competing theoretical positions were understood as competing interpretations of our situation, including interpretations of the status, nature, and authority of reason. Philosophy as the development of rationally necessary conclusions that the authority of reflection imposes upon all, with no decision necessary, no free posit to make, and only the holy light of reflection to be followed with clarity—because supposedly thought and being were identical—would be lost; but philosophy as the elaboration of possibilities, with the limits of reflection clarified, would remain intact. The entire burden of this section may be captured in the suggestive words of Paul Eluard, "I must not look on reality as being like myself."[18]

Metaphilosophy and the Faith-Reason Controversy

The metaphilosophical suggestions just indicated radically transform the classical faith-reason controversy. Traditionally in this controversy the idea of faith involved faith in God, the transcendent, and the issue then centered upon the relationship of such a faith in God to human rationality and reflection. If there is an initial decisional posit, conviction, assumption, presupposition, or leap of faith at the initiation of *any* theoretical position, then this would be the arena of faith in that position and would not necessarily have anything to do with the presence or absence of God. In addition, if theoretical reflection occurs on the

18. Quoted in G. Bachelard, *The Psychoanalysis of Fire* (Boston: Beacon, 1964), p. 1. It should not be concluded that the act of will to halt reflection is necessary only for the religious mind or the believer. This applies, Kierkegaard affirms, to the skeptic as well, who "wills to doubt." "Belief and doubt are not two forms of knowledge, determinable in continuity with one another, for neither of them is a cognitive act; they are opposite passions." Kierkegaard, *Philosophical Fragments*, trans. D. Swenson (Princeton, N.J.: Princeton University Press, 1942), p. 69.

grounds of and within that initial posit or presupposition, regardless of the direction the reflection takes, and regardless of the direction of the initial assumption, then the faith-reason controversy would involve the analysis of the dialectic between that initial posit and the reflection that occurs within its limits and upon its foundation. Consequently, the faith-reason controversy would be relocated and placed at the very foundation and heart of *any* theoretical position, regardless of its content and regardless of how theistic or nontheistic it might be. To see faith as a crucial aspect of the initiation of any philosophical position is obviously vastly different from the conceptualization of faith usually held, which limits it to the sphere of religious concern as if faith always meant faith in God and as if the autonomy of reason removed any attributes of faith from philosophical positions. It is time, in fact it is way past time, for philosophy to deal with clarity and honesty with the assumption, posit, conviction, faith, that may lie at the root of its endeavor, and then to deal with the relationship of reflective life to that presupposition. It is time, in fact way past time, to remove the faith-reason controversy from its usual religious context and place it where it most seriously lies, at the very foundation of philosophical positions as such. It is time for philosophers to make clear, especially in an age crying for clarity, the existential decisions that may undergird the very foundations of their theoretical constructions. By no means am I suggesting that there is any inappropriateness in such decisions. Quite the contrary. It does seem, however, highly inappropriate to have them posited and affirmed by implication but seldom if ever ackknowledged and to continue to pretend that they do not exist. This is the crucial metaphilosophical impact of the Kierkegaardian insights and the question he poses for contemporary philosophy.[19]

It will be difficult for most philosophers to approach this question, as they often consider themselves purely rational men who are not elaborating positions grounded in leaps of faith. Kier-

19. See W. M. Alexander, *Johan Georg Hamann Philosophy and Faith* (The Hague: Nijhoff, 1966).

kegaard proposed that reflection was to be halted by an act of the will and thus by something other than reflection. His proposal calls for an inspection of our theoretical lives, that rational form of life that is philosophy, to see what besides reason may be involved, and to question whether or not, as theoreticians, we are creatures of conviction, assumption, and loyalty as well as creatures of reason. We also need to debate directly the question of the validity of the intended presuppositionless character of many philosophical positions and to face squarely the issue of the entrance to such positions, if they do in fact stand without presuppositions. In Kierkegaard's terms, this would be to inquire how they begin with nothing, or with the immediate. In view of the persuasiveness of "presuppositionless" philosophers to contemporary theoreticians, is it not appropriate that we enter a period of intense discussion of the relationships between presuppositionless rationalisms and Kierkegaardian voluntarism? The judgment that Kierkegaard's profound perceptions were correct might usher in a new Augustinianism regarding the relationship of faith and reason, a position that might be much more relevant than modern philosophers are inclined to think.

It is not surprising that the idea of the prereflective, the convictional initiation of an orientation, is recognized by many religious thinkers, for such thinkers especially have been aware of the role of faith in human existence and have been equally conscious of the tyranny of reason and the eternal temptation to make an idol of the authority of reason itself. Furthermore, in a period when the idea of the death of God has been quickly followed by the philosophical thesis of the death of man, they, among modern theoreticians, may be uniquely prepared to retain the idea of the presence of the self and thereby may be especially sensitive to the intimacy of the self with the theory it produces. They are likely to be aware not only of the reason and its accomplishments but also of the human being whose reason and heart are both at work in those accomplishments.

It is also not surprising that such religious thinkers have been aware of the dangers and limits of systematization, for above all others they have been conscious of philosophical attempts to capture God in the philosopher's system, and have been prepared to protest that the Gods of such philosophers were never their God. Thus, they have been especially aware of both the tyranny of reason and the tyranny of the rational system.[20] The system of totality, which tries to encompass all, becomes a Hegelian demon to be avoided at all cost. Once the tyranny of totalization is recognized, it can be developed in the modern mind well beyond the confines of the religious mind. So Roland Barthes, in characterizing his reflections upon the text, can write:

> ("the endless text"), actually (secretly) aims at denouncing the monster of totality (totality as monster). Totality at one and the same time inspires laughter and fear: like violence, is it not always *grotesque* (and then recuperable only in an aesthetics of Carnival)?[21]

Apprehension concerning the danger of identifying decisional foundations for philosophical orientations reflects the constant threat of arbitrariness and self-contradiction, and such danger ought not to be minimized. The ultimate reliance upon rational conclusions, established upon the premise that reason was identifiable with and intimately related to the real, has offered the hope, ever since Parmenides, of objective rational authority and truth. Recognition of voluntaristic decisional foundations would dissipate such authority, and along with it the possibility of "rationally" overthrowing any particular world view. Kierkegaard was well aware of this danger and, with his proposal that "truth is subjectivity," was quite prepared to run the risk.[22] One would apparently be left with philosophical orientations offering alternative modes of "living the world," which might well provide an

20. For a most useful discussion of the problem of totalization see E. Levinas, *Totality and Infinity* (Pittsburgh: Duquesne University Press, 1969), and H. A. Durfee, "Emmanuel Levinas' Philosophy of Language," in B. Blose, H. A. Durfee, and D. F. T. Rodier, *Explanation: New Directions in Philosophy* (The Hague: Nijhoff, 1973).

21. Barthes, *Roland Barthes*, p. 180.

22. He even recognizes the intimacy of such a position with madness (*Postscript*, pp. 173–74).

appropriate blend of both Kierkegaardian and Wittgensteinian concerns. It is reasonable to expect that in the face of such a rigorous critique of the classical rational authority and the objectivity it supposedly involves, an especially strong defense of reason and its autonomy will be forthcoming. This but reflects the crucial character of the relocating of the faith-reason controversy and philosophical initiation in Kierkegaard's shadow.

Kierkegaard's Shadow in Contemporary Philosophy

I wish now to move beyond Kierkegaard to propose that concern over the authority of reason, including the Kierkegaardian proposals as to the philosophical foundations, pervades nearly every contemporary philosophical position. In what has come to be known as phenomenology, Husserl's attempt at a presuppositionless philosophy was a unique continuation of the theme of the authority of reason. Pure consciousness was to read off its contents and thus describe what is given. But the elaboration of existential phenomenology leaves quite ambiguous the extent to which it intends to continue the "presuppositionless" motif of its ancestry. Heidegger's world of care, Sartre's world of particular "thises" as the function of the *pour-soi* in relationship to the *en-soi,* and Jaspers' "philosophical faith" would all seem to have deserted significantly the Husserlian theme, although the relationship of existential phenomenology to the Husserlian thesis of a presuppositionless philosophy has not been seriously explored to date. Furthermore, even the meaning and nature of phenomenology itself as a presuppositionless position remains highly ambiguous among the Husserlian commentators. It should also be noted that the existential movement was a blending of two quite incompatible themes, Kierkegaard's analysis of the foundational act of decision and the leap of faith and Husserl's thesis of the presuppositionless reading off of the given phenomena. In some strange way, yet to be explained and clarified, these fathers of the twentieth century have been merged, but great tension remains in the merger, and in time it will surely be dissolved. Even in Paul Ricoeur the tension between the effort of the will and his existential interests rests uneasily, although fascinatingly, with his serious appropriation of Husserl.

In addition to phenomenology, a comparable tension pervades recent analytic philosophy, which also remains ambiguous as to the voluntaristic and decision features that may lie at its foundation. With regard to analytic positivism, Ayer's initial presentation of the much-debated verification principle offered it as an analytic proposition. But by 1973 he is prepared to say about the verification principle: "Afterwards, when this question was put to me, I said it was a stipulative definition. And of course if it is a stipulative definition, it's always open to anyone not to accept the stipulation. But one has to start somewhere."[23] The apparent change in the status of the principle, even within the thought of one of its own most distinguished proponents, seems to me to indicate one version of the tension I have been discussing.

Although the verification principle, or some comparable formulation of a rational principle establishing validity, has been regularly proposed, Frederick Waismann has made a series of unique suggestions regarding such rationalism in philosophy: "In philosophy there are no proofs." "Proof, refutation—these are dying words in philosophy, though G. E. Moore still 'proved' to a puzzled word that it exists. What can one say to this—save, perhaps, that he is a great prover before the Lord?" "However, there is no way of proving him wrong or bullying him into mental acceptance of the proposal: when all is said and done the decision is his." "What it comes to in the end is that the asker of the question, in the course of the discussion, has to make a number of decisions." "All the proofs, in a good book on philosophy, could be dispensed with, without its losing a whit of its convincingness. To seek, in philosophy, for rigorous proof is to seek for the shadow of one's voice." "But if I were asked to express in one single word what is its most essential feature I would unhesitatingly say: vision. At the heart of any philosophy worthy of the

23. Quoted in B. Magee, *Modern British Philosophy* (Herts: Granada, 1973), p. 77.

name is vision, and it is from there that it springs and takes its visible shape."[24]

Surely the difference between Ayer, especially the early Ayer, and Waismann indicates a crucial division regarding the role of rationalism and the role of decision in the foundation of philosophy.[25]

A comparable tension is evident in more recent analytic philosophy. In Trigg's *Reason and Commitment,* a serious defense of reason as crucial in philosophy, he is uniquely aware of and deals explicitly with the challenge posed by the more existential concern with decision, conviction, and commitment. He attempts to show that the philosophical enterprise cannot be based upon the basic commitment of the self, as others have suggested, and that such a proposal would lead in the end to self-contradiction. He writes, "Although this notion of an 'ultimate commitment', which is in principle unjustifiable, is attractive to many, it involves a basic misunderstanding of the nature of commitment."[26]

Trigg appropriately realizes that the challenge to the authority of reason needs defense at the very point where commitment even to reason challenges the autonomy of reason itself. His position is a fine implicit example of the continuing concern with the metaphilosophical implications of Kierkegaard's position.

As Trigg knows, however, some of his most influential colleagues offer a quite different analysis. For example, Trigg discusses the significant work of R. M. Hare, and the central role that Hare offers for commitment as logically prior to reason. Hare's famous "blicks" surely provide a serious limitation to the supremacy of reason.

One of the most interesting suggestions to set beside Trigg's

24. F. Waismann, *How I See Philosophy* (New York: St. Martin's Press, 1968), pp. 1, 18, 21, 31, 32.

25. I have neglected all consideration of the distinction in linguistic meaning between decision and vision, although this difference is not without philosophical importance.

26. R. Trigg, *Reason and Commitment* (London: Cambridge University Press, 1973), p. 43.

proposals has been offered by Lange in his study of the claims of philosophy. A concluding section of Lange's book, where he deals with the dialectic of *proposal* and *cognition* in the interpretation of philosophy, further illustrates the centrality of the issue raised by Kierkegaard:

> Let us say simply that the cognitivity of philosophy seems to be proposal-dependent, and that proposals are normally thought to lack truth values, and accordingly that philosophy's self-construal as cognitive, lacking a truth value, is non-cognitive. It is then suggested that proposals may have derivative cognitivity from the cognitivity of value judgments. . . . But that the cognitivity of value judgments may itself be proposal-dependent complicates the issue. Is it merely another proposal that such judgments can be cognitive? Perhaps, but if it is the *best* proposal, then what? And so hierarchies begin to ache upward, and one feels that a decision of passion must be made, that one must choose. So one chooses for cognitivity. And wonders if one has made the *best* choice.[27]

It would be difficult to find a clearer example of my theme—the metaphilosophical impact of the Kierkegaardian issue as to the initiation of the foundations of philosophy itself.

In these illustrations of the current debate within phenomenology and analytic philosophy, the name of Kierkegaard may never be mentioned, but his attention to the role of decision in the life of philosophy itself has contributed greatly to the discussion. The evidence is sufficient to indicate that the tension on the current scene is not confined to a lone Dane, or to European existentialists, or even to theologically minded theoreticians, but rests rather in the very heart of contemporary metaphilosophy and offers seed for a most significant debate. I suspect that even Holmer, in spite of his obvious willingness to make great use of the late Wittgenstein and his appropriation of

27. J. Lange, *The Cognitivity Paradox* (Princeton, N.J.: Princeton University Press, 1970), p. 116.

ordinary language philosophy, would not attempt to argue that that philosophical position was itself presuppositionless.

Let me also suggest that this consideration is an appropriate occasion for analyzing further the relationship between analytic philosophy and phenomenology. The role of conviction at the root of philosophy is not a matter over which those two current major philosophies would be neatly divided as opponents but is rather a focus of attention in which one could find compatabilities within each movement with corresponding aspects of the other position, with regard to both the more voluntaristic interpretation and the more rationalistic interpretation.[28]

Finally, let me pose the issue of the contrast between the metaphilosophy of Kierkegaard and the metaphilosophical interpretation of much of Western philosophy in a slightly different manner, in order to focus the issue as directly and clearly as possible. In the second section of this essay I indicated at some length the centrality of the thesis of the identity of thought and being in classical philosophy, and emphasized that Kierkegaard isolated precisely this as the central aspect of the tradition that must be attacked if he was to oppose Hegel in the most significant manner. It is especially important to be aware of these themes in the light of the increasing Neohegelianism in contemporary philosophy, appearing partly in opposition to the more Kierkegaardian and existential philosophies that dominated the mid-twentieth century. As before, the philosopher attempts to authenticate reason's authority *from within,* by showing that reason can offer its own self-certification, self-authentication, and self-justification. Trigg's proposal that the very conditions of language itself evidence the authority of reason, that the *a priori* of language justifies reliance upon reason and refutes the attempted reliance upon commitment as the final court of appeal, is but one current instance of a classical defense of and self-justification of reason from within.

28. In "Analytic Philosophy, Phenomenology, and Consciousness," I attempted to analyze the fundamental diversities between these two movements (in Smith, *Thought, Consciousness, and Reality*). See also H. A. Durfee, *Analytic Philosophy and Phenomenology* (The Hague: Nijhoff, 1976).

The theme of self-certification was elaborated clearly by Kant, although it appeared well before him. In the preface to the first edition of *The Critique of Pure Reason* he writes: "It is a call to reason to undertake anew the most difficult of all its tasks, namely, that of self-knowledge, and to institute a tribunal which will assure to reason its lawful claims," and "What reason produces entirely out of itself cannot be concealed, but is brought to light by reason itself immediately the common principle has been discovered."[29]

This Kantian program of rational self-certification, self-inspection, and self-justification becomes a major theme of Western reflection and becomes the burden of the German idealism to which Kierkegaard is so deeply opposed. Highly influential upon Hegel, this theme is elaborated superbly by Fichte. As Surber comments:

> This, for Fichte, is nothing other than pure self-consciousness itself, and it can be expressed in the form of the proposition $A = A$, which is the formal representation of "I am absolutely what I am." Such an absolute *Tathandlung*, which might best be translated as "fact-act," establishes, in the most general and primordial way, the basis for all knowledge, if we understand knowledge as a unity of knower and known or of concept and being. For in self-consciousness such an identity is immediately established in the very act of self-apprehension. Subject and object thus are immediately identical, inasmuch as what is being apprehended, the object, is none other than that which is in the process of apprehending, the subject. I am at the same time both conscious and the object of consciousness. Further, this primordial identity of self-consciousness must lie at the basis of all else which we call knowledge, since any knowledge can only appear as a delimitation and specification of this unity which is my own self-consciousness. Without this ultimate unity-constituting act, there could be no knowledge, since knowledge is always a

29. I. Kant, *Critique of Pure Reason*, trans. N. K. Smith (London: Macmillan, 1929), A XII, A XX, p. 9, 14.

synthesis or unification and there is no other ground for this except in the act of consciousness itself. . . .

Rather, it is the non-discursive ground for any subsequent capacity of differentiating "content" and "form" themselves within consciousness. On the other hand, it is no mere concept or form of synthesis, since it is a *fact-act* which accompanies all discursive knowledge. Intellectual intuition thus provides the absolute starting point for philosophy, since, as intuition, it is immediately and necessarily present as the *ground* for all other acts of consciousness. . . .

It is this principle of the identity of subject and object that Hegel sees as the genuine principle of philosophical speculation.[30]

To bring this principle up to date, let me note one of the most recent statements illustrative of the same idea within the phenomenological movement. In a discussion of the relationships between analytic and phenomenological theories of meaning, J. N. Mohanty writes, "what I'm suggesting instead is that a theory of meaning bestows a foundation upon itself."[31]

Hidden in the heart of contemporary metaphilosophy, in a wide variety of orientations, is a basic dialogue between (1) philosophers who conclude that self-authentication of reason by itself, and thus the bestowal of its own foundations, is possible—a doctrine Kierkegaard would call immediacy, and (2) the more Kierkegaardian theoreticians, who insist that the task cannot be accomplished and that any such foundation must be "proposal-dependent," a matter of conviction. It is most desirable that the doctrine of "self-bestowal," and the logic thereof, be elaborated in some detail. We need to understand how it is that reason is able to proclaim its own authority, if it can, and thereby escape the poten-

30. J. P. Surber's introduction to G. F. W. Hegel, *The Difference Between the Fichtean and Schellingian Systems of Philosophy* (Reseda, Calif.: Ridgeview, 1978), pp. xliv, xlv.

31. K.-O. Apel, J. N. Mohanty, and A. Quinton, "Theories of Meaning in the Analytic and Continental Traditions," *Graduate Faculty Philosophy Journal* 7 (1978): 82.

tial arbitrariness and convictional ground of which it has been accused. It is obvious that this concern with and suggestion of self-authentication is not confined to some narrowly identified Hegelianism for, as we have seen, the general proposal that reason can found its own authority by self-inspection has been offered by a wide variety of positions. We need much clearer elaboration than has been offered to date of a presuppositionless reason bestowing its own authority. Whether this analysis be offered in a more linguistic, more phenomenological, or more Hegelian manner makes little difference to the metaphilosophical issue. In all cases it would be an attempt to complete the Hegelian program holding that reason, by its own authority, can both discern the real and justify itself.

The idea that philosophy rests on its own foundations and thereby on purely rational and objective foundations, rather than on decisional grounds, is now seriously challenged. Hegel's program will not and should not die quickly, if at all. But it is imperative that in the face of the challenge of the more voluntaristic proposals as to the initiation of reflective life, the strongest possible case be made for reason's authority. That is the issue raised by Kierkegaard's shadow, for Kierkegaard is convinced that rational men have fooled themselves, albeit in a very clever way, into concluding that they are pure intellects and that those intellects can certify their own operations, with no voluntaristic, decisional, and convictional affirmations at their initiation.

Most branches of philosophical reflection need to debate the self-reflexive character of the enterprise if the discipline is to understand its own deep recesses of initiation. Here is a recovering by memory to parallel the role of deep memory penetration with which psychoanalytic theory is already very familiar. But this remembering and overcoming would not merely overcome some neurosis, unless theory itself be a neurosis, but would ground the very theory that is both philosophical and psychoanalytic theory itself. If Kierkegaard should prove to be accurate in this matter, then not only in religion but in philosophical and psychological theory as well modern man would have to walk by faith much more than *humanitas philosophicus* has realized. If that were established, Kierkegaard would have initiated a grand deconstruction of a great tradition and a grand reconstruction of the very foundation of man's reflective life. This, it seems to me, is the central dialogue fostered in contemporary metaphilosophy by Kierkegaard's shadow.

5

Superego in Kierkegaard, Existence in Freud

WILLIAM KERRIGAN

How might Freud and Kierkegaard be made to confront each other? Although it would be easy enough to find homologies between the two, the display of similarity is in the end an empty demonstration. After their juxtaposition, psychoanalysis can go on being psychoanalysis, and Christian existentialism can go on being Christian existentialism, both of them feeling, perhaps, that they have been vaguely "enriched" by this brief encounter. In pure comparison, nothing is at risk.

Should we drop the restraints of intellectual politesse, allowing a genuine interaction between the two, one of them would seem necessarily to be subsumed in the other. Kierkegaard might become yet another conquest in the missionary project of "applied" psychoanalysis—that hearty colonialism in which the ability of Freudian thought to interpret other thinkers is, explicitly or implicitly, taken as proof of the superior explanatory power of psychoanalysis. This is highbrow folly. That a hermeneutic can produce, in any given instance, a coherent interpretation, proves nothing whatsoever about the validity of its assumptions. The coherent interpretation is generated as a result of the assumptions, not as a test of them. There is, for example, no reason why the Neoplatonic prejudices of Origen and Gregory of Nyssa, who approached the Old Testament as allegory, could not have served the exegetical task of Christianity precisely as well as the typologi-

I would like to acknowledge the value of conversations with Reginald Bell in the writing of this essay, especially the passage on the autonomous authority of reason in the last section.

cal hermeneutic sketched by Paul and perfected by Augustine; with respect to the ability to encompass all the details of the Bible in a unified reading, there was no choosing between them. Christianity, of course, invented missionary colonialism. It would be comparably gratuitous for Christian existentialism to annex psychoanalysis, as it has, for instance, in theorists such as Wilfried Daim (1963), for whom the psychiatric cure melts into the promise of salvation. Is the only alternative to sever Kierkegaard from Freud as radically as Holmer does in the paper that opens this volume?

If not, we need something more than the bloodless exercise of homologizing and something less than the empty victory of appropriation. I will try to formulate a question of mutual concern in such a way that some fundamental commitments of Freud and Kierkegaard become subject to reciprocal correction. By intruding Freud into the drastically elusive subjectivity of Kierkegaard, I hope to contribute, if not a new problematic, then a new intonation to a familiar problematic in the tradition of Christian ethics; reversing this procedure, I hope to show how an accommodation with existentialism and its chosen enemy, the metaphysical tradition from Plato to Hegel, might clarify the metapsychology of the ego and the superego. But I cannot pretend to equal tolerance. The location of my own concern is psychoanalytic, and the aspect of Kierkegaard capable of assimilation with psychoanalysis, which aspires to be a universal psychology, necessarily has more to do with existentialism than with Christianity. For this reason, the attempt at rethinking psychogenesis in this essay relies on the systematic extension of Kierkegaard's strictly philosophical ideas in Heidegger. I have kept Christianity in view, however. I want to understand, insofar as it is possible to understand within a philosophical psychoanalysis, that moment in Kierkegaard when faith, realized in silence and solitude, passes over into the irrefutable.

Specifically, how can the dialectical movement from the ethical to the religious in *Fear and Trembling* be articulated with the theory of the superego? I feel that the old question of the fatherhood of God has again become a timely one. It is my impression, gathered in part from the plain discomfort of Ricoeur (1970, pp. 524-51; 1974, pp. 468-97) over this matter, that psychoanalysis has weakened the metaphor of God as father in the academic tradition of religious studies, perhaps in religion generally. Students of Christianity have tended, unlike Ricoeur himself, to retreat from the old paternal deity to a God of "mystery," substituting for the "way of analogy" up-to-date versions of the *via negativa*. Ironically, in contemporary psychoanalysis the superego also appears to have lost much of its former stature in diagnosis, treatment, and theory. The internalized father is no longer the *mysterium tremendum* he was for Freud; the blinding insight of Oedipus has given way to the enraptured gaze of Narcissus. As Freudianism in the English-speaking world moves steadily toward a psychology of the self, it may be especially appropriate to consider the work of Kierkegaard, the great prophet of the self, for whom the authenticity of selfhood is clearly to be sought in the lived knowledge of Oedipus, not the Arcadian deceit of Narcissus.

The Immaturing of the Superego

For Kierkegaard, man exists in the intensity of his subjectivity. His essence is to have no fixed essence. When the ethical will embodies a universal principle of duty, man has gained an essence but lost his existence. Benevolent though he may be in acts of charity, trustworthy though he may be in the keeping of promises, he must win back from the deadening circumscription of essence the precious interiority of his existence (Wyschogrod, pp. 24-50, 78-100). If, in the *cogito* of Descartes, the ego has the audacity to confer birth and being upon itself, then ego in the form of ethical will, subject to a system of universal laws, has the hubris to confer value and even salvation upon itself. Whether in philosophy or in life, the price of such self-definitions is existence.

Choosing existence, Kierkegaard aimed the fierce energy of his dialectic at overcoming the religious superego in what was for Freud—and, differently, for Kant—its most sublime form. Having identified religion as the illusion of a collective neurosis,

Freud worried that the demise of faith would impair our willingness to renounce instinct and cooperate with civilization. The
problem arose from his conviction about the amorality of the ego
per se. God, allotting rewards and punishments in a transcendent
world, was the creature of the superego; but having exposed God,
Freud could only entrust the future of morality to a lessened
superego. The goal of psychoanalysis with respect to the id could
not be transferred to the superego without abolishing the moral
life: replace the superego with the ego and society would collapse,
for in his metapsychology there was no impulse in the ego alone to
assume the burden of ethical self-determination. When Freud
spoke of the "categorical imperative" of the primitive superego
(1923, p. 48), he was ironically taunting the autonomous rationality of Kant's ethics while at the same time laying the groundwork
for an eventual solidarity with Kant. Heir to an irrational drama
of fantasy, symbol, and affect, the bare imperative of the
superego—"Thou shalt" and "Thou shalt not"—might one day be
filled with no higher authority than "impersonal" respect for
mankind (1926b, p. 223).

Freud would doubtless have admired the sustained effort to
choose oneself and become thereby the father of oneself
(Reinhardt, p. 242) that Kierkegaard urged throughout his work.
The ethic of psychoanalytic treatment, as Loewald has asserted
(1978a, pp. 1–26), can be understood existentially as a becoming-
responsible for one's past in the form of a project for one's future.
Still, however deftly we draw out the moral implications of Freud,
it will be difficult to clear a place of honor in psychoanalytic thinking for the melodramatic Christianity of Johannes de Silentio in
Fear and Trembling. Passing beyond the dialectic of the repressed
despair of the aesthetic man and the acknowledged despair of the
ethical man explored in Either/Or, Kierkegaard's pseudonymous
exegete finds the genesis of the religious man in a "teleological
suspension of the ethical" (1843, p. 67). Abraham is his archetype.
When God enters the family triangle of the father of faith, the
blessed progenitor of a great nation whose blood will flow in
Jesus, duty collapses and alarming paradoxes unfold. Abraham
exists in raising his knife over his son, and Isaac *exists* beneath the

knife of his father. At just this moment of shared sublimity, God determines that the willingness to sacrifice is sufficient unto faith—and all is returned.

Faith discovered in the deliberate suspension of the ethical does not, in any obvious way, serve civilization. Shoham (1976) reveals how the "Isaac Syndrome" and its ideal of sacred infanticide may in fact turn civilization against itself. Surely it is no part of Kierkegaard's intention to underwrite charitable impulses with promises of eternal reward and punishment. He dwells rather on the affront to social piety. Beyond ethics, Abraham is beyond community, choosing himself in an incommunicable moment known only through the involutions of irony and silence. This faith disturbs because its exemplar is so insistently *concrete*. The Abraham of Kierkegaard is not a symbol or a fable but in every particular the man of faith. We are not allowed to domesticate faith by translating the dilemma of Abraham into more quotidian settings. This existential equation of what Abraham means with what Abraham is constitutes the major crisis for a Freudian reader of *Fear and Trembling*. Meeting this crisis with the boldness of the text itself, we must declare that *the very concretion of Abraham makes him a symbol*. To say otherwise would be to deny Freud from the outset. The revelation specific to psychoanalysis lies in its demonstration that thought must continuously be wrested away from a great store of unconscious energy distributed in a network of deeply affective symbols—among them the killing of a son by a father. Whatever else Abraham may mean, he means the Oedipus complex at least. So the question arises, does this faith sublimate the instinctual life, or, masking a desire for "suspension" with the *Verneinung* of "teleological," encourage its release?

It is important to realize that, unique as his exposition of this faith may be, Kierkegaard stands squarely in the Christian-Protestant tradition. In the *Concluding Unscientific Postscript* Socrates properly appears as the archetype of the ethical man, for the movement from ethics to religion, Socrates to Abraham, does in fact encapsulate the difference between the ethic of autonomous reason in Plato and the voluntarism of biblical Christianity; in this respect, *Fear and Trembling* contains a dialectical history of value in Western culture. One commentator has summarized the difference as follows:

> To know God means to stand in a personal relationship to him.
>
> . . . The idea of divine commandment is as characteristic of Christianity as it is remote from Platonism. A commandment has validity not in itself, but derives authority from the commander, i.e. the person who stands behind the commandment. The Platonic principles are not backed by any person and their validity rests within themselves. The Platonist feels obliged to fulfill them since his reason tells him that they are just.
>
> The Christian obeys divine commandments, but not because he has examined their fairness and found them equitable; he knows that God's thoughts are inscrutable (Isaiah 55, 8–9; Rom. 11, 33), he obeys because of his love of God. To love God does not mean to understand or to admire Him but to turn one's entire being towards Him (Deut. 6, 5; Matt. 22, 37). . . . The image of the father and child is here of essential significance: the believer is a "child of God" (Eph. 5, 1) whose "hand is held" (Deut. 31, 6; Hos. 11, 3). A child does not yet feel the need to examine his father's instructions critically, just as the father feels no need to justify them. Thus the prophets and Jesus never appeal to human reason or to human conscience; they simply say: "He has showed thee, O man, what is good; and what doeth the Lord require of thee" (Mic. 6, 8), and "Not every one that saith unto me, Lord, Lord, shall enter into the kingdom of heaven; but he that does the will of my Father which is in heaven" (Matt. 7, 21). The child, refusing to submit to the father's will, struggles not so much against the content of his instructions as against the father's entire personality. Thus, as Steinbuchel has said, Christian sin is "more than a transgression of the divine law, it is the hardening of the self's I against God's Thou. . . ." [Verdenius, 1963, pp. 24–25]

Will, not rationality, is the primal phenomenon in the cosmos of Christian value. God does not will the Good; his will *is* the Good. With the priority of volition, ethics dissolves into the "personal relationship" of faith. There are ways of resisting this dissolution—by arguing, for example, that God wills a rational system of ethical universals, in which case the distance between Plato and Paul lessens considerably—but these are not the ways of the tradition leading to Kierkegaard. From the casuistry of scholasticism, Luther recovered the force of divine volition, and Calvin spoke of the "special decrees" (1957, pp. 91–92), incomprehensible to universalizing human reason, issued by this sovereign power. If we were to subtract from the theology of Calvin everything that deals with predestination, little would remain. But exactly there, in the paucity of the sayable, Kierkegaard professes his existential faith.

His dialectical movement from Socrates to Abraham is a playing out, in reverse, of the typical formation of the superego. All men gain internal regulation by acquiescing to a superior will whose dictates cannot be grounded rationally. Our usual strategy for domesticating the archaic "voluntarism" of the superego is to construct a rational ethics, absorbing the superior will by making our duties both explicit and internally consistent. As geometry succeeds our earliest intuitions of space, so ethical principle gradually organizes our first intuitions of value. Emphasizing the transformation of ego submission into ego function, Hartmann speaks of this process as "value testing" (1960, pp. 45–64). Following Freud's own equation of "mental health" with a "sufficiently impersonal" superego (1926b, p. 223), the "maturity" of the superego in psychoanalytic discourse is almost always placed in the direction we have defined as Platonic (see, for instance, Ticho, 1972). Rapaport once remarked that there remains at bottom an irreducible "absurdity" about the imperatives of the superego, and went on to outline another strategy of accommodation by which the ego arrives at a benign *credo quia absurdum est,* comfortable at last with the very absurdity of this tyranny, even treasuring it as such: the arbitrary impositions of conscience may become, in time, *my* absurdity (1959, pp. 464–65). But Kierkegaard pierces through the sediment of the Oedipus complex to the relationship of wills, the drama of power and forfeiture, at its source. The faith of Abraham brings dread to this expositor, not comfort or stability.

The shadow of a raised knife falls across the entire text of *Fear and Trembling*, as the argument moves, via a logic familiar to psychoanalysis, from the threatened son to the many narratives of thwarted love: the knife of Abraham divides men from women. We know from the *Journals* and *Papers* that this book in particular was to have explained to the abandoned Regine why she had to be sacrificed by her baffling fiancé (Heiss, p. 244). What might she have learned from this indirect communication?

One decoding of the cryptic message of *Fear and Trembling* would concern the ecstatic fusion of father and son, sacrificer and sacrificed. In this return to the threshold of the superego, the father, even as he raises his knife, is represented as suffering the same fate as the son. The first movement of faith is to concentrate, like Abraham, "the whole content of life and the whole significance of reality in one single wish" (p. 53). Abraham has achieved this concentration in his wish for a son; Silentio has even rearranged the biblical narrative so that Abraham will have received from God the promise about the blessing of all nations in his seed (Gen. 22:18) *before* he receives the command to sacrifice (Dietrichson, p. 242), a rewriting that equates the concentrated desire of Abraham for his son with the hopes of all mankind. As the first fruit of a covenant marked by circumcision, Isaac is literally his "seed." From the old penis of the father of faith has come at last a new penis, conduit for a line of seed destined to produce the mother of Jesus. So Abraham must sacrifice the son who is his own envoy in salvation history. The same commandment that makes Abraham the literal embodiment of an oedipal father also makes him, in the sacrifice of his focal wish, an oedipal son.

Throughout the Middle Ages and the Renaissance, this story was glossed as a prefiguration of the sacrifice of Christ. Kierkegaard would probably have rejected the quick application of this interpretation as yet another way of undermining the paradox of faith, encouraging the dread of Abraham to be hidden from us in the assurance of redemption. Yet the ancient *figura* unfolds the psycho-logic of Silentio's redaction: as Abraham raises the knife over Isaac, God raises the knife over Abraham. The will of God reigns supreme over every son in this oedipal tableau. When Silentio shifts from the dread of Abraham to the agony of Mary (pp. 75 ff.), we realize that the symbolic sacrifice of Abraham's seed is, when viewed retrospectively from the eventual fulfillment of the covenant, a genuine sacrifice, preenacting an oedipal gesture of submission to the privileges of paternal deity. God will supply the seed. The seed of Abraham, in the form of Mary, will only present a maternal vessel. And the knife of vengeance will fall indeed on that son.

The representation of the oedipal father as an oedipal son reminds us that the drama of the superego is self-perpetuating. Sons are threatened because fathers, when sons, were threatened. Searching for the origins of this psychic ritual, an infinite regress opens before us. Freud (1913, pp. 125–61) tried to break this conundrum with his Darwinian myth of the primal horde, as his concluding quotation of Goethe's "in the beginning was the Deed" (p. 161) would suggest: there must have been, at some time, an absolute father, a father without the complex, who gave birth to the first oedipal father. The unimaginable father outside the violent history of oedipal fathers and oedipal sons is, for Kierkegaard, God. God is unconditioned will. The complex derives a posteriori from his volition. He arbitrarily shapes the history of salvation into a covenant that founds and perpetuates oedipal relationships. Yet God, being pure fatherless father, does not exist. Bound by the covenant, Abraham and Isaac exist.

Their union is complete, utterly exclusive. In the narrative of Abraham, the concentrated desire of the father for his son replaces the desire of the father for his wife and, insofar as Abraham comes to stand for Isaac, replaces also the desire of the son for his mother. This implosion of the family triangle into a relationship between males (three of them, if we count God) can also be discerned in the dialectic itself. Here Silentio defines the paradox at the heart of his dread by superimposing the ethical upon the religious: "The ethical expression for what Abraham did is, that he would murder Isaac; the religious expression is, that he would sacrifice Isaac; but precisely in this contradiction consists the dread which can well make a man sleepless, and yet Abraham is not what he is without that dread" (p. 41). The ethical sense of things (that this is murder) resists submission to the religious sense of things. If, psychoanalytically, the ethical is equivalent to the autonomous or "Platonic" superego, the superego absorbed into the sphere of ego autonomy, then its resistance to the sheer force of paternal will expressed in the commandment of God must be equivalent to the love of the mother in the original drama of obedience. The antipathy between sexuality and obedience in the Oedipus complex proper gets transposed, through the movement of Silentio's dialectic, to an antipathy between the ethical and the religious, autonomy and submission. Instead of severing son from mother, the knife of religious faith suspends the acquisition of the archaic father by the "mature," ethical ego: these are the lovers who must be divided. The knife does not signify, as in the Oedipus complex proper: "Internalize me!" It rather signifies: "Your value depends on *never* internalizing me entirely!"

Later we will return to the separation of the superego from the ego as a precondition for religious experience. Now, however, we must note that unless the ego can in some sense usurp the authority of the primitive superego, it can never fulfill the promise of taking a woman. This was the hope that, along with the dread of castration, motivated its submission to the oedipal father in the archaic situation. But Kierkegaard broke the covenant of secular love. The sacrifice of ego autonomy in this text entails the sacrifice of woman; there was no place left for Regine, the entire erotic life having been drawn into the history of paternal configurations. On the question of whether marriage could be anything more than the satisfaction of an instinct, and therefore a diminishment of authentic consciousness, Kierkegaard wrote in his *Journals:* "Rubbish! Either simply and solely the satisfaction of an instinct, or spirit" (1834–55, p. 242).

Something is sprung, something is missing in this dialectic of

dread. For what is so mysterious about Abraham? Again and
again Silentio dwells upon the incomprehensibility of Abraham.
He cannot understand this man; this man has vacated the universal of humanity in the faith initiated by his "infinite resignation"
(p. 48 ff.). By addressing the dread inspired by this ineffable
Abraham, which can "well make a man sleepless," our
psychoanalysis of *Fear and Trembling* approaches the position of
this text in the history of religious ethics.

Janik and Toulmin (pp. 25-26, 160-61, 177-79) have argued,
and Holmer (1953) has implied, that the critique of ethics in
Kierkegaard foreshadows Wittgenstein. Since values are anchored in subjective acts of conviction, they are in principle beyond the reach of rational demonstration; we cannot stipulate
criteria for values as we can for facts that are the case, embedded
in a *Bild,* or state of affairs. "What we cannot speak about we must
pass over in silence" (Wittgenstein, p. 151). But it must be remembered that, for Wittgenstein, religion itself lies within the
realm of the silent, whereas the Silentio of Kierkegaard poses
questions with religious horizons. If there is a profundity in the
philosophy of ethics consistent with the absurdity at the ground of
the superego in psychoanalysis, then Wittgenstein, not Kierkegaard, articulated this insight consistently. There *is* a criterion
of value in the Danish existentialist, albeit one that could never be
applied empirically. No longer the correspondence between particular act and universal law of duty, value becomes the correspondence between human act and divine commandment—a
harmony of wills. True to the voluntarism of Christian tradition,
there can be no value without the intervention of a supernatural
edict.

It is now clear why the existential value of faith can only be
found in the deconstruction or "immaturing" of the superego.
Authentic value requires two wills. In the normal development of the
superego, the will of the Other is progressively hidden by the
internalizing ego. This structure of the self must be dismantled
and the will concealed there repositioned externally—as Abraham for Isaac, as God for Abraham—in order to create the only
situation from which authentic value can spring. If we cannot

know that there is a difference between the will of Abraham and the will of God, we cannot tell a murderer from a man of faith— and we cannot, indeed, *know* this. If we grant on faith that this man, or any man, raises his knife in harmony with divine command, then the source of dread would seem to lie more naturally in the supernatural decree than in the human obedience. What sort of God is this? Why is there no either/or in the case of God? Abraham remains incomprehensible to Silentio because his reflections about this man of faith have been displaced from their natural object. What Silentio is silent about, in all his talk of dread, is God.

There are no serious gestures toward a theodicy in the works of Kierkegaard. Theodicy, of course, presupposes the ethical universals that this theologian has abandoned. But does not the absence of a theodicy, or at least of the questions that invite a theodicy, open a lacuna in the dialectic of dread? In a voluntarism as strict as this one, nothing whatsoever can be said about the value of God. Shaftesbury seems to me definitive on this point:

> For whoever thinks there is a God, and pretends formally to believe that he is just and good, must suppose that there is independently such a thing as justice and injustice, truth and falsehood, right and wrong, according to which he pronounces that God is just, righteous, and true. If the mere will, decree, or law of God be said absolutely to constitute right and wrong, then are these latter words of no significancy at all. . . . Thus if one person were decreed to suffer for another's fault, the sentences would be just and equitable. . . . But to say of anything at all that it is just or unjust on such a foundation is to say nothing, or to speak without a meaning. [1900, vol. 1, p. 264]

Commanding murder, God has obviously questioned the absoluteness of the ethical. But the dread of this suspension arises in part because God has simultaneously questioned the ethics of the absolute, compelling us to formulate an urgent "either/or of deity" that we are—such is the difference between the finite and the infinite—impotent to pursue. The truncated dread of Silentio never moves from *what* God wills to the *moral character* of this will.

Because of an unanalyzed injunction *not* to pose the question of theodicy, the labor of justification slides from the will of God to the obedient will of faith: Abraham, rather than his God, is incomprehensible. The indictment of God cannot even be spoken in order to be dismissed. This law, generating the deepest silence of Silentio, reminds us that the crime Michael Kierkegaard revealed to his son on the traumatic twenty-second birthday was, in the judgment of one of his biographers, the sin of cursing God (Lowrie, pp. 67–78). The theology of Søren, in both the assumptions he articulates and those he cannot, seems designed to make this crime unrepeatable.

One cannot question, on purely psychoanalytic grounds, the validity of any discourse. There may be all sorts of pathological reasons for discerning the truth, including the psychoanalytic truth. Yet Kierkegaard, having suspended the metaphysics of knowledge, leaves us within his own thinking no grounds for any sort of validation: either we consent or we move outside him for a ground of assessment, in which case we have already denied his claim. This circularity is hardly unknown in the Christian tradition. But it is the peculiar distinction of Kierkegaard, I think, to have radicalized the suffering of faith while at the same time forsworn the task of theodicy. Summarizing his work in the *Concluding Unscientific Postscript,* he spoke of how easy it was to know what Christianity is, the problem being how to become a Christian. The positive achievement of Kierkegaard may be said to invert the situation he began with. As essence disappears in the concretion of existence, as becoming replaces knowing and "how" supplants "what," the movement of the individual toward Christian faith stands manifest before us. But the penalty exacted by this manifestation is that we no longer know what Christianity is. Indeed, we no longer have, in the perfect submission of faith, a warrant to inquire.

A Procedure for Reconciliation

My psychoanalysis of Kierkegaard has tried to locate his related notions of value, existence, and faith at the formative moments of the superego. As we prepare to rethink these moments under the guidance of Kierkegaard, we must impose still another outrage on the body of his work. Psychoanalysis evidently cannot operate at the level of metapsychology within the closed circle of faith; the guiding concepts of existentialism must be broken loose from Christianity. This suspension will be temporary, however, for we will return to Kierkegaard's moment of faith with a more congenial understanding of its symbolism.

In the history of philosophy, the seminal contribution of Kierkegaard lies in opposing the concretion of subjective existence to the great essentialist systems of transcendental idealism. Holmer clearly feels that he is carrying on in the spirit of this opposition by attacking general "theories" of "human nature," including psychoanalysis. But if one could, as a matter of principle, deny validity to the stages of psychic life formulated by psychoanalysis, would the existential dialectic of Kierkegaard be immune to refutation by the very same principle? For subjectivity is not unsystematic *simpliciter* in Kierkegaard: the word "unsystematic" in a strong sense would be triply prejudicial, since existence is not to be understood as the deficiency of formal ontology, is in fact prior to formal ontological thinking, and is not without a "system" of its own, as the dialectical stages reveal to us. Even as Kierkegaard exposes such an array of nuance in his various tales and examples that they cease to be illustrative of transportable generalizations, becoming instead "philosophical fragments," his dialectic moves on. I do not think that the relationship between the nonexemplary density of Kierkegaard's individuals, their antipathy to universalization, and the structure of his dialectic is different in kind from the *ideal* relationship between case histories and metapsychology in the Freudian tradition (see Ricoeur, 1977).

About to embark on the analytic of Dasein, Heidegger also confronts this problem. Either the Being of Dasein is resistant in principle to the generalizing of philosophical discourse, or else the philosopher of Dasein must allow some concession to the metaphysics of essence. The distinction he offers—without which *Being and Time* could not proceed—seems true to the procedure of Kierkegaard as well:

Dasein always understands itself in terms of its existence—in terms of the possibility of itself: to be itself or not itself. Dasein has either chosen these possibilities itself, or got itself into them, or grown up in them already. Only the particular Dasein decides its existence, whether it does so by taking hold or by neglecting. The question of existence never gets straightened out except through existing itself. The understanding of oneself which leads *along this way* we call "existentiell." . . . This does not require that the ontological structure of existence should be theoretically transparent. The question about that structure aims at the analysis of what constitutes existence. The context of such structure we call "*existentiality*." Its analytic has the character of an understanding which is not existentiell, but rather *existential*. [1962, p. 33]

There is concrete existence (the "existentiell"), recalcitrant to abstraction; it can be conceived as the fullest, most detailed answer to the question "Who am I?" There is also an "ontological structure of existence" common to every Dasein (the "existential") and accessible therefore to philosophical analysis. How can existentialism refuse privileges to psychoanalysis that it must extend to itself? If, unlike Holmer, we acknowledge the concession to essence in existentialism and proceed toward psychoanalysis, we find that the Kierkegaardian tradition has issued a challenge to Freudian thought, rather than rendered it obsolete.

My answer to this challenge will be an effort to purify through phenomenological analysis the sequence of genetic moments in psychoanalysis, the progressive articulation of consciousness *in* a structure and *as* a structure. Trying to expand rather than discard the metapsychology of Freud, my general orientation is close to that of the American ego psychologists and distinct from the "classic" attempts to replace Freud with a psychologized existentialism, such as the Daseinanalysis of Binswanger and Boss (see Spiegelberg, pp. 193–232, 333–42); but whereas Rapaport and some of his students have opened psychoanalysis to cognitive psychology, especially to Piaget, I am pursuing the more general issue of how the insights of metaphysics and existentialism might still, at this late date, reverberate creatively in psychoanalytic thinking.

When Ricoeur, trained in the phenomenology of Husserl, came to Freud, he disowned the "eidetics" of the will elaborated in *Freedom and Nature* (1966), proclaiming the philosophical lesson of psychoanalysis to lie in the recognition that the overcoming of the false narcissim of the *cogito* must be accomplished through a hermeneutic act of self-interpretation, not a directly introspective one (1970, p. 458). Having made this moving and defensible capitulation to the power of those masterful inferences by which Freud leads us to the unconscious, Ricoeur proceeded to limit psychoanalysis in a number of questionable ways: it is a "hermeneutic of suspicion" (pp. 32–36); it is locked into the "space of fantasy," equipped to deal only with repetition (pp. 439–51); it is to be kept entirely distinct from phenomenology (pp. 375–418). These conclusions set in motion the dialectic of archaeology and teleology, repetition and novelty, system and epiphany, characteristic of all of Ricoeur's thinking. They derive, in my opinion, from his equation of psychoanalysis with the texts of Freud, and they suggest the pitfalls of a philosophy that conceives its fundamental act to be the interpretation of texts. The disciplines acquired thereby tend to remain within the horizons of their initial formulation; the guiding pronouncements of the text are generously reexplored so that they may, in the end, be transcended rather than improved. The "psychoanalysis" considered in *Freud and Philosophy* is essentially a finished product that can therefore be "placed" vis-à-vis the "openness" of Ricoeur's own hermeneutic philosophy. But does not the concept of the ego potentially open psychoanalysis to whatever transpires in this ego—and not as knowledge to suspect but as knowledge to reconceive itself by virtue of?

I will argue that the conflict between metaphysics and existentialism is "announced," in the psychoanalytic theory of development, as the tension between two states of the ego—Narcissus and Oedipus, the ego in its genesis and the ego as reconstituted by the superego. Although unable to resolve the conflict between these philosophical positions, psychoanalysis does provide another sort of reconciliation by allowing us to conceive of them as strata in a psychogenesis of insight. Producing a life history shorn of the merely existentiell, psychoanalysis would be contributing something uniquely its own to the interaction of disciplines sought by modern humanism.

Again and again, in their search for first principles, the great modern thinkers have acknowledged the complex unity of the a priori, networks of irreudicible structures that are "there" as such and cannot be analyzed by resolution into elements that then combine to form the whole relationship. The "egology" of Husserl promises to explicate "*the all-embracing Apriori* innate in the essence of transcendental subjectivity," providing a "systematic unfolding of the *universal logos of all conceivable being*" (1973, p. 155)—a task given empirical form by the gestalt psychologists. Though far from the immanent Kantianism of Husserl, Heidegger, too, finds that because Dasein has a preontological understanding of Being, "the constitution of Dasein . . . is primordially a whole" (1962, p. 236): "These existential characteristics are not pieces belonging to something composite, one of which might sometimes be missing; but there is woven together in them a primordial context which makes up that totality of the structural whole which we are seeking" (pp. 235–36). The modern study of language also began with a recognition of the primacy of system. Under the influence of linguistic structuralism, anthropology has pretty much abandoned the effort of its founders, preeminently Lévy-Bruhl, to elaborate a history of consciousness. As we discover, in these and other contexts, the fullness of the a priori, we also encounter a limit: rich though it may be, the ground of our thinking is opaque as well, and we must curb our yearning for a more constructivist understanding of "first things." Here the distinctive features of psychoanalysis suggest their power and potential in interdisciplinary thinking.

Freudian psychology rests upon a history of psychic structure. Its explanations tend to be interchangeably genetic and structural, since a synchronic cross section of the mind at any given moment will constitute an organization of the past keyed, etiologically, to summary events still transpiring in the timeless "now" of the unconscious. Yet there are also past events, such as the genesis of the ego and the superego, that repeat themselves, not only in the "symbolic forms" known to symptomatology but in the persistence and character of psychic structure. Treating these events as both binding *and* revelatory, psychoanalysis can enter into the synthesis of cognate fields by reinstituting the old constructivist analysis in a newly critical form. We can, after a fashion, "take apart" the seamless network of the a priori, animating the givens of other disciplines within an expanded account of individual history. We can try to capture the wholenesses of our Being as they come into Being. If there are, behind the ways of man, no first principles pure and simple, we may still hope to discover through psychogenesis some rough drafts.

Metaphysics, Reflexivity, and the
Truth of Narcissus for Psychoanalysis

The metaphysical tradition scorned by the Christian Kierkegaard, the atheist Nietzsche, and the indefinitely religious Heidegger took as its central theme the act of knowledge by which a subject determines the essence of an object. Insofar as knowledge stood as the explicit issue of this philosophy, not merely as its result, self-consciousness was both thematic and methodological. One of the crucial links between the eidetic ascent of Plato, the god of Aristotle, the Nous of Plotinus, the *cogito* of Descartes, the transcendental subject of Kant, the Absolute Mind of Hegel, and the transcendental ego of Husserl is the triumphant, generative position accorded to reflexivity. The knowing of knowing was often rapturous as well, and something of the inebriation of Plotinus returned to Western philosophy when God as the transcendent guarantor of certain knowledge, the sustainer of essences, gave way to the transcendental a priori of the Enlightenment. Hegel ordered all ontology about the "immediate mediacy" of our self-awareness. Since whatever we are conscious of cannot be that consciousness itself, the objects of our awareness are necessarily Other. Yet mind is self-aware: the self I am aware of immediately, then, is the mediation of I and not-I. Hegel undertook on this basis the extraordinary task—the philosophical equivalent of apotheosis—of demonstrating that both nature and culture develop logically toward the perfect transparency of self-knowledge, that the structure of reflexivity inherent in our knowing, by mediating I and not-I, folds into its own ontology the antinomies that will appear, as Kant had shown, whenever the mind poses ontological questions concerning the not-itself. "The *goal*," Hegel wrote, is "Spirit that knows itself as Spirit" (1979, p. 493).

It is, I suspect, clear already to my psychoanalytic readers that the essentialist tradition addressed problems rooted in the early life of the ego. But how are we to explain this association? How account for the conviction arising, when we turn from the "self-objects" and "grandiose selves" of Kohut's pre-oedipal children to notions such as the Absolute Mind of Hegel, that the *same issues* remain in play? Certainly the metaphysics of the ego is not, as Ricoeur has come very close to arguing, a deceived and alienated reenactment of narcissistic states experienced during the psychogenesis of the ego. On the contrary, metaphysics *is* the drama of ego formation. For when is the drama over? When is there, strictly speaking, a "formation" rather than a "forming"? Because we tend to think of the history of the individual as segmental, punctuated by moments of lucid closure, theorists such as Mahler (1972) and Loewald (1978b) must now and again remind us that the problems of forming an ego or a superego are not so much solved as re-solved throughout life. Those analysts, on the other hand, who write with numb confidence about the regular achievement early in life of a normative separation between mind and world should endeavor, for the enlightenment of mankind, to make this norm explicit. Even among psychoanalysts who disparage the simplistic metaphors of "internal" and "external," such as Meissner (1977, pp. 168–72, 199–200), there is an unwillingness to admit that psychoanalysis, by positing the theory of differentiation, has erased the boundary between itself and traditional metaphysics. Is space the not-me? Read Kant and others. Is time the not-me? Read Husserl and others. If we are not to languish in the differentiation that happens to be given to us by cultural and historical circumstance, our effort to discern how we are situated in the world and the world situated in us must become a lifelong project.

The metaphysical tradition may be considered the science of ego differentiation. The emphatic pursuit of the nature and meaning of reflexivity in this tradition leads me to suppose that psychoanalysis, too, should have something to say about the matter. Reflexivity, after all, must be the definitive novelty established in the prephilosophical drama of ego genesis, if only because there is no criterion for the possession of an ego other than our awareness of possessing one. I will begin by following Lacan, who formulated his "stage of the mirror" (1977, pp. 1-7) in full awareness of the metaphysical tradition.

In Lacan's theory of ego genesis, the three poles of consciousness articulated by Western metaphysics—knowing subject, known object, and reflexive "observation" of this relationship—are structured simultaneously, yet in such a way that the subject and the reflexive awareness of the subject are collected in, even hidden in, the authority of the object. A coherent figure leaps out against a ground. There is the Other; here am I, the image of the Other. There is no pure determination of the self through its own reflexive awareness. Awareness flows back, as it were, from the pole of the object. Later, when the child tries to charm the figure in the mirror or cries when his playfellow stumbles, we understand in a more concrete fashion that reflexivity has occurred primordially at the pole of the object. For Lacan, then, the genesis of the ego transpires with the first in a series of "alienating" identifications. The ego, from the beginning, is the site of an estrangement (Lemaire, pp. 74, 81).

We shall not follow Lacan and his fellow alienists down this shadowy path to captivity. I once examined one of Lacan's Parisian pamphlets, on the cover of which was a drawing of a woman gagged by a leather device, a tear streaming from her eye: that futile, wordless tear is the perfect emblem of Lacan's notion of anything we might wish to call a "real self," while the bondage device conveys with equal precision his idea of the ego—an idea formed by combining the Freudian half-truth that the ego silences us with the structuralist half-truth that language speaks us. Despite the Hegelian allusions in his stage of the mirror (see the *Phenomenology of Spirit,* pp. 104–18, on the master-slave dialectic), Lacan's ferocious deprecation of the ego is due in no small part to the fact that he is writing within a post-Heideggerian tradition for which the metaphysics of the ego, as I have called it, has lost its revelatory power. In my view, the value of his work on ego genesis lies in its consistency, on a philosophical plane, with the largely clinical studies of narcissism published in America in recent years. How vulnerable this early ego is to the reflection of itself in, the recognition of itself by, the parental imagoes! We often speak of this dependency as a mirroring of the subject by the Other, yet as experienced by the child and by the true or borderline psychotic, the situation is just the opposite: the subject is the image or reflection, caught in the irreality of a looking-glass world and desperately in need of the presence or regard of the object in order to be whole, in order to be at all.

These patients, we are told, "lack autonomy." But if we try to elucidate the concept of autonomy "from the inside," with a positive phenomenology, we are thrown back on the themes of Descartes and Hegel. Autonomy resides in the feeling that the self is given to the self. It is the nameless affect of strength and security that accompanies the continuous self-giving of reflexivity. Reflexivity, our relationship to the subject-object relationship, constitutes our grip on our own wholeness; by virtue of this primordial unity in the structure of the psyche, the self is both "me" and "mine." Here we may note that in the definitive myth of ego genesis the tragedy of Narcissus derives from his ignorance that the image in the water, the object of his love, is indeed himself: he is the youth who has not made the transition from object-as-himself to himself-as-object. The psychotics and quasi-psychotics we name after Narcissus have also been unable to move emotionally from the primal object-relation, where the self is but the reflection of the Other, to the solitary companionship of reflexive consciousness, where the self is an Other unto itself—truly and positively Narcissus. Asserting as a metaphysical principle that the fundamental being of the ego involved the constant appropriation of Otherness as self-knowledge, Hegel was also unveiling the first tenuous victory of the prephilosophical life. A lived ontology underlines, as indeed it should, the formal one. For the relative weakness of reflexivity in the formative moments of the ego initiates psychic life at the greatest possible distance from the truth of *cogito ergo sum.* The Other is, therefore I am. If the primitive ego can feel, in times when the absence of the object does not engender peremptory need, the self-sustaining hold of reflexivity, then "all is returned." Ego does not require an Other in order to be, for ego mirrors itself in the doubling constitutive of consciousness. The affective ownership of reflexivity is differentiation. From this base unfolds the entire system of "object-selves" or self-representations.

As all theorists realize, the advent of language solidifies the fluid self-delineation of the early ego. But to the familiar stress on the cognitive and communicative advantages of language, we might add, in this context, that language facilitates a pronounced strengthening of the reflexive structure of the ego. Plato defined thought as a silent conversation with oneself. It may be, as Gadamer has suggested, that our thinking does not *intend* this familiar experience of an internal dialogue: "A person who thinks something . . . means by it the thing that he thinks. His mind is not directed back towards his own thinking when he forms the word" (1975, p. 385). Still, the *impression* of a conversation with oneself, if only a by-product of linguistic cognition, has a genuine psychological importance: more perfectly than before, the ego grasps the autonomy of its constant self-givenness. It seems obvious that the typical psychotic hallucination of hearing voices, of the "influence" or "flowing into" of the Other, duplicates at the level of language the same submergence of reflexivity in the object-relation found at the stage of the mirror. The self-given experience of interior language is transmuted into a message given by the Other.

But the early weakness of reflexivity does not result only from the biological dependency of the infant or from the simple fact that infants, those arrivals from Nonbeing, must somehow "come into awareness." Our primitive vulnerability to the object stems also from the essential articulation of mind as revealed especially in the egology of Husserl. Transforming the observation point of reflexive knowing into a method for exploring mental acts, the first phenomenologist laid bare the inherent limitations of reflexivity. He began with the postulate, derived from Brentano, that all consciousness has the structure of intentionality. It is always consciousness-of, whether of a perception, a memory, an idea, or so forth; in the phenomenological version of object constancy, the flow of consciousness can be analyzed as the stable correlation of the unity of the meant (intended) with the self-sameness of the meaning (intending) ego.

Let us call the I-pole of this relationship the "ego-source," following Strasser (cited by Meissner, 1967, pp. 194–95). As we have said, this ego-source is doubled-over or bifurcated: I am aware of my intending of the object. But can the ego-source have itself as an intentional object? Whenever in introspection the ego-source attempts to grasp itself, it always intends something else—a memory of itself, an idea of itself. The ego-source "is not the content of a lived experience, but the ego living the experience" (Meissner, 1967, p. 195). Since its essence is always to think an object, the ego-source can never *be* an object. Meissner suggests that for this reason the ego-source must be acknowledged as the limit to any conceivable psychology (pp. 200–01). Reflexivity furnishes an awareness of the ego-source but not a knowing of it. The ego comes with an orientation, turned away from itself and toward the object intended. Like light, to which the mind has often been compared, the ego-source is "visible" only in making something else "visible." The one possible way of describing the ego-source is by inference back from its determinations of the object: in the project of transcendental phenomenology, Husserl declared, the object must be our guide (pp. 35–43, 50–53).

Phenomenology as the egological science of Husserl clearly represents a violent dislocation of ordinary consciousness. Because the mind is oriented by nature toward a beholding of the world, we fall into the "natural standpoint": "we grasp . . . the house and not the perceiving," convinced that we stand "on the footing of the world already given as existing" (Husserl, pp. 33–34). But if mature egos can regularly experience the world in the posture of "this is real, and therefore I am aware of it," nearly blind to the constitutive and synthetic acts of the ego-source, then it is hardly surprising that an infant, in the primordial structuring of consciousness, will be "lost" in the object. *For there is*, as we learn from Husserl, *a kind of "unconscious" at the center of the ego itself.* The stage of the mirror is one model in psychogenesis for the concealment of the ego-source; hallucination in the absence of the nourishing object, where the ego must turn away from itself as a source of gratification, is another moment in the early construction of the natural standpoint (Kerrigan, 1980). The two sciences of the ego support each other. A psychoanalysis of the ego unveils the weight of symbol and affect favoring the cognitive naiveté unveiled by a phenomenology of the ego. Mind is displaced onto the world and its objects, as the various myths of its descent into an alien place would indicate. The psychoanalytic interpretation of these myths as representations of the fall from primary narcissism stands parallel to, and ultimately presupposes, a metaphysical interpretation.

In the regular course of things, decline from the narcissistic position crystallizes as novel psychic structure with the dissolution of the Oedipus complex. Something of the antagonism between these two phases can be discerned in the existentialism of Kierkegaard and Heidegger, who abandon the metaphysics of the self-generating ego for questions rooted in the advent of the superego. The goal of their thinking is not apodicticity, a world of determinate essences, but authenticity. Knowing becomes subordinate to deciding and acting. In place of the "know thyself" of Plato and Hegel stands "choose thyself." Existentialism is a philosophy of individuation, not differentiation. As the metaphysical concern for essence leads us back to the origin of the ego—to the primary circumscription, the determination of me and not-me— so the existentialist concern for the unique individual leads us to the origin of the superego. Pursuing the authenticity of the individual, the dialectical stages of Kierkegaard and the "care-structure" of Heidegger attempt to delineate another sort of "awareness." Even the extremes of the two traditions betray their association with different moments of psychogenesis. The persistent danger in the metaphysics of the ego, for example, has been solipsism, the postulate of an infinite and absolutely self-sufficient mind, while the abiding danger in the existentialist tradition has been relativism, a respect for declarations of subjectivity beyond rational dispute. If solipsism, for a Husserl, represents an extreme denial of the natural standpoint of the mature ego and, as our analysis would suggest, a way back to a truth lost early in the history of the ego, then perhaps the subjectivism of Kierkegaard and Heidegger can be shown to represent a comparably extreme denial of the systematic laws of the mature superego that allows us to reclaim the first structure of existence.

Conscience, Death, and Individuation

When the coming of the superego is spoken of as a "dissolution" or "destruction" of the Oedipus complex (Freud, 1924), a unique identification that transforms "oedipal object relations" into "internal, intrapsychic structural relations" (Loewald, 1978b, p. 9), this event presumably results in a modification of consciousness accessible to description. What, then, is the phenomenology of the presence of the superego? Judging from the clinical literature and from my own introspection, the presence of this new master of the ego may be described as a sense of being addressed by a "voice" (see Walsh on "ordinal language") or watched by an "eye," both of which are experienced as to some degree Other. When accusatory, this voice and this vision produce that anxious depletion of self-esteem we call "guilt" and often distinguish from its precursor "shame." Shame, having its source in external accusation, can be assuaged by the flight reflex, whereas the frustration of the flight reflex in the case of conscience registers as anxiety. But is the anxiety of conscience specific only in being a goad to repression or reparation? Freud, in tracing the genealogy of anxiety, connected the castration complex with "moral" and "social" anxiety (1926a, p. 139), and proposed in the same context that the fear of death was the "final transformation" (p. 140) of this affect. Since "Anxiety is an affective state and as such can, of course, only be felt by the ego" (p.

140), is the death of the ego somehow announced in the phenomenology of conscience?

Drawing upon Kierkegaard's treatment of dread, Heidegger argued in his complex and remarkable analytic of the "care-structure" (pp. 225–44, 279–348) that the anxiety of conscience calls us to the authentic resolution of Being-toward-Death. This is the keystone of his ontology of Dasein, for conscience is precisely the *existentiale* that makes Dasein the Being for whom his Being is an issue. Like Kierkegaard, Heidegger begins with the fact that anxiety has no distinct object. Indeed, this mood appears to represent a violation of the intentionality otherwise constitutive of consciousness. Love is love-of and fear is fear-of. But the special mood of anxiety stemming from "bad conscience" drives deeper than a specific accusation of failure to bring before us our primordial existence. The objectless call of conscience, then, manifests our authentic Being-in-the-world, not as an object of knowledge, but in a moment of vision. Coming before our authentic Being-in-the world, we grasp that which in every case (you as you read, I as I write) we are concerned about, if only in the mode of forgetting it. The authentic self called forth by anxiety is marked by *lack* (p. 328): Dasein is in a situation of practical involvements whose structure it has not chosen, including among these unchosen contingencies its mood or state-of-mind; it has, on the basis of this situation, a range of possibilities, the last of which is death; the primordial mood of our vision of this existence is anxiety, because anxiety bespeaks the "thrownness" we have not chosen and the "projection" of possibilities that must end in death; anxiety is therefore the affect of the "uncanniness" of our Being-in-the-world—which is to say that, since any "there" in which we find ourselves (you as you read, I as I write) will open out toward the past as a world we did not make and toward the future as a world we must leave, Dasein or "There-being" is fundamentally *not at home.* This authentic self is regularly hidden from our concern by practical involvements in the social world of the "they-self," whose everyday interpretations of life provide, among other distracting comforts, a *"constant tranquillization about death"* (p. 298).

We are not far from Freud here (see Smith, 1964). In the second theory of anxiety, this mood was understood as a response to absence and separation (1926a, pp. 133–38). Although jargon phrases such as "separation anxiety" encourage us to think of separation as the *object* of the anxiety, it is clear that, for Freud as for existentialism, anxiety occurs in the ego *upon* loss or separation; anxiety is the affect of the ego cast back upon itself, and may be thought of as a primordial demarcation of the solitude of the ego when that solitude can no longer be denied or forgotten. Moreover, even as he placed anxiety among the vicissitudes of pre-oedipal life, Freud continued to assert (1926a, p. 130), as he had in *The Ego and the Id* (p. 58), that the fear of death is a phenomenon occurring between the ego and the superego. But how might we comprehend, psychoanalytically, the bond between conscience and death asserted by Heidegger? Does not the differentiation of the ego, organized about the absence of the object, also take shape in the context of death? The death of unfulfilled need from which the nascent ego turns in its cry to the absent object cannot be felt as a "death of the ego," for there is as yet no ego coherent enough in its reflexivity to predicate death of itself. Rather, the "death" of ego formation must be registered as a possibility of unremitting emptiness as the one-and-only object of unremitting attention—the silent awareness of a nothingness at the ground of consciousness, in the phrase of Joseph Smith (1976, p. 405). As the hallucination is generated and, in its ruins, the object is cried out for, the child "turns" from this first and primitive death. If this "turning" constitutes primal repression (Smith, 1977), then the scene of anxiety in the drama of ego formation has been banished to the unconscious. Primordially we forget.

The difference between the death in ego formation and the death in superego formation is the difference between "nothing" and "the ego-as-nothing." Death in the generation of the superego is not an undifferentiated lack at the ground of consciousness, but death in a form that presupposes both individuality and a relationship to this individuality—a death of the subject of desire. Parallel to ego formation, the castration threat will be repressed. But here it is crucial to ponder the implications of the fact that there *is* a phenomenology of the presence of the superego, that the very experience of consciousness has been transformed by the superego. Theorists emphasizing "precursors" of the superego tend to think of the Oedipus complex as a symbol for the themes of narcissism. In part this view derives from the character of the theorizing itself, which offers a generous account of the complexity of pre-oedipal life and then poses this account against a constricted and unmysterious notion of the oedipal period.

But even the more sophisticated emphases on pre-oedipal guilt, such as that of Modell (1971), who allows for the binding and focusing powers of the superego identification, fail to come to terms with the unprecedented redefinition of the *being* of the ego affected by the superego.

I feel that Freud was correct to think of the Oedipus complex as a genuine transformation, reshaping the ego's mode of existence in such a way that all prior themes become symbolic of this new articulation. Like the primitive acquaintance with anxiety, the castration threat gets repressed. But the novel presence of the superego, for which there is no parallel in ego formation, establishes an otherness in the field of consciousness *that will not let the ego forget.* As a guide to authenticity, the superego takes over at a new level the function of the primary object in the stage of the mirror; it also restores to the conscious ego the very source of anxiety banished in primal repression. As Other and as source of anxiety, the superego constitutes the ego as a dying object, binding this "return of the repressed" into the structure of psychic life. Now the ego exists in its concern for the dying object "heard" in the call of conscience. Attunement to the anxiety of conscience, unlike the attunement of the manic-depressive to the primitive death of nothingness, acquires a revelatory force. Opposed, through its attack on oedipal love, to the infinities of narcissistic wish, conscience summons us to the finitude of existence as a possibility certain to occur, not as a nothingness already accomplished at the ground of the ego. Anxiety becomes the goad of authenticity. Reflexivity is transformed from the process of differentiation, the issue of me and not-me, to the process of individuation, the newly temporal issue "how shall I be?"

In a sense, the ego has made destiny its choice, acquiring the *memento mori* of the superego through a process of loss, internalization, and mourning. Heidegger states that death is "non-relational" (p. 294). I experience the death of others as an absence or a loss, as Freud himself confirmed, but I do not experience their death: death is something that can only be *mine.* As I cannot know experientially the death of others, they cannot know mine. Whenever Dasein stands before death authentically, then, "all its relations to any other Dasein have been undone" (p. 294). Death extricates the self in its pure individuality, insulating Dasein from its submergence in the they-self. It is possibly the most arresting paradox of the Oedipus complex that one moves through object relations and their interiorization in order to discover, through a relationship to the guiding otherness of conscience, a self that utterly transcends relatedness.

Yet thus far our description of the superego seems to present us, to some degree, with a "disarticulation" of the experiencing ego. Insofar as conscience is felt as Other, the superego appears to be something *added on* to the ego. To be sure, the internalization of the castration threat does invest the ego with a new unity of temporal structure: mortality is not a fact learned, but the testimony of internal experience for the post-oedipal ego. Yet have we done justice to the "something novel" that "comes into being" (Loewald, 1973, p. 16) with the dissolution of the complex? Sandler maintains an apparently orthodox position in defining the superego as "a consistent organization which stands apart from the other constituents of the ego" (1960, p. 133). Nonetheless, if the Oedipus complex is "the point of junction from which . . . all later developments proceed" (Freud, 1925, pp. 55), there would be reason to suspect that the complex does not, when internalized, "stand apart"—that some modification occurs in the ego itself homologous to the reflexivity we found at the first genesis of the ego.

The possibility of an oversight in our usual understanding of the oedipal dissolution is clearest when we approach the problem from the economic point of view. Freud posited that the choice of the oedipal child for narcissism over love had its energic counterpart in the restitution of object-cathexes as narcissistic-cathexes, supplying the ego with a pool of relatively neutralized energy:

> If this displaceable energy is desexualized libido, it may also be described as *sublimated* energy; for it would still retain the main purpose of Eros—that of uniting and binding—in so far as it helps towards establishing the unity, or tendency to unity, which is particularly characteristic of the ego. [1923, p. 45]

Is this "uniting and binding" to be found only in the new intrapsychic situation of the post-oedipal ego—solely a matter of the "stability" dispensed by its new master? Is the formation of the superego but a restaging of the genesis of the ego, in which the priority of the object becomes internalized as the not-ego authority of conscience? The superego, of course, draws its energy from a deep alliance with the id; this collaboration is reasonable enough, since the superego is primarily the representative of the same-sex parent who, in the Oedipus complex proper, became a rival through occupying the same libidinal position as the child himself. But here Freud is talking about a desexualized energy bound in the ego, not in the superego. As his italics reveal, any attempt to specify this new unification of the post-oedipal ego must lay some stones for the theory of sublimation that, many have noted, Freud hypothesized without making fully comprehensible.

The aspect of sublimation I have in mind would mean, for psychoanalysis, a theory of the will. Metapsychology is not encouraging in this respect. "Volition and will," as Spitz declared (pp. 136–37), "are terms which appear rarely in psychoanalytic literature. Indeed, it is difficult to find a place for these terms in the framework of psychoanalytic concepts." One difficulty resides in the unpromising mechanism of Freudian energics. Should we bypass this difficulty, there would remain the problem of how a will, even if we call it "overdetermined," could be squared with what is fundamentally a depth psychology. Moreover, if we follow Freud in searching for the origin of sublimation at the internalizing of the Oedipus complex, our theory of will would have to involve a clear differentiation of the sort of "will" exemplified during Mahler's "practising period" (1972), when the child explores his environment, stages games of separation with his toys, and collides against the boundaries of things, from the sort of "will" specific to the acquisition of the superego. These are formidable problems indeed, and I will not be able to offer a thorough solution to any one of them. But Freud has pointed the way: what goes out as oedipal desire somehow returns as a binding energy in the ego. Let us suppose that the ego, regenerated in subjecting itself to the law of the superego, gains in no spectral way the wherewithal to engage this law.

Will as the Reflexivity of the Postoedipal Ego

My beginning is an unlikely one. Yet the reflections of Ralph Cudworth, a British Neoplatonist of the seventeenth century, direct us toward a broadly symmetrical relationship between the reflexivity of the first ego structure and the willing of the second. In his early work this philosopher opposed the materialism of Hobbesian psychology by seizing upon the "doubling" or "echoing" of consciousness. I see a tree. There may be an object in nature to which my tree-perception corresponds, but clearly no object corresponds to my awareness of seeing the tree: immanent in all perception is a reflexive "echo" that cannot be reduced to the effect of a "sensation." Building on this idealist foundation, Cudworth left at his death an enormous manuscript on problems of moral psychology (Passmore, pp. 51–67). Here he was able to expose a fundamental error in some ancient (and some modern) conceptions of will. Predisposed by the metaphysical tradition to find *res cogitans* in essence indivisible, Cudworth insisted that will must not be considered a "faculty" or a "power" distinct from the wholeness of our mentality. Will is not a *part* of the mind. Known to us in our capacity for self-direction, will must lay hold of our entirety. It is a redoubling or second-order reflexivity—"the echo of an echo." I see a tree, I am aware of seeing the tree, and I am aware of willing to see the tree.

With the notion of will as a folding-over of the primary

folding-over of reflexivity, we shall continue our investigation with the work of the Munich phenomenologist Alexander Pfänder. Like Cudworth, Pfänder recognizes that thinking, willing, and feeling always occur together in "intimate interpenetration" (1967, p. 4). Accepting the difficulties of this "hermeneutic circle," in which the specific act we hope to define is always embedded in the whole of mental action, he moves toward a phenomenology of willing by first distinguishing this act from what he calls "striving."

Three movements constitute a striving (pp. 16–18). An object—an orange, let us say—registers in consciousness. This is felt as centrifugal. Physically or mentally, I can "reach out" toward the orange, inspecting it and determining its characteristics. But should the orange arouse a striving, this arousal would be felt as centripetal—an "ignition, a lighting of an *impelling* striving, which issues from the object which confronts us" (p. 17). (In the case of a counterstriving, the centripetal motion would be felt as repulsion.) Finally I renew, in the form of consent, the centrifugal relationship: I grasp and devour the orange. While a striving must capture, to be successful, the "ego-center" (Pfänder's term for what I earlier called the ego-source), the appeal of the object flares somewhere in the periphery of the ego. At this point Pfänder's analysis begins to converge with a psychoanalysis of the ego:

> For this ego has a characteristic structure: the ego-center (*Ich-Zentrum*), or the ego-core, is surrounded by an ego-body (*Ich-Leib*). And the strivings can arise in the ego, but outside the ego-center in the ego-body, and hence, in this sense, can be experienced as eccentric strivings.
>
> ... Now, like all strivings, these eccentric strivings have by themselves a centrifugal direction pointing away from the ego. But at the same time they have a tendency to shift from their eccentric location into a central one, or to seize the ego-center and pull it inside.... The central ego can be quickly seized and held down without its will, now by this, now by that striving as it emerges eccentrically. [pp. 18–19]

Freud, we know, defined the ego as a precipitate of the id—which might be thought of, in this context, as striving in the absence of an ego-center—whose first form was that of a "body-ego" (1923, p. 26). Pfänder suggests the possibility of a concrete phenomenology of the early ego. Striving would be the primal stratum of the will, the first stage in the development of motivation. Dominated by objects, the primitive ego-center would be "pulled inside" strivings aroused in the ego-body, as objects appeal with centripetal force to the mouth, the stomach, and the hand. The ego-center would be regularly and often violently dispersed in these eccentric arousals. Children in the "practising period" still seem to act predominately in this mode—haphazardly attentive, forever distracted by eccentric strivings and drawn inside this or that arousal. During the anal period, strivings—the imposition of the pleasure principle—would begin to yield to the executive hegemony of the ego-center, as the rectum and bladder of the ego-body become subject to the decrees of will.

Pfänder declares that although the object may still be felt as "attractive," willing seems to our awareness purely centrifugal:

> The act of willing differs from striving, too. It differs from eccentric striving by the fact that it is always central, ... performed by the ego-center itself. ... Here the ego-center is not only the subject and origin but also the original performer of the act.
>
> Although the act of willing agrees with striving, inasmuch as it has centrifugal direction, it is, nevertheless, in complete contrast with striving, not blind per se but containing in its essence a consciousness of what is willed. [pp. 20–21]

In order that willing transpire, the ego-center must possess a reflexive awareness of itself *and* the sure power of controlling the entire ego:

> The act of willing refers to one's own ego. If it is not to be one of those pseudo-acts of willing which refer to a severed

fantasy ego, . . . then one's own ego must not be merely thought about but must itself be immediately grasped and must be made a subject-referent of a practical proposing. Thus willing, but not striving, includes the immediate consciousness of self. . . . It is an act of self-determination in the sense that the ego is both the subject and the object of the act. [pp. 22–23; cf. Husserl, pp. 57–58, 66–68]

The authentically willing ego must discover itself, not as an object of knowledge but as a self cast forth into involvements. Its project is the determination of itself: implicit in every act of will is the will to will, the disowning of the wishful "fantasy ego." Willing seems to be the one possible exception to the law that prevents the ego-center or ego-source from being an object unto itself.

The discovery of the authentic and central ego presupposed by willing is the new articulation of consciousness wrought by the dissolution of the Oedipus complex. Abandoning the fantasy ego of oedipal object relations, we come to ourselves in another mode. This is not the primal reflexivity by which we are aware of objects intended in the flow of thought. This is rather the reflexivity of Heidegger's Dasein, the Being concerned with his Being. In our analysis of conscience, we saw how anxiety is the affect of the ego thrown back upon its solitude and its situation. Conscience, in this way, provides the ego-center with a vision of itself to be responsible for. Surely we imply this vision of "self as object in the mode of authenticity" in the concept of an ego ideal residing in the superego, for what is an ideal but something against which we measure ourselves as an object of our concern? The superego does, to this extent, "stand apart." Indeed, the relationship of will and conscience repeats after a fashion the relationship of ego-center and ego-body in striving. I hear its call; I am accused; guilt draws my ego-center "inside" the accuser, compelling me to strive for obedience and to embody the ideal.

But the superego is felt as genuinely Other—not as a "part" of the ego, like the peripheral field of the ego-body. The ego can only constitute itself as an object by adopting toward itself the point of view of the Other. Standing apart, the superego permits the ego to envision itself. It is precisely the function of the felt otherness of conscience to supply the "object" for acts of willing that require the ego-center to be both subject and object. Willing is solidified, made habitual, in the correlation of superego and ego. The "subject" in the secondary reflexivity of willing is the creative response of the ego-center to the "object" manifested by conscience. The existential attitude of willing represents an extraordinary turnabout from the metaphysical attitude of knowing. In the correlation of intentionality, the intended remains in a state of flux while the ego-center in its anchored selfsameness performs acts of synthetic unification. In the correlation of willing, the otherness of conscience exerts a constant stabilizing pressure while the ego-center remains in a state of fluctuating self-determination. Knowing is rooted in the constancy of the subject, willing in the indeterminacy of the subject.

The mystery of this sublimation returns us to oedipal love as the bridge in psychic development between striving and willing. Like striving, love is experienced as demanded by the lovableness of the object. Need, the earliest precursor of oedipal love, would be felt as a "seduction" of the ego-center by the ego-body, which is in turn "seduced" by the impelling object, whether present or imagined: the mouth and stomach desire the breast. When satisfied, however, the peripheral strivings of the ego-body would tend to disappear in the wholeness of well-being, permitting, as it were, a radiant diffusion of the ego-center toward the object that has both caused and fulfilled the need: satisfaction confirms the centripetal power of the object that ignited the striving. This dialectical interplay between need as the eccentric seduction of the ego-center and gratitude as the centric "relaxation" of the ego-center continues to mark oedipal love. The penis of the boy desires the mother. The regularity with which the ego-center is "pulled inside" this eccentric striving is manifest not only in the castration complex, but also in the penis-body equation—which is inseparably a penis-ego equation, a symbolic equivalence of part and whole that mirrors exactly the phenomenology of erotic striving.

But ideally, in the period of oedipal love, part-objects and their counterparts in the ego-body have relinquished something of their priority to the organization of the whole. Need (the whole of the ego claimed by its parts) and gratitude (the parts of the ego reclaimed by its whole) have managed a reconciliation. The mother as a whole is wholly desired. The very indefiniteness of the "sexual act" that the boy hopes to perform with his mother suggests a break with primordial strife. In the *Symposium* Socrates defines Eros as the mediating power by which we move from the many particular beauties to the one concept of the beautiful. This pattern holds true in psychic development, except that the dispersal of many eccentric strivings must first cohere into a particular unified love for a particular unified object. The oedipal child must, like the Abraham of Kierkegaard, concentrate all of reality into a single wish. His love must be in essence a *centric* striving.

How might this centric striving be converted into will? We can edge toward that dark issue by trying to coordinate our phenomenology of striving with the economic point of view. It seems reasonable to assume that the ego-body aroused in striving enjoys a more direct access to the sources of psychic energy than the ego-center; strivings initiated within the peripheral field of the ego betray a mode of action closer to cause-effect, stimulus-response, than to the purposeful and rule-governed adjustment of ends to means characteristic of motive (on this distinction, see Peters, pp. 27–52; Ricoeur, 1966, pp. 66–72). But the ego is by nature intentional. Even as it experiences the pressure of the ego-body, it experiences the impelling pressure of the object. It feels, at least, that the pressure of the object was *prior to* the arousal of the ego-body. The striving of love, too, is experienced as demanded by the intrinsic value of the object, a lovableness that we have in no sense created. If the economic concept answering to this phenomenology is "object-cathexis," then the energics of psychoanalysis impinge upon the conscious ego as the very structure of its relatedness to the world. William James suggested that "the sentiment of reality with which an object appeals to the mind is proportionate (amongst other things) to its efficacy as a stimulus to the will," adding that this proportionality "is a tale that has never yet been told" (vol. 2, pp. 546–47). Phenomenologically, I can only make sense of object-cathexis as the felt passivity of the ego, its attachment of centrifugal strivings to the prior "reality" of centripetal ignitions.

Such a view would bring the psychoanalytic theory of cathexis into line with the "mythical thinking" of Cassirer and Langer. Cassirer (1946, 1955) argued that in myth the symbolic forms by which we organize the world are subjected to a characteristic "hypostasis." Mythical consciousness beholds its own construction of the world as not-ego, as realities that impress themselves upon the ego from the object-pole of knowing. Feeling "awe" in the presence of something, I invest that something with an "awesomeness" existing apart from my feeling and by virtue of which my feeling is compelled: "the spark jumps somehow across, the tension finds release, as the subjective excitement becomes objectified" (1946, p. 33). Is this not, as Langer (pp. 394–400) has implied, an accurate description of the fateful creation of the parental imagoes and the self-representations? Cathexis ignites the spark. It gives a physical name to that cognitive form by which the vicissitudes of love and dread are felt as required and wholly motivated by the "powers" of primary objects. The same form dominates the volitional life. As the reifying or substantializing of affect, object-cathexes "command" the ego to strive. But in the special case of oedipal love, what goes out as strife returns as will. When the object-cathexes of the Oedipus complex have been shattered and assimilated into the ego as narcissistic-cathexes, the consequence is the "uniting and binding" of will: it is as if the libidinal energy "hidden" in the commanding power of the object became, when reacquired by the ego, the power of self-command. The destructive force of the rival is transformed into an ideal that stands apart. Answerable to its call, the erotic force of the beloved is transformed into an ego-drive of willing able to deploy the self manifested by this ideal.

The differentiation of the ego, in summary, is a lived *cogito*. There is a formalism about the first unity of the ego. I am I, not Thou: in the circumscribing of myself through differentiation I do in fact gain something like an essence—a periphery and a center, mine with a constancy of self-givenness. But if the ego is found in the delineation of being, the superego is found in the indeterminacy of becoming. After the Oedipus complex, the unity of the ego is in every way temporal. The father internalized as conscience, more than a code of laws or an imperative to obey, is a model and a future. When I renounce my wish to reunite with my alter ego from the mirror phase, "all is returned" as my futurity. The boundaries of preoedipal self-discovery, marked by the reflexive knowing of my essence, get thrown open to a radically futural existence. I no longer simply *am*, for from this *am* emerge temporal "ecstases," in Heidegger's sense (pp. 370–80). I am Being-toward a future, that is, because I have owned in the deepest way the past imposed on me: severing the maternal tie a second time, I have chosen the differentiation that has already occurred. Though surely not freed, my desire has been distanced from its first and unchosen object, returning to me as the power of self-determination. The Being of this second ego, the ego of individuation, lies in possibilities, and its boundary is death.

My assumption throughout this discussion has been that any psychological theory, even the cathectic energy of psychoanalysis, must ultimately derive from, and refer back to, the phenomena of conscious experience: the term itself is tautological, since there is no other experience. If psychoanalysis were actually, as Ricoeur maintains, incompatible with phenomenology, it would be nonsense. In this regard, all psychology is ego psychology, and as such, must set about trying to understand the essence and existence of the ego. A psychoanalysis developed along these lines would contribute more to philosophy than its hard-won knowledge of the unconscious, for among the possibilities open to an authentic ego is the task of restoring to its reflection the history by which it came to be.

The Authenticity of Kierkegaard

What is really at stake in Kierkegaard's deconstruction of the superego in a moment of submission to divine authority? We have emphasized that will is a reflexivity at the center of consciousness, the ego acting upon itself, whereas conscience is experienced as

Other. If we were to complete the symmetry implied in our analysis of the ego and superego, will in its autonomy could permit a freedom from the internal object of conscience parallel to the freedom from the determining power of the external object affected by primary reflexivity in the drama of ego formation. Self-determination, after all, entails the capacity to dispute and to disobey. Obedience, moreover, could be seen as a more subtle road to the abolition of conscience. Embodying the ideal, the ego progressively diminishes its otherness. But Abraham is obedient to a God whose otherness is absolute and never to be diminished. The paradoxical faith of Kierkegaard contains at once a liberation from conscience *and* a refusal to lessen in any way the phenomenological tension between autonomous self-determination and the otherness of a commanding voice. We can authenticate this faith by discussing other strategies of the willing ego for securing its own liberation.

Normally, of course, the superego will evolve through those "socializing" identifications that constitute the system of ego ideals, progressively diluting the primitive authority of the first parental ideal. "The validity of morals," Gadamer has written, "is based on tradition. They are freely taken over, but by no means created by a free insight or justified by themselves. This is precisely what we call a tradition: the ground of their validity" (p. 249). The faith of Kierkegaard leaves this ground. The command given to Abraham strikes at the fundamental unit of social life, compelling him to discover a self he values more than his most treasured bond of kinship. When conscience can be reduced to "everyone should do this," there is no longer any important difference between conscience and ego-center, or one ego-center and another. Tradition is the morality of the they-self. "Everyone is the other, and no one is himself" (Heidegger, p. 165).

The commandment licenses a revolt against matured conscience. It serves as an epoché or "suspension" of all law that applies to more than one person. The clearest of ordinary values, the love of father for son, is seen as such—as ordinary. In effect, the voice of God reveals that every law applicable to more than one person cannot be authentically self-determining. Forcing

Abraham to liberate from civilizing conscience an utterly singular self, a self to be valued above every engagement with the human Other, God proposes the definitive test of authentic individuation. No wonder Abraham is silent, for the self called forth by God necessarily resides outside of language as a means of relatedness to other people. Choosing to sacrifice Isaac, Abraham sacrifices the genealogy of his social being—everything we term "object-relations" in psychoanalysis. Before the superego, he is also beyond it.

If the ethics of social tradition was, for Kierkegaard, one false liberation from the otherness of conscience, a liberation that compromised the authentic self, philosophy was another. The ethics of autonomous reason developed by Kant, like Hartmann's description of the absorption of the superego into the ego, projects the ultimate sufficiency of the self-determining ego-center. "Rational will" advises itself; ethical acts are entirely centric; reason has authority not only over strivings but also over the promptings of conscience. As our analysis of the superego would lead us to suspect, the appearance of this autonomous ethic was a genuine revolution in the history of philosophy. Only those philosophers whom we might call, after Harold Bloom, "strong" philosophers, such as Kant, have been able to contain the sphere of ethics solely within the ego-center. Before and after Kant, the point of crisis in the unfolding of a systematic ethics has always come at the moment when reason, at the center of the ego, realizes that *it is itself the author of the law.* Free from the call of conscience, the ego has committed a sort of patricide. This moment of sublime self-determination has often been felt, I think, as narcissistic excess—as anxiety, in fact—and the inscription of this anxiety can be read in the redundance characteristic of some ethical systems. In Aquinas, for instance, reason can apparently ground the law within the enclosure of itself, showing by necessary argument that the Decalogue is its own voice. Nevertheless, his system falls back on a correspondence between the "order of reason" and the "order of being" sustained by God: were reason not sufficient, its determinations could rest upon a revelatory ontology. There is the ghost of an otherness in ethics, if only in the form of a redundancy.

Kierkegaard viewed the captivity of conscience to the universalist ethics of the ego-center as an empty formalism of identity. Perhaps our psychogenesis of the superego implies the truth of this concern. What is the relationship between conscience and will? Their correlation in the volitional life is the transformation of precisely that—a relationship. The obliteration of the superego in the ego may be the subtlest totalitarianism of all, diminishing the *meaning* of a superego. When the trace of oedipal object relations is lost in the assimilation of conscience into the ego-center, the existential project regresses into the essentialist realm of ego formation, and the ethical life deteriorates into the drawing and redrawing of definite boundaries of the ego, a consistent reaffirmation in dutiful behavior of the frozen essence of one's goodness. Becoming lapses into repetition. But the voice of conscience, opened to infinity, speaks as Wholly Other to Abraham, and turns with irresistible authority against any form of the conscience known to social tradition or philosophical ethics. God calls forth from Abraham a self as absolute in its mineness as the self posited by Hegel is absolute in its ubiquity. With the voice of law both Wholly Other and perfectly specific in its address, the religious ego has rescued the intuitive adventure of becoming—an adventure predicated on submission and sacrifice.

The last act of autonomous will is to play its own Oedipus. Structurally, the moment of faith is the exact opposite of the philosophical moment at which reason emerges as a law unto itself, born into the heavy freedom of complete self-determination. Here God acts as autonomous will, not the ego-center. His law is pure unreason, a non-ideal. When God reveals his irrationality before the gaze of centric reason, faith is the "condition" in light of which reason abdicates, understanding itself as refuted, not God: "When the Reason and the Paradox encounter one another happily in the Moment, . . . the Reason sets itself aside and the Paradox bestows itself" (Kierkegaard, 1844, pp. 72–73). Unreason becomes a law unto reason. As the two states of the ego we have defined are placed against each other in an either/or, faith seals the victory of an order rooted in the second genesis over one rooted in the first. This new death of the ego is the death of the metaphysics of the ego.

It is also, as I have argued, the nullification of Kierkegaard's love. When the central will coalesces in psychic history from the remnants of shattered love, this love is transformed at the core of the will into a guiding hope: obedience seeks the restitution of this love in another. We may now appreciate once again how Kierkegaard came to discern in the faith of Abraham, with its willed renunciation of autonomous will, a parable signifying the disavowal of marriage. In this particular, faith reaffirms the oedipal prohibition. But that is not all, even for psychoanalysis. For the complex is also being reworked, so to speak, in another dimension. The Father asserts himself to the father of faith in such a way that the dynamics of the oedipal drama can be rewoven into a strange negation, a negation that is simultaneously a confirmation, of its first and profane closure.

Psychoanalytically, faith's moment presents itself as a third genesis of the ego. Kierkegaard understood, profoundly I think, that the law of conscience cannot be rational, for if it were, conscience would not be either other than or Other to the reasoning being of the ego-center: *only the irrationality of the law can guarantee the felt otherness of conscience.* Now if, like Kierkegaard, one must at all cost preserve this otherness as the sole basis of authentic value, what would be the most terrible moment conceivable? The moment when the ego becomes the superego. But that is precisely the moment of faith: directed to sacrifice his son, *Abraham is commanded to become the superego.* The act whose symbolic meaning is the self-extinction of the rational and metaphysical ego has as its overt form the absorption by this ego of the authority of its first master. Ordering the ego to become the equivalent of its own primitive conscience, the Wholly Other frustrates this equivalence by the very act of commanding it and establishes itself as a new transcendent master of the ego-as-superego. Successor to the superego, God outthinks the logic of the Oedipus complex, contriving his investiture as the undoing of the superego. If faith is born through the self-sacrifice of the ego, then we might say that

God offers himself to faith through the self-sacrifice of the superego.

My earlier suggestion that the oedipal father and oedipal son were condensed in Abraham can now be seen as the crux of faith's paradox, the point from which its emotional authority derives: a triumph over the first oedipal submission is at one and the same time the act of submission in a new enactment of the complex at the level of faith. Just as the Oedipus complex transforms the themes of narcissism into symbols of authenticity, so faith would transform the themes of the Oedipus complex into symbols of sacred authenticity. *The complex is the condition of faith's condition.* There is, after all, a canniness, a psycho-logic both ironic and necessary in the apparently irrational Word of Abraham's God. Extricated from all profane entanglements, Abraham performs with Isaac a ritual symbolic of the instituting of the superego, vehicle of civilization. The act that liberates him from the social order also founds and perpetuates the social order, enabling his seed to transcend this institution because their father has inserted them into the epigenetic sequence that leads from the authentically willing ego to the authentically faithful ego, and from the precarious otherness of the superego to the unassimilable Otherness of God. Abraham completes the symbolism by initiating the symbolism. He lowers his knife: the seed is now in the son. "All is returned."

Kierkegaard wrote in *Philosophical Fragments* that faith "is not a form of knowledge" (p. 76) and "not an act of will" (p. 77). After the suicide of the rational ego and the submission of the willing ego is there a third-order reflexivity in my concern for an ego unbounded by death? I am not the one to attempt its phenomenology. What can be said, from the worldly position of this essay, is that psychoanalysis abandons much of the mystery and complexity of our existence when the Oedipus complex remains almost unrealized in the work of many of its fashionable theorists, who obscure its unique ontological structures by attempting to reduce them to the narcissistic order of "internal object relations." This is no way to think the self. Everything has its precursors, but psychic development is transformational as well as incremental: in order to understand the man who lives on a borderline, we must grasp what lies on *both* sides of him. A similar narcissistic collapse has occurred in the psychoanalysis of religion. The faith of Abraham, however, bears no resemblance to the "faith" that Erikson and others have unearthed at the deepest stratum of Christian desire. Here is no reuniting in primary narcissism with the trustworthy mother. Abraham exists, far from the placid nirvana of an equilibrated pleasure principle. The imaginative excitement of this man springs from the paradoxes that are his choice and his risk. A genesis indeed, the Oedipus complex—where rival becomes ideal, love will, castration freedom, and impossible fantasy true authenticity—is the Paradox par excellence of the psychological world.

REFERENCES

Calvin, J. *On the Christian Faith.* Edited by J. T. McNeill. New York: Bobbs-Merrill, 1957.

Cassirer, E. *Language and Myth.* Translated by S. Langer. New York: Harper & Row, 1946.

————. *Mythical Thinking.* Vol. 2 of *The Philosophy of Symbolic Forms.* Translated by R. Manheim. New Haven: Yale University Press, 1955.

Daim, W. *Depth Psychology and Salvation.* Translated by K. Reinhardt, New York: Frederick Ungar, 1963.

Dietrichson, P. "Introduction to a Reappraisal of *Fear and Trembling.*" *Inquiry* 12 (1969): 236-45.

Freud, S.
Standard Edition of the Complete Psychological Works. London: Hogarth, 1953-74.
Totem and Taboo (1913), vol. 13.
The Ego and the Id (1923), vol. 19.
"The Dissolution of the Oedipus Complex" (1924), vol. 19.
An Autobiographical Study (1925), vol. 20.
Inhibitions, Symptoms and Anxiety (1926a), vol. 20.
The Question of Lay Analysis (1926b), vol. 20.

Gadamer, H. G. *Truth and Method.* New York: Seabury Press, 1975.

Hartmann, H. *Psychoanalysis and Moral Values.* New York: International Universities Press, 1960.

Hegel, G. W. F. *Phenomenology of Spirit*. Translated by A. V. Miller. Oxford: Oxford University Press, 1979.

Heidegger, M. *Being and Time*. Translated by J. Macquarrie and E. Robinson. New York: Harper & Row, 1962.

Heiss, R. *Hegel Kierkegaard Marx*. Translated by E. B. Garside. New York: Dell, 1975.

Holmer, P. "Kierkegaard and Ethical Theory." *Ethics* 58 (1953): 157–70.

Husserl, E. *Cartesian Meditations: An Introduction to Phenomenology*. Translated by D. Cairns. The Hague: Martinus Nijhoff, 1973.

James, W. *Principles of Psychology*. 2 vols. New York: Dover, 1950.

Janik, A., and Toulmin, S. *Wittgenstein's Vienna*. New York: Simon & Schuster, 1973.

Kerrigan, W. "Husserl's Epoché and the Genesis of Imagination in Psychoanalysis." *Psychoanalysis and Contemporary Thought* 3 (1980): 55–83.

Kierkegaard, S.

   The Journals of Kierkegaard [1834–55]. Edited by A. Dru. New York: Harper & Row, 1959.

   Fear and Trembling and The Sickness unto Death [1843, 1849]. Translated by W. Lowrie. Princeton, N.J.: Princeton University Press, 1967.

   Philosophical Fragments [1844]. Translated by D. Swenson. Princeton, N.J.: Princeton University Press, 1967.

   Concluding Unscientific Postscript [1846]. Translated by D. Swenson and W. Lowrie. Princeton, N.J.: Princeton University Press, 1968.

Lacan, J. *Ecrits: A Selection*. Translated by A. Sheridan. New York: Norton, 1977.

Langer, S. "On Cassirer's Theory of Language and Myth." In P. Schilpp, ed., *The Philosophy of Ernst Cassirer*. La Salle, Ill.: Open Court, 1949.

Lemaire, A. *Jacques Lacan*. Translated by D. Macey. London: Routledge & Kegan Paul, 1972.

Loewald, H. "On Internalization." *International Journal of Psycho-Analysis* 54 (1973): 9–18.

———. *Psychoanalysis and the History of the Individual*. New Haven: Yale University Press, 1978a.

———. "The Waning of the Oedipus Complex." Address, Plenary Session, Annual Meeting, American Psychoanalytic Association, 1978b.

Lowrie, W. *A Short Life of Kierkegaard*. Princeton, N.J.: Princeton University Press, 1970.

Mahler, M. "On the First Three Subphases of the Separation-

Individuation Process." *International Journal of Psycho-Analysis* 53 (1972): 333–38.

Meissner, W. W. "Spirit and Matter—The Psychological Paradox." *Journal of Existentialism* 8 (1967): 179–201.

———. "Cognitive Aspects of the Paranoid Process—Prospectus." In J. H. Smith ed., *Thought, Consciousness, and Reality, Psychiatry and the Humanities,* vol. 2. New Haven: Yale University Press, 1977.

Modell, A. "The Origin of Certain Forms of Pre-oedipal Guilt and the Implications for a Psychoanalytic Theory of Affects." *International Journal of Psycho-Analysis* 52 (1971): 337–46.

Passmore, J. A. *Ralph Cudworth: An Interpretation.* Cambridge: Cambridge University Press, 1951.

Peters, R. S. *The Concept of Motivation.* London: Routledge & Kegan Paul, 1960.

Pfänder, A. *Phenomenology of Willing and Motivation.* Translated by H. Spiegelberg. Evanston, Ill.: Northwestern University Press, 1967.

Rapaport, D. *Seminars on Elementary Metapsychology.* Vol. 3. Edited by S. C. Miller. Mimeographed transcripts, 1959.

Reinhardt, K. *The Existentialist Revolt.* New York: Frederick Ungar, 1960.

Ricoeur, P. *Freedom and Nature: The Voluntary and the Involuntary.* Translated by E. Kohak. Evanston, Ill.: Northwestern University Press, 1966.

———. *Freud and Philosophy.* Translated by D. Savage. New Haven: Yale University Press, 1970.

———. *The Conflict of Interpretations.* Edited by D. Ihde. Evanston, Ill.: Northwestern University Press, 1974.

———. "The Question of Proof in Freud's Psychoanalytic Writings." *Journal of the American Psychoanalytic Association* 25 (1977): 835–71.

Sandler, J. "On the Concept of Superego." *Psychoanalytic Study of the Child* 15 (1960): 128–62.

Shaftesbury, A. A. C. *Characteristics.* 2 vols. Edited by J. M. Robertson. London, 1900.

Shoham, S. G. "The Isaac Syndrome." *American Imago* 33 (1976): 329–49.

Smith, J. H. "The Heideggerian and Psychoanalytic Concepts of Mood." *Journal of Existentialism* 4 (1964): 101–11.

———. Review of E. Bär, *Semiotic Approaches to Psychotherapy* and M. Edelson, *Language and Interpretation in Psychoanalysis. Psychiatry* 39 (1976): 404–09.

———. "The Pleasure Principle." *International Journal of Psycho-Analysis* 58 (1977): 1–10.

Spiegelberg, H. *Phenomenology in Psychology and Psychiatry: A Historical Introduction.* Evanston, Ill: Northwestern University Press, 1972.

Spitz, R. *No and Yes.* New York: International Universities Press, 1957.

Ticho, E. "The Development of Superego Autonomy." *Psychoanalytic Review* 59 (1972): 217-33.

Verdenius, W. J. "Plato and Christianity." *Ratio* 5 (1963): 15-32.

Walsh, M. "Ordinal Language and Superego Genesis: A Hitherto Unnoticed Influence of Language on the Formation of Psychic Structure." *International Journal of Psycho-Analysis* 52 (1971): 115-26.

Wittgenstein, L. *Tractatus Logico-Philosophicus.* London: Routledge & Kegan Paul, 1961.

Wyschogrod, M. *Kierkegaard and Heidegger: The Ontology of Existence.* New York: International Universities Press, 1969.

6

Psychology and Society: The Social Falsification of the Self in *The Sickness unto Death*

BRUCE H. KIRMMSE

Kierkegaard's most perfect book is *The Sickness unto Death*, his justly celebrated masterpiece of psychology, in which an ideally clarified or healthy self serves as the standard against which various forms of sickness or falsification are measured. Yet, for a work that deals with the psychology of the individual, and that is supposedly setting forth the unchanging theoretical architecture of the human spirit, *The Sickness unto Death* contains a number of striking references to the effects of society upon the individual in his task of self-realization, as well as some very pointed allusions to the political situation in mid-nineteenth-century Denmark. Coming as they do in the middle of a work on the psychology of the spirit of the human individual, these references to supposedly nonessential social factors and transient political events seem curious, and they have not received the careful attention and interpretation they deserve.

This essay will explore *The Sickness unto Death* and will attempt to relate its general theoretical framework to the specific references to social types and political influences that it contains. This should be helpful not only in illuminating the particular issues in this work but also in providing the rudiments of the general Kierkegaardian understanding of the interaction between individual and society. Furthermore, the investigation attempted in this essay will, I hope, be a useful tonic that will help to dispel the unfortunate notion that Kierkegaard was an asocial, ahistorical individualist who had no real interest in the ramifications of the social and political realities in which every individual is implicated.

It is no accident that *The Sickness unto Death* was composed during the first five months of 1848, those months of extraordinary upheaval in Europe that in Denmark witnessed a revolutionary and apparently permanent change of regime from monarchical absolutism based upon narrow elites to liberal constitutionalism resting upon popular sovereignty. The months following the completion of *The Sickness unto Death* in May 1848 were tumultuous ones, both for Denmark in general and for Kierkegaard in particular, and we know that he perceived a great deal of his agitation as rooted in the social changes and political events taking place around him, which he followed very closely. In the middle of 1849 came a breathing space, both for Kierkegaard and his society; in June 1849 the new liberal democratic constitution that was to regulate postrevolutionary Denmark was officially promulgated, and the following month, after more than a year's hesitation, Kierkegaard published *The Sickness unto Death,* itself a statement of the spiritual constitution of the individual.

Although constraints of space compel this essay to view *The Sickness unto Death* more or less in isolation, its treatment of the relationship between the individual and society is actually a link in a chain of Kierkegaard's works, extending back at least as far as his review of *Two Ages*[1] from the spring of 1846, and including *Christian Discourses,* published in 1848; *Training in Christianity,* published in 1850, which shares with *Sickness* its claim to pseudonymous authorship by "Anti-Climacus"; the two series of discourses "recommended to the present age," *For Self-Examination,* written and published in 1851, and *Judge for Yourselves!,* written in late 1851–early 1852 but published posthu-

1. Part of Kierkegaard's review of *Two Ages* has been published in English as *The Present Age,* and the entirety of Kierkegaard's review has recently been republished, in a new translation, as *Two Ages: The Age of Revolution and the Present Age. A Literary Review,* ed. and trans. Howard V. Hong and Edna H. Hong (Princeton, N.J.: Princeton University Press, 1978).

mously; and culminating, of course, in the famous "attack on Christendom" with which Kierkegaard ended his career, a rabid attempt to influence public opinion on questions of church and state and "Christian society." This outburst has hitherto eluded successful interpretation or has been ignored, the same fate that has been accorded the less striking but still significant social and political aspects of *The Sickness unto Death.* The present essay will begin by examining the conceptual vocabulary developed in *The Sickness unto Death,* and will then turn, first, to the social-historical correlatives of the various sorts of "sickness" described and then to the notions of politics and "health" that are also present in the book.

The Conceptual Vocabulary of "The Sickness unto Death"

On its title page, *The Sickness unto Death* is further qualified as a "Christian psychological exposition for awakening and edification," by which Kierkegaard[2] wishes to differentiate the book from ordinary, profane scholarship, which is characterized by an "indifferent" scientific detachment that claims to be humanistic "heroism" but is actually "inhuman curiosity." Genuine Christian knowledge, Kierkegaard contends, is not at a distance but is engaged, "concerned," and genuinely serious in that it relates to "the reality of the personality" and involves true heroism, which is not the stoical neutrality of scholarship but a "daring entirely to be oneself, an individual person, this particular individual person, alone before God, alone in that enormous effort and that enormous responsibility" (p. 117).[3] As Christianity understands matters, Kierkegaard writes, there is no neutral, scientific ground. Thus, it is not a "natural" psychology but a "Christian" one with

2. I am naming "Kierkegaard" as the author of *Sickness,* with the warning that the "real" author is Kierkegaard's pseudonym Anti-Climacus, whose radically absolute views Kierkegaard did not—in 1849, at any rate—dare to set forth as his own.

3. All page citations in the text are from Søren Kierkegaard, *Sygdommen til Døden (The Sickness unto Death),* vol. 11, *Søren Kierkegaards Samlede Værker,* 1st ed., ed. A. B. Drachman, J. L. Heiberg, and H. O. Lange (Copenhagen: Gyldendal, 1905). All translations are by the present writer.

which we are dealing. Everything that is not "edifying"[4] is thereby un-Christian. This is Kierkegaard's formulation of Romans 14:23, "Everything which is not of faith is of sin," a scriptural citation that appears numerous times in the book and that is a principal leitmotif.

The "sickness unto death," Christianly understood, is a sickness worse than any physical ailment and involves a death worse than any physical death. It is a sickness of the spirit, and it leads ultimately to the death of the spirit. The self, Kierkegaard explains, is spirit, that is, a self-reflective or self-conscious relationship between necessity and possibility, finitude and infinity, body and mind; that is, the self is *that* this relationship between two elements of a synthesis *can also* reflect upon itself; and, in addition, since man's self is posited by God, the self is also *that* this relationship can relate itself to God (pp. 127–28). The sickness unto death, which is a sickness of the spirit or of the self, is a misrelationship within the self and is known generically as despair and within specifically Christian categories as sin.

Because of the complex structure of the self-system, there are three fundamental forms of despair, which vary in intensity according to the level of complexity at which the misrelationship has fastened itself. The lowest form of despair is that in which one is unconscious that one has a self, that is, that one is a spiritual and not merely a physical or mental-physical being. This is to fail to realize that one is capable of reflection, to fail to reflect upon the fact that one is a synthesis, and to fail to realize not only that one can reflect upon *this* but that reflection can reflect upon *itself*. This lowest form of despair is *"spiritlessness"* (*Aandløshed*).

The next form of despair is that in which the self is aware that it is a self but wishes, despairingly, not to be itself; the self wishes to escape the self that it is aware it is. It wishes to abandon its humanity. This is the despair of *weakness.*

The third and highest level of despair is that of the self that is aware of being a self and that wishes, despairingly, to affirm itself

---

4. "Edifying" = *opbyggelig,* which literally means "upbuilding," that is, that which builds up one's soul in the personal, Christian sense.

as the human self it is, but to affirm itself without at the same time recognizing the relatedness and ultimate dependence of that human self upon God. This the the despair of *defiance.*

Thus, the three levels of intensification of despair correspond to the three levels of increasing complexity within one's consciousness of the structure of the self: at the lowest level is *spiritlessness*—unconsciousness of being a self-reflective synthesis; at the next level is *weakness*—consciousness of being such a human self, combined with the desire to escape from that condition; and at the highest level is *defiance,* in which the self proudly affirms its self-consciousness and its humanity but wishes to end its systematic understanding of the self while still on the purely human plane of self-sufficiency and without acknowledging any transcendent relationship to God. If, on the other hand, one is the (hypothetical) "healthy" individual, one "relates oneself to oneself, and in willing to be oneself, the self grounds itself transparently in the Power [God] Which posited it" (p. 128).

Thus far the forms of the sickness unto death have been sketched from the point of view of natural man and have been defined as forms of *despair.* However, if one examines the forms of this sickness from the specifically Christian point of view, the sickness itself can be seen to be the revealed, dogmatic state known as *sin,* and the individual types of despair (*Fortvivlelse*) can be seen to be various intensifications of "offense" (*Forargelse*).[5]

Because man is not a static essence but a *capacity*, that is, a relation that relates (or misrelates) itself to itself and that also relates (or misrelates) itself to God, sin is not an individual action or a series of individual actions or "sins" but a misuse of a capacity, an ongoing misrelationship or posture. Similarly, Kierkegaard continues, the opposite of sin is not, as the pagans thought, the individual right action or series of right actions called "virtue" but rather the proper use of one's capacity, the ongoing relationship

5. "Offense" is understood in the sense that the individual recoils from and rejects or takes offense at God's approach to him, as when Christ says "Blessed is he who is not offended in me" (Matt. 11:6), or when St. Paul writes, "I preach Christ crucified, an offense to the Jews and a foolishness to the Greeks" (1 Cor. 1:23).

of health, which is *faith*. Thus the Socratic definition of sin, for example, corresponded to the static, heathen view of man, and sin was seen as ignorance of the good. This Socratic conception, Kierkegaard contends, was too naive to grasp the situation as it really is. The categories of ordinary human thought, of which the Socratic philosophy was the best representative, "lack a dialectical category appropriate to the transition from having *understood* something [the Good] to *doing* it" (p. 204, emphases added). Here Christianity comes in and illuminates psychology with the notion of will, of defiance, and with the revealed dogma of original sin.

Modern philosophy, Kierkegaard insists, has not come essentially beyond the Socratic position. The motto of modern philosophy is *cogito ergo sum*, for in timeless ideality, as in Socratic thought, thinking is identical with being; there is no time elapsed between *knowing* the good and *doing* it. In Socrates, the greatest of all heathen philosophers, this error was excusable, but the crime of modern-day philosophy, Kierkegaard writes, is that it repeats this error while passing itself off as "Christian" (p. 205).

The "modern philosophy" Kierkegaard has in mind is Hegelianism, and in particular the Hegel-tinged speculative dogmatics of H. L. Martensen, which in lecture form had been the wonder of the Danish theological world in the 1840s and which were published in their definitive book form as *Christian Dogmatics* in the summer of 1849, almost simultaneously with *Sickness*. Martensen was a brilliant and suave intellectual who managed to become the protégé both of the august Bishop Jakob Mynster, who was primate of the Danish church, and of the scintillating tastemaker and playwright Johan Ludvig Heiberg, himself the leading apostle of Hegel in Denmark and as such an aesthetic philosopher of no mean talent. Mynster and Heiberg, representing Church and Culture respectively, were pillars of the conservative cultural establishment that dominated Danish intellectual, artistic, religious, and political life during the so-called Danish Golden Age in the first half of the nineteenth century. Martensen, with his "speculative Christianity," could plausibly be presented as the apotheosis of this Golden Age, the producer of an intellectual synthesis that stretched from the Cathedral to the

Royal Theater, from Christianity to Culture, binding them together in a higher unity of Christian Culture or "Christendom,"
the marriage of heaven and earth. It was certainly as such that
Kierkegaard perceived Martensen: the champion of "speculative
Christianity," the arch-representative of the refined, elitist Golden Age of Danish culture, the spokesman for and the personal
embodiment of "Christendom."[6]

Speculation, Kierkegaard complains, claims to have an orthodox Christian understanding of sin, but at the same time it
gives up the paradoxical quality of this Christian concept and
makes Christianity "comprehensible" by "going further"[7] than
Socrates, understanding "the highest," and rolling everything up
into a synthesis called "the result" (p. 203). No, Kierkegaard insists, Christianity says that man is in sin and cannot understand
the Good because *he does not want to,* and that he requires God's
revelation even to show him that he is in sin (p. 206). Sin itself is
thus a revealed, dogmatic, Christian category; it is one of the two
key concepts in Kierkegaard's Christian psychology, forming the
negative, "real" counterpart to the positive, "ideal" notion of the
self's "transparent"—that is, consciously accepting—grounding
in the God Which posited it. So pivotal is this concept of sin to
understanding the Christian psychology of the self, that Kierkegaard daringly insists that it is in fact not the doctrine of the
atonement but rather that of sin which separates Christianity
from heathenism (p. 201).

"The Christian doctrine of sin is sheer impudence against
man," Kierkegaard writes (p. 206), and may be rejected as an
"offense," which is the specifically Christian form of despair. All
sinners are to a greater or lesser extent offended, Kierkegaard
writes, and those who try to defend Christianity by removing
offense do it a disservice by minimizing or overlooking its radically heterogeneous demands. The enemy here is again the op-

6. Nor is it any accident that Martensen's elevation to the primacy of the Danish
church in 1854 was the final event that caused Kierkegaard to unleash his career-
end "attack on Christendom."

7. "Going further" is a jibe at Martensen, who in his speculative theology
claimed to "go further" than Hegel.

timistic Golden Age notion of Christendom in general and Martensen's reconciling speculative dogmatics in particular. Rather than defending Christianity and reconciling antitheses in higher syntheses, Kierkegaard writes, we should call attention to offense and warn against it (p. 195). Sin, thus, is not Socrates' lapsus, or a negation, but an existential state, a willed condition, a *position,* as Kierkegaard calls it. Kierkegaard's presentation in *The Sickness unto Death* of his scheme of a Christian psychology rests upon his defense of his identification of the sickness unto death with his version of the Christian category of sin, a defense that in turn becomes an attack upon the speculative philosophy and theology which set the intellectual tone for the Golden Age of the 1830s and 1840s; as we shall see shortly, this attack upon Golden Age Christendom will have a very concrete function in Kierkegaard's diagnosis of the political expression of the sickness unto death.

Despair (or sin) is man's never-ending, impotent attempt to be quit of his own spirit, his own connection with the eternal, "an impotent self-consumption" (p. 132). Because of his peculiar constitution, the *capacity* to despair (or to sin) is a sign of the eternal in man, the sign of man's greatness. The *reality* of despair, however, is man's greatest misfortune. Because man is posited by God, despair is an objective condition that can exist without one's being conscious of it, and to be unconscious of being in despair is a particular—and the lowest—form of despair, spiritlessness. The other forms, in which one is in varying degrees conscious of one's condition, are higher, more intense forms of despair, in one sense at a greater remove from health, while in another sense, that of potential energy or consciousness, closer to health. All people, Kierkegaard writes, must have had some sense of being at least a bit ill, or they have not awakened. There is no *immediate* form of spiritual health (p. 139); the immediacy of the child or the animal, for example, is not a category of spirit, for spirit is precisely *mediacy* or consciousness. Kierkegaard thus says of a relatively intense form of despair that it is "precisely because this despair is more intense that [it is] in a certain sense nearer to salvation" (p. 174). He who without affectation admits to having this sickness is closer to being healed than those who do not believe they have it. It is the greatest misfortune never to have had this sickness, but at the same time it is the most dangerous sickness when one refuses to allow oneself to be healed from it. To win health, one must come to the highest level of consciousness, to the realization that one is spirit and that one exists as the individual one *is*, before God; *this* *"prize of infinity is never won except through despair"* (p. 140, emphasis added).

When trying to find one's way amid difficult concepts such as these concerning the dialectical relationship of sickness and health, one is often best served by taking a cue from the metaphorical language. In discussing despair and its Christian correlative, offense, *The Sickness unto Death* frequently employs metaphors borrowed from astronomy and physics, and one is thus directed to think in terms of points in space and of absolute and relative motion in relation to these points. The *forms* of despair are in themselves "neutral" (Kierkegaard would call them "dialectical") *points*, while sin and its opposite, faith, are directions, or, rather, *movements*. The viewpoint generally adopted in the book is that the forms of despair are mileposts on the road of sin that leads away from self-realization and the affirmation of the God-relationship;[8] however, if one is moving in the opposite direction, the various forms of despair can be seen as mileposts on the road of health or faith. "In the life of the spirit everything is dialectical," Kierkegaard writes in this connection (p. 226 n.). Thus, for example, despair over the fact that one is a sinner can be the first moment of faith, when one is moving in that direction, but when the movement is in the opposite direction, despair over one's sinful condition is merely new sin, a confirmation and consolidation of one's position on the road of perdition (ibid.).

If one is self-aware and moving in the direction of faith but is repelled by offense, that is a form of sin, but an even worse situation is to be so distant from oneself that one cannot even be offended by Christianity. Thus, too, one can believe oneself to be

---

8. Cf. the foreword to *The Sickness unto Death* (p. 218). Anti-Climacus' other book, *Training in Christianity*, follows the development in the opposite direction, that is, the way of faith.

healthy and happy and in motion in the direction of self-fulfillment, but the motion one perceives by virtue of one's limited consciousness of the self is, in effect, only relative and not absolute; in order to be the movement of faith it must be in the direction of realizing one's ultimate dependence upon God. One may believe oneself to be rising but in fact be sinking (p. 102). Only when motion is perceived in relation to an absolute, fixed grid or ground is it perceived properly as absolute motion; only when one's perceptions coincide with absolute and objective reality can they be trusted as indicators of the actual situation. As in the Newtonian physics of relative and absolute movement, where all motion is ultimately referred to the absolute gridwork of the Universe that Newton calls "God's sensorium," so also in the Kierkegaardian "physics" of perceived and actual health, is all motion ultimately referred to God, or to the fact that we all exist, not exactly in God's sensorium, but "grounded in the Power Which posited us." Thus, too, a study of the sickness unto death becomes—in another of Kierkegaard's deliberate allusions to the language of physics—the study of "the law of motion in the intensification [of despair]" (p. 218), where one's perception of one's position becomes increasingly correct in accordance with one's level of consciousness. Increasing intensity in despair does not itself heal, but the increased consciousness of one's real position, which the higher levels of intensity involve, is a precondition of health. Again, we can see that "the prize of infinity is never won except through despair."[9]

9. Thus, Kierkegaard maintains that, in relation to spirit, "everything is dialectical," and therefore even the most apparently devastating properties of modern mass society have no unambiguous qualities about them. Rather, what modern society does is merely to raise the stakes enormously, proffering, at the same time, both easy perdition and also the possibility of purification by ordeal, the refiner's fire, which produces a new simplicity that is beyond the sophistication and blandishments of the modern age—beyond, not because it has circumvented these things but because it has gone *through* them. This point, that the maturity required of man in the modern age can liberate him into a new integration, is one of the principal themes of Kierkegaard's social thought and is found throughout his authorship; nowhere, however, is the point made as well and as trenchantly as in the second half of his review of *Two Ages*.

The Social Typology in "The Sickness unto Death"

Let us turn now to the particular phases of the "sickness" in order to see to what extent they contain a tacit or explicit analysis of particular social types. Because man—viewed logically, according to his components—is a synthesis of finitude and infinity, necessity and possibility, and so forth, man's sickness can be described according to whether it excludes or overemphasizes one or the other of the moments of that synthesis, and Kierkegaard does sketch the rudiments of such a logical analysis. But man, in addition to being a synthesis, is also, to one degree or another, a conscious being, and the sickness unto death also admits of examination under the rubric of varying degrees of consciousness; it is this phenomenological approach that most engages Kierkegaard's attention.[10] Both sorts of analysis, however, lead to essentially the same result—namely, a tripartite division of the levels of intensity the sickness can take. We shall examine these three levels, or forms, and their social correlatives, in ascending order of intensity of consciousness.

As we have seen, from the point of view of consciousness, the lowest form of despair is "spiritlessness," which is also the condition of the person who, viewed under the rubric of man-as-synthesis, lacks infinity or possibility in his make-up. Kierkegaard explains that spiritlessness is the most widespread form of despair and is precisely and specifically characteristic of the apparently well-integrated and self-satisfied philistine bourgeoisie of Danish Golden Age "Christendom," of the Christian gentlemen. The person lacking the component of infinity in his make-up, Kierkegaard tells us, is the "bourgeois philistine" [*Spidsborger*],[11] a

10. *The Sickness unto Death* in fact forms a parallel to Hegel's *Phenomenology of Spirit.* In Kierkegaard's book, as in Hegel's, the self is described as it passes through successively more adequate levels of self-knowledge until it finally comes to know itself as self-conscious spirit and in its factual relation to God.

11. Unlike the English word "philistine," the Danish word *Spidsborger,* which is usually translated "philistine," contains a built-in indictment of the bourgeoisie (*Borgerskab*) and the respectability that being bourgeois implies. *Spidsborger* itself is allied to the German *Spiesbürger,* and originally meant a free citizen (*Borger*) wealthy enough to be allowed to be a part of the militia for the defense of the city

member of the crowd, characterized by ethical limitedness and
narrowness (p. 146). But this sort of despair is very little noticed in
the world, for it is these people who are most often admired as
successful (pp. 147-48).

   Kierkegaard's use of a specific social group to exemplify a general type of spiritual disorder is very curious and instructive. As a
social group, this "philistine bourgeoisie" of Kierkegaard's Golden Age Denmark can be more precisely defined as members of
the comfortable urban middle class, more likely to be of the world
of business, perhaps, than the other part of the bourgeoisie, the
academically educated intellectuals and professionals who often
held royal appointments and who enjoyed greater social esteem.
Because of their business connections, the "philistines," more so
than the more respected and quite conservative upper crust of
intellectuals and officeholders, were likely to entertain liberal
political notions and to support, if timidly, the revolutionary
changes of 1848-49. However, despite differences in political
outlook, both the "philistines" and the "cultured" upper crust
shared elitist presuppositions about the relations that ought to
obtain between the comfortable urban class as a whole and the
eighty or ninety percent of the population that lived by manual
labor or on the land. The "philistines" constituted the bulk of the
bourgeoisie and of the literate public, yet they were not themselves tastemakers, but rather followers, consumers of the taste or
ideology prepared by their Golden Age superiors in "Culture."
"Culture" was the revered value of "philistines" and "cultured"
alike. The "philistines" sadly acknowledged their shortcomings in
this respect and took their lessons and corrections from their
betters, who, in turn, delighted in serving as schoolmasters in
matters of taste and culture. The deans of this Golden Age school
for philistines were, of course, Mynster, as primate of the church;

---

and as such permitted to carry a spear (*Spyd*). Thus a Spidsborger was a respectable, spear-carrying member of the middle class and came in time to be a term of
contempt. I have therefore chosen to convey the word's full meaning by translating it as "bourgeois philistine" rather than simply as "philistine." The specifically
class-related sense of the term Kierkegaard uses is of interest to this article.

Heiberg, as director of the Royal Theatre; and Martensen, as the protégé and inheritor of both: the brilliant intellectual defender of Christian culture *and* the coming primate of the church. All these paladins of Christendom noted the unfortunate philistine qualities of the bulk of the bourgeoisie and all dutifully berated them in an attempt to bring them up to the level of Culture. The two portions of the bourgeoisie thus lived in mutual dependence, in a symbiosis of producers and consumers of ideology.

The spiritless social type can also be seen as a person whose synthesis lacks possibility, that is, as a person in whom necessity reigns at possibility's expense. If such a person follows his imbalance to its logical conclusion, he is a determinist or fatalist, a frightful state to be sure, but one that at least looks the absence of possibility squarely in the eye and that, precisely because of its uncompromisingness, contains a potential for growth and change. More common, however, is the more stable and "normal" sort of denial of possibility within the self, and this is the condition of the bourgeois philistine. "Bourgeois philistinism is spiritlessness. . . . Bourgeois philistinism lacks every category of spirit and is taken up into the realm of Probability, within which the Possible has its little bit of room . . ." (p. 153). Philistinism, then, operates within the boundaries of shrewdness, of probability, within which it attempts to accommodate "the possible." This is Kierkegaard's description of bourgeois calculation and self-protection, where businesslike methods are presumably transferred into the life of the spirit, with predictably deadly results. Unlike fatalism or determinism, which faces a disquieting reality, bourgeois philistinism tranquilizes itself into spiritlessness with its apparently comforting, compromise notion of "probability." "It leads Possibility around captive in the cage of Probability, exhibits it, imagines itself to be in charge, not noticing that it has thereby imprisoned itself to be the slave of spiritlessness, and the most wretched thing of all" (p. 194).

Viewed specifically under the rubric of consciousness, the spiritless person is one who is ignorant of having a self, or of having an eternal self, and is in despair even though he is not aware of it. That this form of despair can exist at all is possible, as has already been noted, only because man has been posited by God; because, consequently, man's nature and the truth in man has an objective quality independent of all consciousness about it; and because that truth insists on having what is its own, what is its right [*Sandhedens Rethaveri*] (p. 155). All forms of despair are forms of negativity or negations of the God-relationship that is essential to man, and ignorance of one's despair is but another negativity. However, "in order to reach the truth one must go through every negativity" (p. 156), so that the spiritless person, far from being freed from his despair by his ignorance of it, is actually more deeply mired in it and has another layer through which he must go if he is to reach health. In a reference to the dangers of this unconscious despair, Kierkegaard admits that the person who is conscious of being in despair is only closer to salvation in one sense, but he continues by saying that "so far is ignorance from abolishing despair or making it into non-despair, that it, on the contrary, can be the most dangerous form of despair" (p. 157). Spiritlessness, or ignorance, is by far the most common form of despair, and it is characteristic of "the heathen," both those of classical times and, especially, those of Christendom. The classical heathens lacked self-consciousness of being spirit in the simple sense, while the latter-day heathens, the so-called Christian heathens of Christendom, "lack spirit in the direction of being opposed to spirit, or by having fallen away from it, and are therefore spiritless in the strictest sense" (p. 159).[12]

In the second and more specifically Christian half of *The Sickness unto Death*, Kierkegaard pursues his quarry of spiritlessness still further, and it becomes even more forcefully clear that not only is this type a bourgeois philistine but that he is the

12. It is suggestive to note that Kierkegaard's category of "spiritlessness," which is a form of opposition or resistance to "Spirit," is very similar to the metaphysical definition of fascism as "resistance to transcendence" given by Ernst Nolte in his classic *Three Faces of Fascism*, trans. Leila Vennewitz (New York: Holt, Rinehart, and Winston, 1966), pp. 429–54 passim. It is further interesting to note that the social class to which Kierkegaard has typically related "spiritlessness" is the "philistine bourgeoisie," while fascism has been classically associated with the lower middle class.

specialized product of Christian culture, the cautious, respectable, unruffled, middle-class Christian gentleman, a consumer of the ideology of respectable Christianity dispensed by the Heiberg-Mynster-Martensen circle. With respect to the extraordinary claim that Jesus Christ can forgive sins, for example, Kierkegaard pointedly notes that, unless one has faith (full self-awareness), it takes "an unusually high degree of spiritlessness, that is, that which is ordinarily found in Christendom," to avoid being offended (p. 226). But Golden Age Christendom has managed to produce just this degree of blandness. Christendom is in fact so spiritless that, for the most part, in the strictly Christian sense it is not even in *sin,* Kierkegaard asserts. "Most people's lives are, Christianly understood, too spiritless even to be called sin[ful] in the strict sense" (p. 214). Of course, Kierkegaard points out, "to be a sinner in the strictest sense is certainly very far from being advantageous. But on the other hand, how in all the world can one find an essential consciousness of sin (and note, that this is something Christianity indeed wants) in a life which is so sunken in triviality, in silly aspiring after 'the others,' that one almost cannot call it—that it is too spiritless to be called—sin, and is only worth, as scripture says, 'to be spit out'" (p. 212).

Yet we also know, from what we have already learned in *The Sickness unto Death,* that even this self-satisfied ignorance or spiritlessness is a form of sin, for sin—like man's synthetic composition and his God-relatedness—is *an objective condition* that exists independent of one's awareness of it. Man's ignorance of his condition is "*produced* ignorance" (p. 199; emphasis added), as Kierkegaard puts it. This spiritlessness, which makes spiritual concepts simply inapplicable, "like a jackscrew in a bog," is brought upon the individual by himself. "Is it something which happens to a person? No, it is the person's own fault. No person is born with spiritlessness" (p. 212).

Where, then, does spiritlessness come from? Who helps the people lull themselves to sleep? Kierkegaard replies that it is Christendom, Christian culture itself, that is the worst and most clever enemy of Christianity and consciousness. It must be said, Kierkegaard insists, "as unreservedly as possible" that "this so-

called Christendom—in which everyone by the millions is thus
without further ado Christian, so that there are just as many,
exactly as many, Christians as there are people—is not merely a
poor edition of Christianity, full of typographical errors which
distort the meaning, and thoughtless omissions and additions, but
that it is a misuse of it, that it has taken Christianity in vain" (p.
212). Christendom is a demonically stable compound, a self-
affirming and symbiotic relationship of the tastemakers and "the
priests" on the one hand and the "philistines" on the other. In
Christendom, Kierkegaard writes, man typically is only occasionally, only momentarily conscious of being spirit, once a week for
an hour (i.e., in church), a "bestial way of being spirit" (p. 215).
Yet this is the consequence of Christian culture, of "the priests,"
who have so abused the nearness of God in Christianity that
people, when they do go to church, go there in condescension, to
honor God with their presence (p. 225). Thus, too, most people
have become, have been permitted and encouraged to become, so
spiritless that they can avoid the open, conscious (and hence instructive) forms of offense at Christianity, and have instead
shrewdly and tacitly decided to withhold judgment on it. Most
people would indeed not find this to be a form of offense, but
offense, like the other definitions of the sickness unto death, is an
objective fact, whether we wish to dignify such spiritlessness with
that title or not, because Christianity requires us to take a *position*.
The cautiousness of taking no position is itself a position. Indifference is no more permissible a position with respect to God than
it is with respect to the self (p. 239).

The critique of "spiritlessness" has thus broadened from a personality critique of a specific social group, the philistine
bourgeoisie, to an indictment of "Christendom" per se. Both the
"spiritless" philistine followers and the "cultured" leaders of
Christendom—even though the former were likely to be associated with the respectable fringe of the political party of
movement while the latter were likely to be solidly for the party of
order—shared the same notions of elitism, refinement, and a
hybrid Christian culture, and they are seen by Kierkegaard as the

interconnected components of the Christendom that he rejects and blames for nineteenth-century Denmark's decadent spiritual constitution. We will turn later to the specifically political side of Kierkegaard's attack. For now it is sufficient to have established that Kierkegaard's description of the lowest and perhaps most dangerous form of the sickness unto death, spiritlessness, is specifically linked to the philistine bourgeoisie, and that it is through the agency of "Christendom" that this group has been helped to consolidate itself in its ignorance and complacency. Later we shall see that this "misuse" of Christianity has also led to the release of a dangerous virus that threatens to destroy all social, as well as all religious, order. For now, however, we can take our leave of spiritlessness, of the self-satisfied Golden Age "Christian gentleman," Kierkegaard's favorite villain.

A related form of despair that warrants attention is "despair over something earthly," a subform of the despair of weakness, the desire not to be oneself. It often results in driving the despairing person back into unconsciousness or spiritlessness, a condition to which it is closely related. A person in despair over something earthly can grope inwardly for a while, or he may turn outward, toward busy activity, "toward, as it is called, Life, Reality, the active life . . . for many years happily married, an active and industrious man, father, and citizen, perhaps even a great man; in his house his servants call him 'Himself'; in the city he is among the notables; his behavior is that of a respectable person, or with the respect of one who is, as far as one can see, a person. In Christendom he is a Christian (in just the same sense that he would be a heathen in heathendom, and in Holland a Dutchman), one of the cultured Christians" (p. 168). By means of "shrewdness" he has conquered—that is, repressed and rendered unconscious—the despair that had flickered into consciousness, but his shrewdness is really dangerous and profound "stupidity," for it lulls him away from consciousness and self-awareness. Though this form of despair originally contained a glimmer of consciousness, Kierkegaard apparently feels that we should group it in the general category of spiritlessness, for he labels it, too, "the most common form of despair" (p. 169), a term he elsewhere reserves for spiritlessness proper. The types of despair become rarer as they become more reflective.

In order definitively to take leave of spiritlessness, one must look at the more intense forms of the "weak" (but conscious) form of the sickness, namely, the self that is no longer spiritless but is shut up or "encapsulated" within itself. Such a self refuses to call upon the help of forgetfulness in order to slip back into spiritlessness and become "a man and a Christian like other men and Christians; no, the self is too much self for that" (p. 174). Such *encapsulation*[13] can take on a myriad of forms, but Kierkegaard points out that it is quite capable of taking on the incognito of respectability, much like its counterpart, the spiritless bourgeois philistine, though the differences between the two outwardly similar types are instructive. This more intensified type of despairing person plays the role of respectable citizen less convincingly—at any rate to himself.

> Our despairing person is thus encapsulated enough to be able to hold every extraneous person, thus, everyone, away from his self, while, externally, he is entirely "a real person." He is an educated man, a man, father, even an unusually capable official, a respectable father, pleasant to be with, very sweet to his wife, carefulness itself with his children. And a Christian?—well, yes, he is that too; however, he prefers to avoid talking about it, even if he is happy to see, with a certain wistful joy, that his wife occupies herself edifyingly with godly things. He goes to church very rarely, because it seems to him that most of the priests don't know what they are talking about. [p. 175]

Thus, as can be seen from this middle level of consciousness of the sickness, the more consciousness one has of one's condition, the

13. See Kresten Nordentoft, *Kierkegaard's Psychology*, trans. Bruce H. Kirmmse (Pittsburgh: Duquesne University Press, 1978), for an excellent treatment of "encapsulation," which Nordentoft finds to be a key focal point of Kierkegaard's psychology and a concept in many ways similar to the psychoanalytic notion of resistance, which Nordentoft finds similarly central to Freud.

less the church and the official ideology of Christendom satisfy, though, by the same token, the greater is the real but unfilled spiritual need that is opened up.

The final and highest level of consciousness the sickness takes is that of *defiance,* in which the self defiantly and despairingly wills to be itself in defiance of the Power Which posited it. Such a self wishes to "create itself" (p. 179),[14] and its proud and conscious defiance of its own ultimate grounding in God can take two forms, both of which are Promethean. The *active* form is that of the stealer of fire, sheer Byronic energy, the absolute ruler of himself, the inhabitant of the realm of pure possibility, a realm that never becomes anything actual or concrete. He is in fact absolute ruler over Nothing, and the splendid structures he builds are only "castles in the air" (p. 180). The alternative, *suffering,* type of defiance—Prometheus chained to the rock—is a proud unwillingness to shoulder the burden of temporality and positivity that is man's lot, a despairing superiority to the world with its strife and its duties. Thus, the defiant Promethean, according to whether he is "active" or "suffering," tries to abandon the eternal or the temporal component of the self (p. 181), in contrast to the healthy individual, who meets his responsibilities both to eternity and to time (cf. pp. 181–82 n.). As we will see in our examination of Kierkegaard's view of health and politics in *The Sickness unto Death,* both parts of the human synthesis are indispensable, even though the eternal part ought to occupy a superior position; it is just as much a form of defiant despair to desert the world for "eternity" as it is to attempt to forget the eternal for the world. Kierkegaard's presentation of these two forms of Promethean defiance is symmetrical.

The three basic forms[15] of the sickness unto death are thus, in ascending order of consciousness, *spiritlessness, encapsulation,* and *defiance* (*Aandløshed, Indesluttedhed,* and *Trods*), and they correspond to distinct social types. Spiritlessness, or unconscious self-

14. The Danish is *at skabe sig* and is a pun that means both "to create oneself" and "to put on an act."

15. For the sake of simplicity, some of the variations and subforms included in Kierkegaard's rather baroque (but tripartite) presentation have been omitted.

satisfaction, is the special characteristic of the philistine bourgeoisie, while defiance is the property of the highly self-conscious oppositional type, the romantic genius-rebel. These two types correspond to the extremes of unconsciousness and hyperconsciousness that Kierkegaard delineated earlier, in *A Literary Review* (1846), as the self-satisfied burgher of the "present age" and the rebel of the revolutionary age. Encapsulation and the despair of weakness, in which one consciously wills not to be oneself, have a mediating, or middle, position between these two extremes, and a typical representative is the respectable and duti-ful Christian who sees the hollowness of his respectability and fears the emptiness of his Christianity without having anything definite to substitute for them; this troubled individual is perhaps Kierkegaard's ideal intended reader.

Let us turn now to the notions of politics and health contained in *The Sickness unto Death,* which will lead us to an examination of the way in which mankind's sickness demonstrates itself in social action, and, finally, to man's potential.

Politics and Health

We know from his other works and from his entries in his journals that Kierkegaard was very moved by the cataclysmic events of the spring months of 1848 and that he saw those social and political changes as providing him an opportunity to set forth, in *The Sickness unto Death,* his version of what was happening to Christendom—his diagnosis—and also the beginnings of a pro-posed cure. "The fundamental misfortune of Christendom," Kierkegaard writes, "is really Christianity, [namely,] that the doc-trine of the God-Man . . . by having been preached again and again, has been taken in vain; that the qualitative difference be-tween God and man has been pantheistically abolished, first aristocratically, speculatively, then by the mob in the streets and alleys" (p. 227). Elitist intellectual circles—that is, such speculative philosophers and theologians as Heiberg and Martensen—have compromised Christianity by abusing Christian notions of God and the God-Man in order to deify their own aristocratic-conservative notion of a compound Christian-bourgeois culture, and this disrespect for the distance that is nevertheless present in the nearness of God and man in Christianity has carried over from the elite conservative circles to liberals and street revolutionaries. "Of course," Kierkegaard continues, "a good number of the philosophers who participated in spreading this doctrine . . . turn away in disgust when their doctrine has sunk so low that the mob has become the God-Man" (p. 228). However, the elitist conservatism of the leading circles does not acquit them from the charge that the present revolutionary development is their creation. Kierkegaard thus charges that the very same leading spirits who had made such a career out of taunting—and being idolized by—the philistine bourgeoisie, laid the groundwork for the ensuing rampage of spiritlessness under the banners of the deification of the people. This is the ironic result of the symbiosis of the "refined," ideology-producing part of the Christian bourgeoisie and the "philistine" or "spiritless," ideology-consuming portion. Without naming individual names, Kierkegaard is in effect charging Heiberg, Martensen, and their colleagues with having made possible the success of the revolutionary liberal leaders and the rabble behind them.

According to Kierkegaard, what has happened in the political arena of Christendom is the analogue to what has happened in the religious sphere, namely, that "the doctrine of the God-Man had made Christendom impudent." Instead of having limited what mankind claims as its rightful sphere, the Christian doctrine of the God-Man, speciously interpreted by modern speculative philosophy and theology, has fueled an all-consuming pride and ambition, so that the age sees a God who comes close to man as weak, like a king who has been obliged to grant a constitution, and people secretly whisper: "Well, he really *had* to" (p. 228). The speculative interpretation of the doctrine of the God-Man has overlooked or minimized the significance of the absolute and qualitative distinction between God and man that lies at the center of the closeness of God to man. Thus, Christendom has been impertinent in relation to God. It makes no difference that the cultivated aristocrats who started this latest misinterpretation

of the relation of God to man did so in the name of refinement
and the status quo, because their handiwork, in Kierkegaard's
opinion, formed the intellectual and spiritual climate that nurtured the revolutionary forces of leveling and mob rule; the
speculative deification of man in the God-Man became the most
powerful weapon in the arsenal of "the tyranny of the fear of
man." The conservative misuse of the God-Man has led to the
revolutionary notion that the voice of the people is the voice of
God, and it is now believed that when "the public, the highly-
honored, cultivated public, or the people" commits a crime in
collectivity, it is no longer a crime but "God's will" (p. 232).

The only way out of political and religious chaos, in Kierkegaard's opinion, is a firm rejection of both camps, both the
aristocratic Hegelianism of the "cultured" class and the will-o'-
the-wisp notion of absolute, deified, popular sovereignty es-
poused by the bourgeois-philistine "spiritless" class. All forms of
philosophical or political abstraction must be eschewed, and every
person must confront his own concrete individuality and responsibility as an ethical and religious individual. "If order is to be
maintained in existence . . . attention must first and foremost be
given to the fact that every person is an individual person, and
becomes aware of himself as an individual person" (p. 227). Each
person must resist the temptation to be melted down into an
abstraction, the mass, which wishes to combine with the doctrine
of the God-Man in order to deify the totality of mankind, for
whom, by implication, *anything* will be possible if it is done in the
name of the people.

From the very beginning, Kierkegaard continues, Christianity
has protected itself from impertinence and presumption with the
key psychological-anthropological axiom of *sin*, whose category is
the category of *individuality*, which cannot be speculatively
thought (p. 228). Sin and the individual person do not admit of
being thought, and speculation, knowing this, belittles them. The
doctrine of sin brings with it the realm of the ethical, with its
concentration upon reality and the individual, while speculation
cannot hold fast to concrete individuals but merely to abstractions. "The dialectic of sin is diametrically opposed to the dialectic
of speculation" (p. 229). The individual and the doctrine of sin as

the responsibility (and the sickness) of the individual are Christianity's mode of protecting itself against any impertinent familiarity that would abuse the closeness established between man and God by the God-Man. For God, every individual sinner exists in his full individuality, and God has no trouble keeping track of it all. Kierkegaard insists that it is not as a simple equality via the abstract middle term of the human race, but as a sinful individual, and in fear and trembling, under pressure and in humiliation, that man ought to feel his relatedness to God. Unlike the situation with animals, where the example is less than the species, with mankind the individual is greater than the species, "and this definition is again dialectical, signifying that the individual is a sinner, but also that it is perfection to be an individual" (p. 230 n.). Thus, the doctrine of sin not only splits the mass into individuals but also strengthens the qualitative difference between God and man, for in no way is man so absolutely different from God as in being a sinner "before God." The two things—God and man—that Christianity holds together, can be seen all the more clearly, because of their proximity, to be qualitatively different (p. 231).

Thus, man is separated from God by the chasm of sin, while God is separated from man in His ability to forgive sin. Kierkegaard stresses that right here, in the heart of the religion that has most taught the equality of God and man, is also to be found in its most concentrated form the possibility of offense, which is necessary to keep us from confusing God and man (p. 232). And willfully forgetting this difference, in the midst of our likeness, is defiance, the most intense form of disorder in Kierkegaard's psychological scheme of despair/offense. As we have seen, without the possibility of offense, the doctrine of the God-Man would simply be the deification of man and would give man total license. "Christianity's doctrine is the doctrine of the God-Man, of the kinship between God and man, but, be it noted, such that the possibility of offense is, if I dare say so, the guarantee by which God insures that man cannot come too near Him" (p. 235).[16]

Therefore, the possibility of "offense" developed in *The Sick-*

16. "To come too near" = *at komme for nær*, which means both "to come too close" and "to give an affront" (*Fornærmelse*).

ness unto Death is the regulatory notion for Kierkegaard's entire psychology and keeps it from being a "natural" psychology. Kierkegaard stresses that the possibility of offense, which speculation has done so much to minimize with its notion of mediation, must be reemphasized as a corrective both of religious and of social-political confusion. In Kierkegaard's view, this confusion threatened to create an all-engulfing Leviathan in the post-revolutionary era, a Leviathan more terrible than any of the properly pagan cultures precisely because the modern society would derive its unparalleled power and its presumption from its distortion of Christianity's unparalleled claims. "These words— 'Blessed is he who is not offended in me'—are a part of the proclamation of Christ" (p. 237). To reject them straightforwardly as untruth is the highest form of sickness, according to Kierkegaard, the sin against the Holy Spirit for which there is no help. The possibility of this highly conscious, defiant form of the sickness unto death is the irreducible core of Christianity; without this possibility, its opposite, faith—which is the only genuine state of human health—would be rendered impossible.

Almost as an aside, *The Sickness unto Death* contains an incidental description of the state of spiritual health and of the place of social obligation in the healthy individual. At the point where he discusses despair under the rubric of man as a synthesis of infinitude and finitude, Kierkegaard writes that

> the self is the conscious synthesis of infinitude and finitude, which relates itself to itself, whose task is to become itself, which can only be done in relation to God. But to become oneself is to become concrete.[17] But to become concrete is neither to become finite nor to become infinite, because that which must become concrete is indeed a synthesis. The development must thus consist in coming infinitely away from oneself in the infinitization of the self and in coming infinitely back to oneself in finitization. [p. 143]

17. Kierkegaard here uses "concrete" in the ordinary sense of "particular" but also in its original sense of something "grown together."

The self must both be out of the world and in it simultaneously; it must abstract itself *and* return. The self must be

> to the same degree concrete and abstract, so that the more it is infinitized in intentions and decisions, the more entirely present and simultaneous it becomes with itself in that little part of the task which can be done right now, so that it [the self], in becoming infinite, in the strictest sense comes back to itself, so that when it is *farthest away* from itself . . . [it] is at the same instant *nearest* to itself in doing that infinitely small part of the work which can be done even today, even in this hour, even in this instant. [p. 145]

The healthy self, aware of itself as a self-reflecting synthesis and gratefully acknowledging its God-relatedness, avoids both of the Promethean forms of defiance and accepts finitude and temporality, on the one hand, and infinitude and eternity, on the other.

The healthy self also avoids the more common form of despair, at the other end of the scale, the spiritless amiability that Christendom fosters by its tranquilizing refusal to emphasize the possibility of offense. In producing an emasculated version of Christianity, which seeks to circumvent intellectual embarrassment and the real dangers of the highest and most conscious form of offense, Christendom has also ruled out the alternative form of the highest consciousness that is health, and society has been tranquilized into a state of semiconsciousness and sent careening down the road of political disaster. Here, in *The Sickness unto Death* and with increasing intensity in the remainder of his career, Kierkegaard saw his task as the opposite of this tranquilization, namely, to call attention to the qualitative differences that lie at the heart of Christianity, to stress the possibility of offense, and in effect to make Christianity *dis*respectable, so that the Golden Age juggernaut of philosophically and theologically sanctioned Christian culture would come to a halt.

The human spirit is not anything it wishes to be; nor is human culture infinitely plastic. The human psyche, in Kierkegaard's view, has a definite, objective form, a God-positedness, a simultaneous freedom toward the finite and the infinite, which it is man's task to accept and to realize. The programmatic declaration of the structure of man's spirit and of the forms of his unfreedom is Kierkegaard's psychology, which finds its most succinct statement in *The Sickness unto Death*. We have already seen that this work contains social and political material that draws analogies between forms of psychic unfreedom and specific social types. We can now see that there is an even deeper reason for a work that purports to deal with individual psychology to introduce much social and political material. To the extent that it attempts to deal with the freedom and unfreedom of the individual, all psychology—including Kierkegaard's Christian psychology of the individual—is *social* psychology, at least in the negative sense that human institutions, while they may not be able to make man become what he is and can be, can certainly help to *prevent* him from fulfilling his potential, from realizing his essence. Just as the individual spirit has absolute freedom to develop itself but not the freedom to evade itself and its own freedom, so in the social and political sphere there are limits to the plasticity of culture. In Kierkegaard's view it is neither possible not permissible for a Christian psychology to specify what a culture and a society ought to be, for the task of fulfilling the promise of the human spirit is an open-ended and individual one. However, it is possible to specify what a culture ought *not* to be, and this negative, limiting, political prescription took the form of the indictment of Golden Age Christendom, which Kierkegaard necessarily included as an important part of his greatest psychological work, *The Sickness unto Death*.

7

A Ram in the Afternoon: Kierkegaard's Discourse of the Other

Louis H. Mackey

> . . . because it is produced in the locus of the Other, it is first
> of all for the subject that his speech is a message. By virtue of
> this fact even his demand originates in the locus of the Other,
> and is signed and dated as such. This is not only because it is
> subjected to the code of the Other, but also because it is
> marked by this locus (and even the time) of the Other.
> —Jacques Lacan, *Ecrits*

The *Philosophical Fragments* is obsessed with alterity. In particular with the question, how can language give expression to that which is wholly other than language? Although the ostensible subject of the book is Christianity, it is Christianity *as wholly other* that structures its discourse. Since the other than language cannot be uttered, the text of the *Fragments* turns back upon itself and becomes an exploration of the limits of language. But since the limit of language is itself the alterity language cannot express, the *Fragments* neither says nor shows but rather *performs* the "absolute paradox": that the limit of language, its irreducible other, is also its radical source. It is in this sense that the book is an "indirect communication." And it is only in this absolutely indirect way that the book is, importantly, "about" Christianity.

I shall try to substantiate this claim by reading crucial passages of the text.

I

The first chapter of the *Fragments* opens with the question, "To what extent can the truth be learned?"[1] The question is "asked by the unknowing, who does not even know what has given him occasion to question in this way" (*PF* 9A, *PS* 7). The pseudonymous author, Johannes Climacus, contrasts two answers to this question: the "Socratic" answer and an anonymous view he represents as his own "thought-project."

The Socratic view heads up in the doctrine of recollection, according to which "the truth is not introduced into him [the ignorant man], but was within him" (*PF* 11A, *PS* 7). On this assumption the temporal moment in which a man "learns" the truth and the teacher from whom he "learns" it are alike no more than occasional. "Each man is his own center, and the whole world centers only in him, because his self-knowledge is a knowledge of God" (*PF* 14A, *PS* 9). All that concerns me as learner is "my possession of the Truth, which I had from the beginning without knowing it" (*PF* 15, *PS* 10).

> The underlying principle [*finale Tanke*] of all questioning is that the one who is questioned must himself have the truth and must acquire it by himself. The temporal point of departure is nothing; for as soon as I discover that I have known the truth from eternity without knowing it, that moment is hidden in the eternal, incorporated in it in such a way that I,

1. Søren Kierkegaard, *Philosophical Fragments*, 2d ed., trans. David F. Swenson and Howard V. Hong, with introduction and commentary by Niels Thulstrup (Princeton, N.J.: Princeton University Press, 1962), p. 11. All further references to the *Philosophical Fragments* are to this edition and are given in the text in the form *PF* plus page number(s). In this passage and in many others I have adapted the English translation, usually in the direction of greater literalness. In such cases the letter A is added to the page number(s) of the primary reference. The Danish edition I have used is Søren Kierkegaard, *Philosophiske Smuler*, with introduction and commentary by Neils Thulstrup (Copenhagen: Ejnar Munksgaard, 1955). This edition is the basis of the English translation by Swenson and Hong. References to the Danish edition are given in the form *PS* plus page number(s). For this passage the reference is *PS* 7. Page numbers will not be repeated when successive quotations come from the same page.

so to speak, could not find it even if I looked for it, because there is neither here nor there but only an *ubique et nusquam*. [*PF* 15–16A, *PS* 11]

The Socratic presumption (whether it is the view of Socrates himself is of no concern in the present context, for reasons that will soon become clear) is that there exists an eternal and omnipresent structure of truth centering equally in all men and therefore just as much but no more present in one than in another: an *ubique et nusquam* to which time, space, and occasion are strictly irrelevant.

Truth is always and everywhere attainable by everyone. One attains it simply by reverting to its always already presence to himself. That is the meaning of the doctrine of recollection and the presupposition of all inquiry. For which reason it is irrelevant (as Socrates himself would have been the first to acknowledge) whether or not this is the view of Socrates. It is the view (acknowledged or not) of man thinking.

The Socratic answer to the question with which the chapter begins is therefore: truth may only be "learned" if and to the degree that it is always already known by the learner. "Learning" is just the realization of this presence, which is the condition of all questioning. Because its presence in the learner is assumed, the truth is never introduced into him from without.

This presence of truth is a kind of absolute. Therefore, since a man's self-knowledge necessarily incorporates a knowledge of the eternal truth, knowledge of self is knowledge of "God." The title page of the *Fragments* poses this question, thematic for the work as a whole:

Can there be an historical point of departure for an eternal consciousness? How can such a point of departure be of more than historical interest? Can one build an eternal blessedness on historical knowledge? [*PF* iiiA, *PS* 1]

From the Socratic point of view this is a pseudo-question. Not that the answer is No. But rather: the question cannot be asked, since it presupposes what is contrary to the presupposition of all questioning—that one might in a historical moment and by a historical occasion come to know something he did not know before, that in a moment of time and by the agency of a teacher a hitherto simply absent truth might become simply present. Or, if the question (asked by one whose ignorance conceals from him even the source of his questioning) is not to be altogether meaningless, then it merely expresses the inattentiveness to truth (the Socratic forgetfulness) in which inquiry (that is, recollection) begins. The absolute (a knowledge of God, eternal consciousness, eternal blessedness) is always already possessed and known: it is impossible to be absolutely surprised.

What is said *in* the *Fragments* concerning the presuppositions of all inquiry must also be said *about* the *Fragments,* which is an inquiry into the limits and conditions of inquiry and therefore perfectly self-reflexive. More of this later.

Impossibly, Climacus goes on to propose his own "thought-project" as an alternative to the Socratic (the only human) option. Beginning with the moment of learning. "Now if things are to be otherwise" (with respect to the question of the title page), "the Moment in time must have a decisive significance" (*PF* 16, *PS* 11). In this moment the eternal (truth, consciousness, blessedness), *hitherto nonexistent,* must have *come into being.* Were it always already present, the moment would not be decisive. Let us see, Climacus says, what follows from this assumption.

The assumption is that the answer to the question on the title page is Yes. But as we have seen, the question is unaskable. The assumption that it might be both asked and affirmatively answered entails absurd consequences, which Climacus proceeds to unfold.

Prior to learning the truth, the inquirer must not possess it even in principle, as an ever-present recourse. It does not *exist* for him. So alienated from the truth that he cannot be occasioned to recollect it, the learner must be *defined* (*bestemmet*) as *un*truth. He is (not "is in a state of" but *is*) untruth (*PF* 16–17, *PS* 11).

The teacher may, Socratically, serve as occasion to remind the learner that he is untruth. If he is to be more than occasion, he must give the learner both the truth and the ability to understand it.

> The condition for understanding the truth is like the capacity to inquire for it: the condition contains the conditioned, and the question contains the answer. . . . All instruction depends in the last analysis upon the presence of the condition; if this is lacking, the teacher can do nothing. [*PF* 17–18A, *PS* 12]

To save the hypothesis, the teacher must impart both truth and condition. Since this is beyond human capacity, the teacher must be divine.

In the moment of learning, which Climacus calls the "fullness of time," the eternal truth (impossibly) comes into being. The learner experiences the transition from untruth to truth as a transition from nonbeing to being: a second birth by which he becomes a new man.

"But," Climacus asks disingenuously, "is that which is here expounded thinkable?" (*PF* 24A, *PS* 18). Only, he answers, by one who has experienced the second birth. It would be "preposterous" and "laughable" to suppose anyone else (any ordinary human being, here defined as untruth) capable of imagining this passage of eternal truth from the simple absence of nonbeing to the full presence of existence in time. In a deeper than Socratic sense the question of chapter 1—To what extent can the truth be learned?—and the question of the title page—Can there be a historical point of departure for an eternal consciousness?—are asked in ignorance by one who cannot even know what prompted his asking. For Climacus' thought-project proposes what is strictly unthinkable by any human being. It contradicts the presupposition of all questioning—that he who asks already knows the answer—and of all inquiry—that he who seeks the truth already knows it.

The doctrine of recollection expresses both ontological and epistemological necessities. It is necessary to situate the present against the background of the past. The new is only the making explicit of what was implicit in the old, the actualization of a permanent or preexistent potentiality. Likewise for the conditions of intelligibility: the novel must always be understood in terms of the fixed and familiar. But Climacus' hypothesis defines a *radical* novelty, a coming-into-being unfounded and unprepared for, which of course would be unintelligible to anyone who had not experienced the novelty in question. And to him intelligible only in a radically new way, not by reference to an eternal *prius* but (impossibly) as the incommunicable meaning of a unique event in his own being.

Compounding unintelligibilities, the coda to chapter 1 (a dialogue between the fiction, Climacus, and his imagined interlocutor) argues that Climacus' thought-project is self-verifying. It is ridiculous and foolish, which is just what one would expect if it were true. And it is old and well known: every Sunday school child knows that Climacus' project is no more than orthodox Christian doctrine. Climacus is, his interlocutor says, "like the man who collected a fee for exhibiting a ram in the afternoon, which in the forenoon could be seen gratis, grazing in the open field" (*PF* 26, *PS* 19). But at the same time the hypothesis was not invented by its purported author, it was not invented by the interlocutor, and it could not have been invented by any human being. Say what you will about human folly, no man could think up something *absolutely* unintelligible.

The fact that the hypothesis exists, that it is unintelligible, that everyone knows it and also knows that he did not invent it, proves its truth. For that is exactly what the hypothesis predicts. At the very least it is clear that something utterly uncanny is afoot in the world. Something that disturbs and dislodges the norms of truth and meaning. Something no less disquieting because familiar to every man, woman, and child—a sickening uncertainty, a wild insecurity, that undermines assurance with the threat of radical unintelligibility, and which yet, through misunderstanding, carelessness, the force of habit—or bad faith—has come to be taken for granted.

Given a ram in the morning free, what is the point of a ram in the afternoon at great price?

It is instructive to transcribe Climacus' argument in (loosely) semiotic terms. Can there be a historical point of departure for an eternal consciousness? may be taken to mean, Can the historical signify the eternal? The question about learning is a search for vestiges of truth in the ignorant consciousness. Generally: terms like "history," "ignorance," "the learner" stand for signifiers, while terms like "the eternal" and "truth" stand for the transcendent signified. The argument investigates the relation of signification.[2] But since Climacus' text is itself a system of linguistic signifiers, the further question arises, How can language be "about" the eternal and "about" the relation of eternal truth to temporal fact? How can the transcendent signified be implicated in/by the play of signifiers.

To put the matter in this way is to undertake that self-reflection which the *Fragments* demands and itself enacts.

On the Socratic view, the signified is given in and with the signifier. To know oneself is to know God. On this view one is already, in history, out of history, so that to talk about anything at all is a way of gathering oneself out of time (the realm of signs) back into eternity (the always already presence of the signified). Language is pure self-transcendence. Instant recall. The signifiers, revoked as soon as they are uttered, collapse immediately into the signified.

On the Christian view (if that is what it is), time and eternity are simply diverse. There is no passage from time (the signifier) to eternity (the signified), only (on the one hand) the play of signifiers and (on the other) the silent alterity of the signified. Truth is not manifest in history save by a rupture of all the categories. Every Christian concept shatters the logic of signification. The terms of Climacus' thought-project, affirming the unsayable, merely open faults in language.

Hence the irony of the concluding dialogue, in which the absurdity of the Christian hypothesis is made a test of its truth. Ironic because Climacus catches discourse in a double bind. He permits either schizogenic signification or none at all. In order for signification to occur, the signifier must be distinct from the signified. On the Socratic view, therefore, there is no signification,

2. Cf. Søren Kierkegaard, *Concluding Unscientific Postscript*, trans. David F. Swenson and Walter Lowrie (Princeton, N.J.: Princeton University Press, 1944), pp. 86–97, on the relation of accidental historical truths to eternal truths of reason, with special reference to Lessing. Kierkegaard's fascination with proofs of God's existence, in which the same problem arises, is shown by chap. 3 of the *Philosophical Fragments*. Cf. my discussion below, sect. II.

only the prevenient reabsorption of all signifiers into the signified. But if signifier and signified are categorically distinct, as in Christianity (if that is what it is), then signification is contradiction. Every linguistic operation (including the *Fragments*) is doomed, either to nullity or to absurdity.

It is not surprising that Climacus (himself a being of language) splits in two at the end of the chapter. For one of him, the interlocutor, the thought-project is old hat. For the other it is so novel as to be unthinkable. "Better well hanged than ill wed" (*PF* 2A, *PS* 2). But the choice is not a happy one.

II

Chapter 3 of the *Philosophical Fragments,* on the absolute paradox, may be read as an attempt to conceive the Augustinian doctrine of the relation of faith and reason in terms of a Hegelian conception of reason. It argues that reason is fulfilled in faith; that is perfectly Augustinian. But it adds that the fulfillment of reason is the undoing of reason—the crucifixion of the understanding. That is to take "reason" in an idealist sense.

The passion of reason (according to Climacus) is to think what is not thought. Yet is is the fate of reason to think nothing but thoughts. Realist by desire, idealist by destiny, reason is paradoxically situated in its passion. It seeks its own destruction in collision with its other. Being is either a category of thought or an alterity cancelling thought. That reason desires its annihilation is paradoxical. That its annihilation is also its beatification is absolutely paradoxical.

The known is coextensive with the human. That was Socrates' view—all knowledge is implicit in self-knowledge—and it must be taken as normative. The other with which reason seeks collision must therefore be the unknown. "But what is this unknown . . . ? It is the unknown. . . . So let us call this unknown *God.* That is only a name we give it" (*PF* 49A, *PS* 36-37).

The text continues: "It could scarcely occur to reason to want to prove that this unknown (God) exists." This introduces a long digression on—proofs of God's existence. But the digression is to the point, and the point is to seal the unknown as such, to certify the absolute discontinuity of the unknown divine with the human and the known. The argument is as simple as the dialectic that sponsors it. The reality of the unknown (God's existence) cannot be demonstrated, for if it could it would not be other than reason.

The unknown is unknown, and there's an end of it. It could hardly occur to reason to make the unknown a *topos* of cognition. Reason could not even imagine the problem, since one of its terms is *de jure* extrarational. Yet the history of philosophy is virtually coterminous with the history of proofs of God's existence. What *did* put this notion into philosophers' heads?

In the ensuing discussion Climacus manipulates a distinction between essence (ideal being) and existence (factual being) that is equivalent to the distinction between the rational (continuous with the human) and the not-rational (discontinuous with the human). Existence, he insists, is never demonstrated but always assumed in demonstration. It is not part of the structure of ratiocination but a *prius* or an *accessorium*—a datum or a supplement (*PF* 50, *PS* 37). The reality of thinking presumes the thinker's participation in that which is not thought (*PF* 46, *PS* 34). Before he thinks, he *is*, and to this being-before-thought he persistently returns on the other side of thought.[3] But it is never comprehended in his thinking.

Proofs of God's existence, cosmological or ontological, take "God" as a concept (*PF* 51, *PS* 38) rather than a name (*PF* 49, *PS* 37) and proceed to unpack the contents of this concept—among which, of course, is (ideal) being (*PF* 50–52, 51 n., *PS* 38–40, 38 n.). But they do not reach through to (factual) being, which is the nub of the matter. The idea of proving that *this* (other than reason) exists could scarcely suggest itself to rationality.

> He, therefore, who wants to prove the existence of God ... proves in lieu thereof something else, something which at times perhaps does not even need a proof, and in any case needs none better. For the fool says in his heart, there is no God; but he who says in his heart or to men, wait

3. Cf. *Concluding Unscientific Postscript*, pp. 267–82, 293, 296, 314.

> just a little and I will prove it, O what a rare man of wisdom he is! [*PF* 54A, *PS* 41]

He who would know the unknown only proves himself a fool. And yet this folly of reason is not conspicuously different from its paradoxical passion: to encounter that which, in the encounter, will destroy it.

"A project of this kind would scarcely have been undertaken by the ancients" (*PF* 54). Presumably because they were perfectly rational. The thought that something discontinuous with reason might exist had not yet entered the world. Whence then the paradoxical passion of reason and its (decadent?) expression in the foolishness of theistic proof? Cryptically inscribed in Climacus' text is the suspicion that *Christianity* put this notion into reason's head. "What an excellent subject for a comedy of the higher lunacy!" (*PF* 54 n.).

There is, Climacus says, one way a man may get to God's existence via demonstration. By stopping:

> As long as I hold on to the proof (i.e., continue to be the prover), existence does not appear . . . ; but when I let go of the proof, existence is there. But the fact that I let go . . . is indeed my contribution; . . . it is a *leap*. [*PF* 53A, *PS* 40]

One arrives "rationally" at the other-than-reason by abandoning ratiocination. By a leap. A movement across radical discontinuity. Not by summoning all one's powers and venturing into the unknown. Where or what is the unknown? And what good are all one's powers? One "leaps" by letting go, giving up the attempt at proof, no longer demonstrating anything. There, in that abeyance of reason, reality beyond reason reveals itself.

The unknown makes its appearance when reason "sets itself aside" (*PF* 73, *PS* 55). Can reason dismiss itself in this way? No. It cannot abstain from seeking that which, found, will rebuff it.

> Thus the paradoxical passion of reason collides continually with the unknown, which indeed exists, but is also unknown, and in so far does not exist. Reason gets no farther, yet it

cannot in its paradoxicality refrain from coming to this point and concerning itself with it. . . . [*PF* 55A, *PS* 41]

It will not do for reason to deny the existence of the unknown, for the denial itself would affirm a relationship between reason and (that which reason conceives as) the nonexistent. To say that the unknown simply cannot be known, and that if it could it could not be expressed, correctly interprets the unknown as a limit. But the cognizance of the limit does not satisfy reason's passion for encounter, it only incites it.

What then is the unknown? It is the limit to which reason continually comes, and insofar . . . it is the different, the absolutely different.

Because it is the absolutely different, there is no mark [*Kjendetegn*] by which the unknown may be recognized: it is not signified by any sign. To call it the absolutely different may seem close to revealing what it is: it is the negative of everything rational. Not so. It is simply diverse from reason, and "reason cannot even think the absolutely different."

The unknown is no more than a limit. Unless it is left as such, the simple notion of difference turns into a profusion of monsters and ludicrous fantasies: the pantheons of polytheism and the wilder speculations of religious philosophers.

But this difference cannot be held fast. . . . If the difference cannot be held fast, because it has no distinguishing mark [*Kjendetegn*], then difference and likeness are identical, as is the case with all such dialectical opposites. The difference, which fastens itself to reason, has confounded it so that it does not know itself and quite consistently confuses itself with the difference. [*PF* 56A, *PS* 42-43]

Paradoxically, the attempt to conceive—or even to postulate—the absolutely other than reason leads to the absolutely paradoxical indistinction of reason and its other. But this, the paradoxical satisfaction/frustration desired by reason, is indistinguishable from idolatry. "Deepest down in the heart of piety lurks the mad caprice which knows that it has itself produced the God" (*PF* 56).

> Thus God has become the most terrible deceiver, because reason has deceived itself. Reason has brought God as near as possible, and yet he is just as far away as ever. [*PF* 57A, *PS* 43]

The paradoxical passion of reason—to be consumed in collision with the other—leads to the paradoxical impasse that reason cannot distinguish its salubrious immolation in the other from the idolatrous generation of the other in the vanity of its own imagining.

The absolutely different is indistinguishable from the absolutely same. There is no mark by which it may be known and therefore none by which it may be discriminated. The other-than-reason is that which in principle is contained in no rational category and which nonetheless is categorized as nonrational by this statement. With respect to any set of signs, "reality" is that which is included by exclusion and excluded by inclusion. The meaning of a text is the unwriteable inscription, and all discourse (*pace* proposition 7) is about that which cannot be spoken.

By Climacus' argument the Hegelian dialectic is made to generate the ultimate un-Hegelian conclusion. Not the unity of the rational and the real, subject and substance. And not simply their difference. Rather, their *indistinguishable* difference. The paradoxical issue of this paradoxical labor of reason is the interminable dialectical oscillation of the same and the other, the irresolute alternation of reflection aiming at being and recoiling into itself. The inconclusiveness is the conclusion.

At the end of chapter 3, Climacus' alter ego appears to protest that this discourse about the absolute other is so ludicrously absurd that "I must exclude from my consciousness everything that I have in it in order to hit upon it" (*PF* 57). Granted. And from this it follows that

> if he is to know anything in truth about the unknown (God), man must first know that it is different from him, absolutely different from him. Of itself reason cannot get to know

this . . . ; if it is to learn this, it must learn it from God, and if it
does learn this, it cannot understand it, and therefore cannot
know it. For how should reason understand the absolutely
different? [*PF* 57A, *PS* 44]

Reason itself, which cannot even imagine the absolutely different,
cannot be the source of its own passion nor of the undecidable
dialectic of likeness and difference to which it is thereby brought.
Christianity is offered as the origin and the interpretation of this
predicament of reason. For it is Christianity alone that discovers
in man his absolute difference from God (the untruth of sin) and
effects the absolute likeness of atonement.

Christianity resolves the residual Socratic perplexity about
human nature[4] and in so doing makes the paradox of reason
absolutely paradoxical. As Kierkegaard might have said, poten-
tiates it infinitely[5] by declaring humanity both monstrous (by sin)
and divine (by adoption). In order to make himself understood by
man, God (the unknown) himself became man.

> Thus the paradox becomes even more terrible, or rather the
> same paradox has a duplicity that shows it to be the absolute
> paradox; negatively by producing the absolute unlikeness of
> sin, positively by proposing to sublate [*ophæve*] this absolute
> unlikeness in absolute likeness. [*PF* 59A, *PS* 44-45]

Christianity is literally unthinkable, and "reason will have much to
urge against it" (*PF* 59). And yet

> reason in its paradoxical passion desires its own destruction.
> But the paradox also wills this destruction of reason, and so
> they understand one another. [*PF* 59A]

Precisely because it is unthinkable (the destruction of reason)
Christianity is the satisfaction of that passion of reason (for self-
destruction)—of which it is, aboriginally, the origin.

Exceeding in its paradoxicality even the paradoxical indistinc-

---

4. Cf. *PF* 58, *PS* 44. Also, Plato *Phaedrus* 230A.
5. Cf. Søren Kierkegaard, *The Sickness unto Death*, trans. Walter Lowrie (Princeton, N.J.: Princeton University Press, 1954), part 2.

tion of the same and the different, Christianity (if that is what it is) is the absolutely absolute other than the Hegelian absolute knowledge. The Absolute Paradox (the capitalization is at last necessary) propounds the consubstantial union of reason (the human) and its other (the divine). A union absolutely unintelligible, to be sure, signed and sealed only in the "moment of passion" and the "passion of the moment" (*PF* 59). Whatever that may be.

There is no doubt that Climacus' conclusions are paradoxical. Yet one might, in the spirit of his interlocutor, question the dichotomies on which his dialectic is strung. For example, why does he regard existence (factual being) as absolutely different from essence (ideal being), so sundered that there is no rational transition from one to the other? It is not strange or unprecedented to define ideal being as the realm available to thought, or simply as the realm of thought; nor to define factual being by opposition as being independent of thought. In which case reason, by definition restricted to one side of this duality, could not reach across to comprehend its contrary. Existence is in principle incomprehensible.

But there is more than stipulation at stake. Thought, as Climacus points out,[6] is never pure. It is always the thinking of a thinker who in his thinking is not just his thought. Thinking presupposes and intends the other than thought. Just as a ghost of significance—a phantom of reference—plays about the margins of even the most self-contained text, so the edges of thought are haunted by the ghost of reality. A ghost that can neither be laid nor made to materialize.

Climacus' text enacts the ambivalent relationship of text-as-such ("reason," "humanity," "self-knowledge," etc.) to its extratextual presuppositions ("God," "the unknown," "the absolutely different," etc.). This beyond-the-text cannot be comprehended or even adumbrated in the text without becoming itself textual: everything in the preceding parentheses—both of them—is a signifier and no more. In that sense there is nothing

6. Cf. *PF* 46, *PS* 34. Also *Concluding Unscientific Postscript*, pp. 269-70, 273-79, 292, 296-99.

outside the text. And yet it is this "nonexistent" *hors-texte* that all texts are "about." That is paradoxical enough. The absolute paradox is that the nontext is the source and meaning of the text, the extrastructural foundation, fulfillment, and frustration of every structure.

In Climacus' version of this paradox, "existence" is a name (like "God" it is only a name, no more than a signifier) for (another signifier!) the nonthought from which thinking starts and departs. Thinking starts and departs from existence; it cannot disavow its origin, nor can it turn and devour it. Thought cannot escape from its escape from its point of departure, nor can it arrive at that which is always already its destiny.

Yet the passion of reason is to do just that: to reach back before the beginning or forward beyond the end and to recover by thinking the presupposition which as thinking it makes and loses. The passion and the paradox of thought is a nostalgia for the primordial but always already sundered unity of thought and being. Which in actual thinking becomes an apocalyptic trajectory toward their always intended but ever unrealized reconciliation.

The passion of thought is as persistent and inescapable as it is desperate. The name for this nostalgia, protended as apocalypse, is the search for truth or the love of wisdom: the signifier "philosophy." It is a desperate passion, because the original unity of thought and existence was never given and is never experienced. There is no such thing as immediate experience and certainly no immediate thinking.[7] All that is given is nostalgia for a primal harmony that is felt as lost but which "in fact" (that is, in reflection) never was. What is experienced is not sameness but difference, not presence but absence.

The desperate passion of reason is desperately self-destructive, for the presence of being would annul thinking by obliterating its difference (both *differentia* and *différance*) and "fulfill" it by engulfing it. The Greek doctrine of recollection is the nostalgia of thought for return to its no-longer-present origin (preexistence), and the modern belief in afterlife (postexistence) is only recollec-

7. Cf. *Concluding Unscientific Postscript*, pp. 101–06.

tion in reverse. Both of them are expressions of the pathos of death (*PF* 11-12, 12 n., 26, *PS* 7-8, 8 n., 19). The passion of reason for reunion with being is simply the present experience of their diremption. *Media vita in morte sumus,* and the attainment of everlasting life, whether a priori or a posteriori, would be the triumph of death. Life is the difference between life and death— and the impatience for its obliteration.

Wallace Stevens wrote, "In the long run the truth does not matter."[8] Truth is at best an external correspondence of signs with realities or a coherence among signs utterly indifferent to reality. Truth would not repair but only perpetuate the breach between thought and existence. In the same vein, "Realism is a corruption of reality."[9] Realism is an act, a form, and a content of thought which derealizes the real by asserting it. "The difference [man] himself produces is identical with likeness, for he cannot get outside of himself."[10] "Thus reason has brought God as near as possible, and yet he is as far away as possible; and this is the most ironical thing thinkable, that God has become pure negativity."[11]

But "the whole thing is a trick."[12] Not just Climacus' suggestion that what man has put asunder God can join together, but the far more irritating insinuation that perhaps it was not man who put asunder in the first place. Man can neither think the absolutely different nor imagine a likeness that is not idolatrous. The absolute paradox is a "metaphysical crotchet" (*PF* 46, *PS* 34). A crotchet so outlandish that a man would have to lose his mind in order to hit upon it. Yet as the name [*Grille*] says, it's all in the head. How did it get there?

Like every chapter of the *Fragments,* chapter 3 ends in a dialogue between Climacus and his other. The repeated emergence

8. Wallace Stevens, *Opus Posthumous* (New York: Knopf, 1957), p. 180.

9. Ibid., p. 166. Cf. also "The ultimate value is reality" (p. 166) and "The real is only the base. But it is the base" (p. 160).

10. *Søren Kierkegaards Papirer,* 2d ed. enlarged by Niels Thulstrup (Copenhagen: Gyldendal, 1968), V B 5, 10.

11. Ibid., V B 5, 8. Cf. below, sect. V.

12. Ibid., V B 5, 5.

of these little dissensions reveals two things. First, that Climacus is divided within, or against, himself by the matter under discussion. And second, that the inner contention which surfaces in them has been present all along, agitating the depths of the argument. The argument is not an argument at all, but an agon between Climacus and his alienated self instigated by the "wholly other" that occasioned (spoke?) their discourse in the first place.

In his preface to the *Fragments* Climacus identifies himself as the frivolous exponent of the absolute paradox, but betrays another, more conscientious and socially responsible self. The former is an idler who writes for his own amusement and hopes that his work will make no contribution to the common welfare or the progress of knowledge. The latter, reflecting that perhaps the life of society and the public mind are already badly confused by their all-too-many and all-too-eager teachers and benefactors, surmises that the example of his self-indulgence—like Archimedes' concentration on his circles or Diogenes trundling his tub (*PF* 3-4, *PS* 3-4)—may be just what the age demands. At least a "kind and benevolent reader" may find something of use in his "piece" (*PF* 5, 3, *PS* 5, 3). But even this modest expectation sustains nothing but ambiguity:

> It is not given to everyone to have his private tasks of meditation and reflection so happily coincident with the public interest that it becomes difficult to judge how far he serves merely himself and how far the public good. [*PF* 3]

The failure to reconcile his public and private egos (the radical of this failure be what it may) prevents Climacus from formulating a doctrine or espousing an opinion:

> But what is my opinion? . . . Let no one ask me that. For next to knowing whether I have an opinion, nothing could be of less importance to another than knowing what my opinion is. [*PF* 5-6A]

To have an opinion would be too much and too little. Too much, because it presupposes the unity and solidarity of the social self—domestic happiness and civic respectability—which the dis-

junct Climacus cannot count on. And also too little, for Climacus'
opinion would be the opinion of a trifler, and

> if anyone were to be so polite as to assume that I have an
> opinion, and if he were to carry his gallantry to the extreme
> of adopting this opinion because he believed it to be mine, I
> should have to be sorry for his politeness, in that it was bes-
> towed upon so unworthy an object, and for his opinion, if he
> has no other opinion than mine. [*PF* 6, *PS* 5-6]

The duplicity of its author, recollected at the (in)conclusion of
each chapter, transforms his work from exposition to enactment.
Climacus himself (whoever that is) describes it as a dance, in the
service of thought, to the glory of God, and for his own enjoyment. A dance, however, in which his partner is (indomitable
thought) the thought of death. A game. But a game played in all
seriousness, in which (for reasons that are beginning to become
clear) his life is at stake (*PF* 6-7, *PS* 6).

The appendix to chapter 3 discusses "offense" (*Forargelse,
skandalon*)—the rejection by human reason of the absolute
paradox—which it describes as an "acoustic illusion" (*PF* 61, *PS*
46). Reason's encounter with the paradox may issue either in
understanding and reconciliation ("that happy passion" [*PF* 67,
PS 51] as yet unnamed) or in scandal and alienation. The latter
Climacus calls offense. The nature of offense, in particular its
linguistic proclivities, shows that the passion of reason, however
paradoxical, does not itself discover the absolute paradox. The
passion of reason, like erotic passion, wants to find its other in
order to be overwhelmed and fulfilled by it. But as erotic passion
is fundamentally self-love and desires to surrender *itself* to *its own*
other, so reason demands that *it* shall meet *its* other and achieve
fulfillment by means of *self*-immolation. Realism, though its accomplishment would mean the end of (idealistic) reason, is to be
the work of reason, its *self*-sacrifice. Hegel might have understood that.

The paradox, however, posits the impossibility of a rationally
motivated encounter of reason with its other. The other is absolutely unlike reason and could not be met by reason in any course
of ratiocination. Thereupon the paradox proposes the abolition

of this absolute difference in absolute likeness: a reconciliation of reason and the paradox initiated, empowered, and enacted by the paradox. This (absolutely un-Hegelian) outcome reason cannot conceive—concerning which it must be said "with all possible ambiguity" that it "did not arise in the heart of any man."[13]

It follows that all offense (like "that happy passion") is passive. Never so passive that reason is wholly annihilated, but never so active that reason can extricate itself from scandal. Reason desires to surrender itself to the other; it cannot desire the dissolution of its autonomy by the other. Offense, like the paradox itself, is paradoxical.

The verbal expressions of offense, while they seem to come from reason, are only echoes of the paradox in the offended consciousness (*PF* 63, *PS* 47-48). Hence the acoustic illusion: the language of offense is nothing but a ventriloquism in which the paradox speaks through the mouth of reason. As his interlocutor notes, Climacus' own characterizations of offense are quotations from Tertullian, Hamann, Lactantius, Shakespeare, and Luther—partisans of the paradox one and all (*PF* 66-67, *PS* 50). As radically other than reason (even its paradoxical passion), the paradox generates its own rejection by reason. "Reason says that the Paradox is absurd, but this is mere mimicry, since the Paradox is the Paradox, *quia absurdum*" (*PF* 65, *PS* 49). In this way offense is an "indirect proof of the validity [*Rigtighed*] of the paradox," of its origin in the absolutely other than reason. Offense is "the mistaken reckoning [*den feile Regning*]" and the "invalid consequence [*Usandhedens Conseqvents*]" by which the paradox repels reason. Offense only "parodies [*bagvendt copierer*]" the paradox—copies it and gets it all backwards (*PF* 63, *PS* 48). Like a mimic, it testifies to the absolute priority of its original and its own absolute unoriginality.

The paradox of chapter 3 is identical with the "moment" of chapter 1. It marks the unmediated transition from the nonbeing of untruth to the being of truth. Because it is unmediated and unmediatable, the incursion of the wholly other into the structure of rationality introduces into that otherwise orderly world an un-

13. *PF* 138, *PS* 105. Cf. I Corinthians 2:7-9.

manageable shiftiness. The appearance of the paradox inaugurates an interminable play of discontinuity and difference. The
mere possibility of the absolutely other and the mere suggestion
of the (impossible) absolute sameness of the absolutely other—the
dialectic of sin and atonement proposed by Christianity—means
that reason can no longer trust itself, not even its distrust. Once a
hole is made—a breach in the continuity of rational structures—
reason is perforated everywhere and always by the irrational. "Is
perforated," because reason did not discover the irrational itself.

> The expression of offense is that the moment is folly, the
> paradox is folly; which is the claim of the paradox that reason
> is absurd, resounding as an echo from offense. . . . [S]ince the
> paradox has made reason absurd, reason's regard signifies
> nothing [*er intet Kjendetegn*]. [*PF* 64–65A, *PS* 49]

A possibility once is a necessity forever. That is what Christianity (if that is what it is) has introduced into the world: the
possibility, once insinuated never eluctable, of an irrationality
unmasterable by reason, an unreason which even the cunning of
Hegelian rationality cannot surround and make its own. The de-
thronement, in principle, of all security. All it takes to destroy the
confidence of reason for good and all is the rumor (which is now
somehow inexplicably abroad in the world) that literally "all
things are possible."[14] That little hint is sufficient to expose
human thought and discourse intolerably to the infinite uncertainty of all things.[15] In Kierkegaard's language these phrases are
names of God. God has become pure negativity. What could be
more ironical?

III

Signed and dated. Signed with the sign of the cross and dated
from the Incarnation. The mark of a unique and decisive histori-

---

14. *The Sickness unto Death,* pp. 173–74. "God *is* that all things are possible, and
that all things are possible *is* God. . . ."

15. Cf. *Concluding Unscientific Postscript,* p. 80: "The Deity . . . is present as soon
as the uncertainty of all things is thought infinitely."

cal occurrence. The temporal point of departure for an eternal consciousness and the historical foundation of eternal beatitude. In chapters 4 and 5 of the *Philosophical Fragments* Johannes Climacus meditates the historicity of the eternal.

That is the gist of the absolute paradox, "the historical made eternal, and the Eternal made historical" (*PF* 76, *PS* 58). The historical coming-to-be of the eternal or the fulfilling of time by eternity could only issue (rationally) in the cancellation of time by eternity or the dispersion of the eternal along the moments of temporality. Climacus' concern is not with the concrete historical event of the Incarnation—historical content is irrelevant to his purposes—but with historicity in the abstract. The absurdity of the Incarnation is its structural (in principle) impossibility (*PF* 73-74, *PS* 56).

To "that happy passion" in which reason and the paradox meet with understanding Climacus gives the name "faith," though as he notes, it is not the name that matters. Faith is the opposite of offense and the God-given condition for understanding the God-given truth. It is also the occasion for a couple of precisions. Faith is not a kind of knowledge. All knowledge is either of the eternal or of the historical, never of their paradoxical conjunction (*PF* 76, *PS* 58). The relation of the sign (history) to the transcendent signified (eternity) is either a continuity in which the sign is absorbed into the signified (Socrates) or a discontinuity whose overcoming is absolutely impossible (Christianity). On the former view, cognition of the sign has no independent epistemic value: it is only incipient cognizance of the signified. On the latter view, cognition of the sign can never lead to cognition of the signified and vice versa, since they are by definition mutually exclusive.

Neither is faith an act of will. It is impossible to will without knowing what one is willing. Lacking this condition, which on the Christian view is the faith imparted by God, there can be no will. On the Christian hypothesis, the capacity both to know and to will is given with faith (*PF* 77, *PS* 59). God is neither immediately knowable (*lader sig jo ikke umiddelbart kjende*) nor conceivable (*lader sig ikke forestille*) (*PF* 78, *PS* 59-60). He is received and known only in the faith that he himself bestows. And faith is as paradoxical as the paradox itself (*PF* 81, *PS* 62).

Climacus' conclusion (he is discussing "the case of the contemporary disciple") is that there is no immediate contemporaneity with the paradox. "Contemporaneity" in this context means immediate presence, either the everywhere always presence of the eternal (with which all men at all times are contemporary) or the presence to each other of beings coincident in time (whose contemporaneity would be a function of the intersection of their spatiotemporal coordinates). A being that is at once historical and eternal, itself the breach with every form of immediacy, can have no immediate contemporary (*PF* 83 ff., *PS* 63 ff.).

The contemporary of the paradox is neither the eyewitness nor the timeless subject of cognition, but the believer. And in the nonimmediacy of the "autopsy of faith," which iterates in the subject the paradoxicality of the Incarnation, every noncontemporary (in the immediate sense) may become a contemporary (in the paradoxical sense) of the paradox (*PF* 84, 87, *PS* 64, 66). The moment of his transition from untruth to truth is identical with the moment of the coming-to-be of the eternal in time: his knowledge of God-in-time is, by virtue of the gift of faith, at once a vision of himself reborn to eternal consciousness.

If the distinction eternal truth–historical occasion be assimilated to the distinction transcendent signified–immanent sign— as it must, since the "Socratic" philosophy simply enunciates the norms of rationality as such—then problems arise concerning cognition of the sign, of the signified, and of their relationship. Knowledge of the temporal sign would be sensuous awareness or historical witness. Knowledge of the eternal signified would be purely intellectual. Knowledge of their relationship (signification) might be either direct or indirect. If it is direct, then the signified is immanent in the sign, and the sign as mere occasion vanishes as soon as the signified is known. If it is indirect, then there is no transition at all from sign to signified; cognition is arrested at the level of the sign, and passage to the signified is indefinitely deferred. Or else—the Christian alternative—the union of sign and signified (the absolute paradox) is apprehended in the absolutely paradoxical passion of faith.

Pace Hegel, there can be no mediation of time and eternity. Mediate cognition of the signified by means of (immediate) cognition of the sign would require the presence of the signified, if not to the sign, then at least to $sign^1$, $sign^2$, or $sign^n$. At some point either the Socratic view is reinstated—the immanence of the signified in the sign—or else the Christian dichotomy stands fast and the absolute paradox is the only escape from the schizophrenia of cognition. Either presence or absence: either the eternal signified is present in the historical sign, or the signified is simply absent and cannot be recuperated save at the unimaginable and unthinkable limit of the "autopsy of faith." A faith whose "objective" condition (the moment of incarnation) and whose "subjective" condition (the moment of conversion) are themselves unthinkably and unimaginably conjoined.

The relation of sign and signified is both a likeness and a difference. The likeness, which at some point must be identity, cannot be preserved without, at that point, denying the difference and fusing sign and signified. The difference cannot be maintained without denying the likeness and converting the difference of sign and signified into their mutual exclusion. A logic of analogy—of likeness-*in*-difference—would fall prey to the dialectic of likeness *versus* difference—every analogy consists of an element of likeness juxtaposed to an element of difference—which would relocate the problem (*ad infinitum*) without solving it. To say that analogy uniquely and unanalyzably merges likeness and difference is to beg off the problem with a plea of ineffable mystery that is conceptually no advance on, though conceivably more ingratiating than, the absolute paradox itself. This side of mystery, either the knowledge of the signified is given with the knowledge of the sign or indefinitely postponed by it.

The absolute paradox is that the temporal sign and the eternal signified are and are apprehended as at once absolutely other and absolutely same.

But of course the very idea of a sign–signified relation—the concept of signification itself—incorporates the paradox. The sign must participate the being of the signified; else it cannot mediate *cognition* of the signified. But at the same time the sign must be distinct from the signified; else it cannot *mediate* cognition of the signified. Although it contains analytically the notion of the signified (to be a sign is to signify the signified), the concept of the sign insists upon the sign's identity with itself and its difference from the signified. Identity and difference alike are affirmed and compromised by the conception of their relation.

The paradox of the sign is the paradox Augustine found in Platonism: the forms are both known and not known in their appearances. A discomforting paradox, which led to the separation, in the subsequent history of Platonism, of Neoplatonic gnosis (a knowledge of the forms that has sloughed off appearances) and New Academy skepticism (an acquaintance with appearances unstructured by form). It was this paradox to which the Christian-revisionist Platonism of Augustine counterposed as resolution the absolute paradox of the Incarnation.

It was the Christian Augustine who discovered the paradox of the sign in Platonism. Is it possible that the paradox of signification is a Christian innovation? Climacus' fascination with the relation of alterity and identity would suggest as much.

In the (unusually long) dialogue that concludes chapter 5 and the book, Climacus finally concedes his identity with his interlocutor, in response to whose opening (and untypically conciliatory) speech he says: "Well said, I would reply, did not modesty forbid; for you speak as if it were myself" (*PF* 133, *PS* 102). As the discourse of *his* other (alter ego) the interlocutor is Climacus' unconscious, at first repressed and rejected, now—albeit somewhat grudgingly and with a certain coyness—acknowledged. He is as Climacus' own depth—the cultural language in which Climacus' self is originally encoded—the one for whom this discourse is designed and to whom it is addressed. At the end of the work Climacus and himself are reconciled.

Alternatively, it is possible that Johannes Climacus is the unconscious voice of his more "normal" interlocutor. The latter remarks:

I have now read your exposition through to the end, and really not without a certain degree of interest, noting with pleasure that there was no catchword [*Stikord*], no invisible script [*usynlig Skrift*]. But how you twist and turn, so that . . . you always manage to mix in a little word [*et lidet Ord*] that is not your own, which awakens disturbing recollections. [*PF* 132A, *PS* 101]

Otherness is a repeater. And it is just possible that this entire discourse—the *Philosophical Fragments*—is the voice of another than both Climacus and his interlocutor: the suppressed language of Western Christendom, still to be heard beneath its song and clang. A song of mockery, unlicensed but inevitable. A "shrill laughter, like the mocking nature-tones on the island of Ceylon." The revenge of the law of contradiction on an age that preferred wonders and wonders-workers no matter what the cost (cf. *PF* 135–36, *PS* 103–04).

Or perhaps—this unspeakably and with "all possible ambiguity"—the *Fragments* is the discourse, unconscious because unutterable, of the Absolute Other, now at last and impossibly reconciled with human speech. The ultimate iteration—and so the closure—of alterity. As the terminal dialogues repeatedly point out, this "did not arise in the heart of any man." Climacus himself—and his other—say so. Is it conceivable that the voice of Johannes Climacus (J. C.) is the voice of God? The historical costume, ill-fitting and unbecoming, is irresistibly proffered.

In which (any) case, while we may not say that the project here unfolded is true, we may at least be certain that it makes an advance upon Socrates. Certain, that is, with all possible ambiguity. For, in conclusion and with respect to the beginning, "'When the question cannot be asked the answer need not trouble us, and the difficulty becomes slight indeed.'—'This does not quite follow; for suppose the difficulty lay in perceiving that one cannot ask such a question.'" [*PF* 111, *PS* 85] That perception may be difficult indeed. Whereof one cannot speak one must keep silent. But how else than by speaking may one perceive that whereof one cannot speak?

IV

Between chapters 4 and 5 of his discussion Climacus inserts an "Interlude," comparable to the entr'acte played during an intermission in the theater. Its purpose is to create the illusion that time has passed, say the 1,843 years that separate the eyewitness of the paradox from the latest generation of noncontemporary disciples. Although there is little more than temporal difference between contemporary and noncontemporary, Climacus' Interlude occupies a tense moment: the moment between acts during which it is possible, among other things, to walk out.

However paradoxical (what else?) its conclusion, the argument of chapters 4 and 5 is the essence of simplicity, based as it is (dichotomies again!) on the strictly exclusive disjunction of time and eternity. The Interlude is meant to clarify this disjunction and pursue its implications so as to substantiate the argument it sponsors. The question it poses is, "Is the past more necessary than the future? Or, does the possible by becoming actual thereby become more necessary than it was?" (*PF* 89A, *PS* 68).

To open this question Climacus distinguishes between qualitative change (*alloiosis*) and coming-to-be (*kinesis, Tilblivelse*). In the former, essence (*Væsen*) changes while being (*Væren*) remains the same. In the latter, essence remains the same while being changes. If essence did not remain the same in coming-to-be, then A could never come to be but would in the process of becoming change into B. Coming-to-be is (just) a change from nonexistence (*ikke at være til*) to existence (*at være til, Tilværelse*), essence abiding. It is, in other terms, a transition from possibility (*Mulighed*) to actuality (*Virkelighed*), where possibility is the being which is still nonbeing and actuality the being which is indeed being.

It is important to note the *pseudo*-Aristotelian character of Climacus' description of *kinesis*. Not quite the movement from potency to act, coming-to-be is the change from possibility to actuality.

By contrast with possibility and actuality, necessity (*det Nødvendige*) cannot change. It cannot undergo anything. Necessity "always relates itself to itself and relates itself to itself in the same way" (*PF* 91, *PS* 70). Necessity simply *is*.

Possibility is annihilated by actualization. Not only the excluded possibility (−A, for example, when A is actualized), but also the actualized possibility (A), which is negated *as* possibility when it is made actual. Possibility and actuality are mutually exclusive. Each is the nonbeing of the other. Wherefore necessity could not be a synthesis of possibility and actuality, the Hegelian unity of *an sich* and *für sich,* since any such synthesis would be contradictory:

> Possibility and actuality do not differ in essence but in being; how could there from this difference be formed a synthesis constituting necessity, which is not a determination [*Bestemmelse*] of being but a determination of essence, since it is the essence of the necessary to be. [*PF* 91–92, *PS* 70]

The discrimination is crucial. Possibility and actuality are categories of being—the only categories of being, and contradictories. But necessity is a "determination of essence." It is that the essence of which is to be and thus escapes the disjunction of possible and actual. There is therefore no transition from the realm of being (possibility-actuality) to the realm of essence (necessity), or vice versa. Necessity "stands entirely by itself" (*PF* 92A, *PS* 71).

Since necessity is excluded from the realm of coming-to-be, the latter (necessarily?) takes place with freedom (*Frihed*). Becoming has no (logical) ground (*Grund*), though it does have a cause (*Aarsag*). And all causes terminate in a freely effecting (*fritvirkende*) cause. It is only in the domain of freedom that anything really *happens*. The realm of freedom is the realm of history.

The eternal, which is also the necessary, has no history in any sense. It sustains no relationship to possibility, actuality, change, or freedom. Nature is pure synchrony (spatiality, *Nebeneinander*), save for the fact that it has, as a whole, come into being. History is pure diachrony (temporality), save for the fact that it presupposes space as its locus. Nature has no "dialectic with respect to time" (*PF* 94, *PS* 72). Strictly speaking, nothing happens in nature. It is always, if cyclically, the same, for which reason there are *laws* of nature. But historical events, for which there are no laws, are the operations of freely working causes terminating in the working of an absolutely free cause.

Climacus' desire to identify the domain of history and distinguish it from the realm of nature prescribes his substitution of the categories possibility-actuality for the Aristotelian potency-act. Aristotle's concern is with nature, which from Climacus' perspective is as a totality not necessary (since it has come to be) but in all its parts is a system of simultaneous nonevents. In potency the act is already contained and will emerge. Every potency, moreover, is rooted in (strictly, *is*) a prior act. But possibility is just the nonbeing of its corresponding actuality. The freedom of history—the unmotivated discontinuity of historical action—is opposed to the quasi-necessity—the explicability and continuity—of natural change.

However, although Climacus' appeal to Aristotle is oblique, the classical allusions strewn throughout the Interlude serve a purpose. By aligning his own discourse with that of the "honest" Greeks, Climacus hopes to ally himself with their integrity and oppose himself to the "mendaciousness" of the Hegelians.[16] This in spite of the fact that he deploys some of Hegel's categories and says things that no Greek could imagine.

The past (to continue with Climacus' text) is necessary only in the sense that what's done cannot be undone. Its "thus" (*saaledes*) is immutable. But because it did happen, the past was not and is not necessary. Its "how" (*hvorledes*) might have been otherwise. The future is no more necessary than the past, but no less so merely for the fact that it has not yet happened. If the past were necessary, the future would also be necessary. If necessity were to be found anywhere in the realm of happening, past and future could not be distinguished. For a strict determinism time is unreal, and the distinction between past and future nugatory. To claim (as Hegelian philosophers of history did) to discern the necessity of the past is no more and no less rational than to claim to predict the future with certainty. If necessity were once to get a foothold in the process of becoming, then past, future, freedom, change, and history would all be illusions.

But there is no necessity in becoming. The past, having come to be, is uncertain. As actualized, however, it annuls all possibilities including its own. In that sense the past is certain. With its duality of certainty (its "thus") and uncertainty (its "how") the past is confronted in wonder and apprehended in belief (*Tro*). Belief is

16. *Søren Kierkegaards Papirer*, V A 98.

an attitude in which (objective) uncertainty is negated by (subjective) assurance. Its epistemological structure corresponds to the ontological structure of the past, which is an actuality that negates a possibility.

What is true of the past is true of all becoming, including the becoming of the present. Even here the conjunction of certainty (annihilated possibility) and uncertainty (the antecedent possibility annihilated in its actualization) engenders wonder. Doubt succumbs to the uncertainty. Belief, comprehending the uncertainty and sublating doubt, affirms the certainty.

Belief is not an act of cognition. All cognition, sensuous or intellectual, is infallible. It apprehends essences, sensible or intelligible, which are constant (necessary). Belief affirms becoming, which is free and fallible. Like its opposite, doubt, belief is a passion, a resolution of the will, not an inference from ground to consequent. In this respect it answers to the free causation that is the instrumentality of becoming.

The contemporary of a historical event has his sensuous or intellectual knowledge of its "what." A noncontemporary has the testimony of contemporaries. Belief follows no more and no less from testimony than from direct cognition. As far as belief is concerned (this is the gist of the argument in chapters 4 and 5), whether one is or is not contemporary with a historical event is a matter of indifference.

Climacus now applies these precisions to the assertion that God has come into existence. As a historical assertion this formula proposes an object of belief (*Tro*) in the ordinary sense. As an assertion that affirms a contradiction—that the eternal (the necessary) has come to be in time (the domain of freedom and change)—it defines the object of faith (*Tro*) in the eminent sense. The Incarnation, as the historical event which in principle could not happen, is apprehended by that faith which is neither an act of knowledge nor an act of will but a divine gift accepted with divine subvention.

The existence of God—properly his eternal and necessary being—cannot be proven, as chapter 3 has shown. Neither is it a matter of faith. The object of faith is the content of the moment:

not that God *is,* but that he *has been* in the past and continually *comes to be* in the experience of the twice born.

For Socrates history as a whole is only an occasion for reversion to the eternal. It is from all eternity continuous with the eternal and from all eternity subsumed into the eternal. The being of time, a diminution of the being of eternity, has no reality outside or against its eternal source. On Climacus' Christian hypothesis (if that is what it is), history is abruptly discontinuous with the eternal and set against it, so that the marriage of time and eternity in the moment is absolutely paradoxical. For Hegel history is continuous with the eternal but more than an occasion of eternal truth: history itself is the reality and truth of the eternal. The conjunction of history and eternity is superlatively the work of reason.

That is the "mendaciousness" of Hegel, that he wants the best of both incompossible worlds. He will have his Socratic cake and also, like a good Christian, eat it. The *Philosophical Fragments* is meant to affront that Hegelian option. In the Interlude Climacus has guaranteed the incommunication of time (freedom) and eternity (necessity) and assured that the allegation of their communication in "the fullness of time" is a contradiction which no cognitive inference or determination of the will can resolve.

But surely words like "guaranteed" and "assured" are devious in this context. What makes the guarantee valid and the assurance trustworthy? Only the assumption that the Teacher has already come and gone (*PF* 89, *PS* 68). Given Christianity, Climacus' definitions and exclusions tell it like it is. Otherwise they are arbitrary and nonsensical stipulations. Only if Christianity is *already there*—by virtue of the absurd, for no man could posit it—does Climacus' very un-Greek diversion of Greek categories and his very un-Hegelian inversion of Hegelian categories make sense. Given that unthinkable presupposition, his analysis is impeccably rational.

Climacus, like Socrates and like necessity, is always "repeating the same things, 'about the same things'" in order to create the "illusion" that time—1,843 years!—has passed. The conjunction of freedom and necessity in the language of the Interlude is no less refractory to reason than the absolute paradox itself. Addressing his reader, Climacus says:

> ... I do not by any means doubt that you have completely understood and assented to the newest philosophy, which like the modern age seems to suffer from a curious distraction, confusing the superscription with the execution; for what age and what philosophy was ever so great as our own—in superscriptions. [*PF* 90A, *PS* 69][17]

If superscription is to execution as possibility is to actuality, then perhaps the Interlude should be subtitled "a possibility." Standing as it does between past and present, the Greeks and Hegel, the Interlude stands also—possibly—between two worlds, one dead, the other powerless to be born. It is—possibly—a piece of becoming in its own right, the coming-to-be of the impossible possibility of the historical coming-to-be of the eternal.

A lengthy footnote coaches this reading of the Interlude:

> The Absolute Method, Hegel's discovery, is a difficulty even in Logic, aye a glittering tautology, coming to the assistance of academic superstition with many signs and wonders. In the historical sciences it is a fixed idea. The fact that the method here at once begins to become concrete, since history is the concretion of the Idea, has given Hegel an opportunity to exhibit extraordinary learning, and a rare power of organization, inducing a quite sufficient commotion in the historical material. But it has also promoted a distraction of mind in the reader, so that ... he may have forgotten to inquire whether it now really did become evident at the end, at the close of this journey of enchantment, as was repeatedly promised in the beginning, and what was of course the prin-

17. Cf. Søren Kierkegaard, *Stages on Life's Way*, trans. Walter Lowrie (Princeton, N.J.: Princeton University Press, 1945), pp. 258–68, "A Possibility," in which the paralyzing terrors of possibility are explored. Also Søren Kierkegaard, *The Concept of Dread*, trans. Walter Lowrie (Princeton, N.J.: Princeton University Press, 1957), passim, on the effects of possibility.

cipal issue, for the want of which not all the glories of the
world could compensate, what alone could be a sufficient reward for the unnatural tension in which one had been
held—that the method was valid. Why at once become concrete, why at once begin to experiment *in concreto?* Was it not
possible to answer this question in the dispassionate brevity
of abstraction, which has no means of distraction or en-
chantment, this question of what it means that the Idea becomes concrete, what is the nature of coming into existence,
what is one's relationship to that which has come into existence, and so forth? Just as it surely might have been cleared
up in the Logic what "transition" is and means, before going
over to write three volumes describing its workings in the
categories.... [*PF* 96 n.–97 n., *PS* 74 n.]

Does Climacus offer his little Interlude as an abstract and undis-
tracting concretion of the categories, a transition in which the
meaning of "transition" is made—clear? Ostensibly the Interlude
connects the past (the actualized and so abrogated possibility) and
the present (the possibility now awaiting actualization by a free
cause). So conceived, the Interlude, entirely in the spirit of the
newest philosophy, is a mediation. As it connects past and present, so also it mediates essence and existence, necessity and freedom, eternity and time, and so forth. A veritable paragon of the
absolute method, perhaps even its paradigm.

   Yet it cannot be an accident that the author never explains the
relationship of the necessary and the possible, the changeless and
the changing. Nor does he clarify the double relationship of essence to the necessary and to the possible. Essence is both that
which is necessarily self-identical (relates itself to itself always in
the same way) and that which comes to be (is actualized) in every
spasm of becoming. These conjunctions are taken for granted but
never accounted for, perhaps even prohibited, in Climacus' singularly well-written, brief, and undistractingly abstract theoretical
resumé.

   The Interlude's "mediation" is ironic. Which is not quite the
same as no mediation at all, but rather: a mediation denied. In

preliminary drafts of the Interlude Kierkegaard says that it is the passion of philosophy to minimize the concrete in order that the "thought" may not be confused or allowed to fall into oblivion. And in order that the reader may not be fooled with diversions and entertainments (*Ordspil og Vittigheder*: "word games and witticisms"), but enlightened with understanding.[18] It is therefore crucial to philosophy to be absolutely clear about the distinction between abstract and concrete, ideal and actual. That would account for the irony of this "mediation," as well as the algebraically abstract language of the *Fragments* as a whole. The point is to guarantee that the essential (abstract) shock of the absolute paradox will not be confused by the rich but distracting (concrete) history of Christianity.

If Climacus' project is to go beyond Socrates without, like Hegel, rushing beyond faith as well, then it must be irrational. Becoming and history themselves must be irrational in a way that no Greek would dream of and no German tolerate: a play of the categories between the no-longer-possible serene rationality of the Greek and the never-to-be-actual synthesis of absolute knowledge. *Must* be? Given Christianity, without which neither these disjunctions nor their reconciliation were (!) conceivable. As Climacus says in another work, reality is an *inter-esse* between the actual and the ideal:[19] a being-between the no longer and the not yet, between the possible which when actualized is no longer possible and the actual which is never possible. The impossible possibility of transforming that *inter-esse*, suspended in abstraction, into the concretion of becoming: that is the awful and consoling thought with which Christianity disturbs and allures the passion of philosophy.

One of Walker Percy's characters has suggested, by not saying so, that Christianity is a technique of reentry from the orbit of transcendence.[20] Irony, once you hit upon it, puts the self into

18. *Søren Kierkegaards Papirer*, V B 14. Cf. also V B 41.

19. *Concluding Unscientific Postscript*, p. 279.

20. Walker Percy, *The Last Gentleman* (New York: Avon Books, 1978), pp. 269, 277, 291.

orbit. Only Christianity can bring it down. That is what Climacus, speaking ironically, says. His Interlude is the ironic moment—the moment of absolute freedom—from which Christianity absurdly promises to save us.

The Greeks defined for Western consciousness the conditions of intelligibility and truth: the "Socratic" view. Christianity has perforated consciousness with the possibility of radical uncertainty, radical insecurity, and radical irrationality. But the inhabitants of that consciousness have, through carelessness, misunderstanding, bad faith, and the force of habit, come to regard this absurdity as a matter of course. His subject matter being what it is—the absolute paradox—Kierkegaard's strategy is to promote not understanding but ineluctable confrontation. His device—the ram in the afternoon—is recommended by the desperate hope that men will pay an exorbitant price to acquire that which they were not sufficiently ironic to recognize as a gift.

V

In 1841 Kierkegaard published his master's thesis, *The Concept of Irony with Constant Reference to Socrates.* From his many characterizations[21] it is possible to conflate a definition: irony is the principle of infinite abstract negative subjectivity. The discovery of this principle is credited to the sophists, who acted on it without knowing what they were doing, but eminently to Socrates, who formulated it *as* a principle and practiced it systematically.[22]

"Infinite abstract negative subjectivity" stands for the liberty of the subject to refuse any determination proposed to him or projected onto him. Absolute freedom: the capacity to say No without limit and without qualification. Which negative capability in a deep sense *is* the subject.

Irony in the literary sense, the figure of speech so-called, is the verbal expression of this negative freedom. Of necessity, an oblique and problematic *modus loquendi.* Infinite abstract negative

21. Cf. Søren Kierkegaard, *The Concept of Irony,* trans. Lee M. Capel (New York: Harper & Row, 1965), pp. 224, 230–34, 238–40, 253, 255, 271–75, 278–79.
22. Ibid., part 1, chap. 3.

subjectivity could hardly be rendered in the finite concrete positive objectivities of ordinary speech. The principle of irony bespeaks itself in words that negate what they say, indeterminately, as they say it.

The textbook examples of irony, like the usual practice of irony, are most imperfect.[23] For instance, "Brutus is an honorable man," with circumflex accent on the "honorable." Antony's statement negates what it says, but not indeterminately. The Roman mob knows that he means exactly the opposite of what he says, that is, "Brutus is a scoundrel." Similarly, the standard textbook definition—"saying one thing and meaning the contrary"—makes irony a special case of allegory: a finite not an infinite negation.

A better example would be the Greek imagined by Kierkegaard, who, invited to dinner, replies: "You can count on me, I shall certainly come; but I must make an exception for the contingency that a tile happens to blow down from a roof and kills me; for in that case I cannot come."[24] The very randomness of the excepted contingency makes it clear that the speaker, though he probably will come to dinner, regards himself as in no position to make any commitments whatsoever.

An even better example would be the pious qualification we often (thoughtlessly) append to our assurances: "God willing." A codicil that tacitly acknowledges the infinite uncertainty of all things; that is, indeterminately and in the abstract ("in principle") disallows all certainty.[25]

Irony—in principle, in fact, and in discourse—is the anomaly of the absolute. Etymologically, the "untied" or the "unbound." Irony is the negative and abstract absolute of subjective freedom, the emancipation of the subject (by which the subject is constituted as such) from every finite ("objective") determination.

The concept of irony instructs the interpretation of Kierkegaard's theory and practice of indirect communication. Indi-

23. Cf. ibid., pp. 264–65.
24. *Concluding Unscientific Postscript*, p. 81.
25. Cf. ibid., p. 80.

rect communication is a "means of expression" wholly self-consuming. It negates not only the said but also the saying. In a word: communication from the standpoint of irony. All of Kierkegaard's texts are written from that standpoint. It is impossible to understand them unless one keeps this constantly in mind. Whether it is possible to understand them *with* this in mind is another question.

A Kierkegaardian text, like any other, is a system of signifiers. It is one thing to find an interpretation of this system. In the case of the *Philosophical Fragments*, the interpretation that is irresistibly insinuated is Christianity. It is another thing altogether to ask about the sense of the words. The former is easy, since Kierkegaard has provided all the clues, everything but the "historical costume" (*PF* 137, *PS* 105). That, he adds, "every divinity student"[26] should be able to furnish. Finding the meaning is much harder but absolutely indispensable. For unless you know the meaning, the interpretation is worthless. It is not much help to know that Kierkegaard is talking about Christianity if you don't know what he is saying about it. And what he is saying about whatever he is talking about is something you get only by deciphering his language. It is illicit to take the formal properties of the interpretation—some system of Christian doctrine—and read them back into Kierkegaard's words. There is no guarantee that what Kierkegaard is saying about Christianity is what anyone else has ever said about it. Indeed, there is massive reason to think otherwise.

Direct (un-ironic) communication is the use of verbal signs to refer to something, thoughts or things, with which sender and receiver are both already acquainted. Or perhaps to direct attention to something with which the sender is familiar and with which the receiver may become familiar if suitably alerted. In any case, this ordinary usage is intentionally referential, and it presupposes on the part of both communicator and recipient a common knowledge or capacity for knowledge of a referent signified

26. *Concluding Unscientific Postscript,* p. 14.

by language, transcendent of language, and in principle public. Meaning, in direct communication, is taken for granted. The order of the signifiers is either determined by the signified or given in advance by the linguistic code, which is itself an object of common knowledge and thus a kind of referent. In direct communication, sense and interpretation tend to coincide. An indirect (ironic) communication is a system of signifiers that obviates reference. When we read, we ordinarily construct hierarchies of signification. At least we project a referent, a transcendent signified, of which the text is signifier. Ordinary uses of language encourage this hierarchizing tendency by offering themselves as icons, indices, or what-have-you of facts or ideas. The order of the sign-surface reflects to us our conventional notions about the order of things and its relation to the order of words. But if the sign-surface is disordered with respect to ordinary usage and conventional notions of meaning, then we are led to reflect upon the signs and the sign-function itself.

The language of the *Fragments* proscribes any hierarchizing of sign and referent. "Christianity" is proposed, by the text itself, as the interpretation of this language. But it does not in any ordinary sense "stand for" Christianity; it does not conventionally describe it, picture it, or point to it. It pretends to elicit Christianity deductively from hypotheses, but the pretense is exposed. It pretends to imagine Christianity fairy-tale fashion, but the imagination fails. And so on. As an indirect communication the *Fragments* is a system of signs that systematically severs its bonds with any referent that it might be supposed to designate. The meaning of the text is therefore to be sought exclusively in the interrelations of the signifiers themselves, their reflection upon each other, and not in their allusion to any transcendent thought or thing.

But there is another turn of the screw. A further irony. Indirect communication not only impedes reference, it also confuses connotation. The relations of the signifiers with each other are deranged, so that meaning is indefinitely postponed. Kierkegaard's texts conventionally violate the conventions of the linguistic codes he works in, philosophical and literary. The movement from signifier to signifier does not yield a satisfactory ordering of the whole. The signifiers invite attention to themselves and to the process of signification. But they do not converge upon a core of sense. The *Fragments* begins several times to propound the unthinkable, interrupts itself to underscore the banality and/or unintelligibility of what it proposes, asserts the superior veridicality of the banal and the unintelligible, and begins again. Only to end (inconclusively) with a dubious "moral"—whatever else this may be, it is certainly different—and the claim, doubly ironic, to have made an advance beyond the master of irony himself (*PF* 139, *PS* 106). The inconstancy of the sign-system, perpetually discounting its implications and cancelling its commitments, prevents the emergence of a stable pattern of meaning.

Indirect communication occurs in the expansion of the interface between sign and referent and in the indefinite deferment of sense procured by the restless play of the signifiers. This is the source of the mystification systematically practiced in Kierkegaard's texts. It is the source, also, of their literary—or as he preferred to say, "aesthetic"—character. For that is what identifies literary language as such: the use of verbal signs to call attention to themselves and to the act of signifying—that is, to block reference and to postpone meaning. Signs as motifs. Poetry and all that.

The pursuit of these exquisite involutions and hermetic introversions prompts an obvious question: why call this a technique of *communication*? Literary language may justify its crypticality and its narcissism by reference to the intrinsic value of the verbal object. But a communication, presumably, communicates something. What is communicated by Kierkegaard's works? In the light of Kierkegaard's own thematic preoccupation with the indecisiveness of reflection it is tempting to suppose that what is communicated is just this indecision itself: the impossibility of halting by reflection the process of reflection and the impossibility of a return by way of reflection to the reality from which reflection is a departure.

The aesthete of *Either/Or* remarks that what the philosophers say about reality is like a sign in a shop window that reads "Pressing Done Here." If you take your clothes in to be pressed, you find that they do not press clothes—they only sell signs.[27] It is tempting to conjecture that what is here said about the philosophers is also true of Kierkegaard. For his own texts are like series of signs, each of which reads "This Way to the Sign." It is tempting, that is, to advance the hypothesis that Kierkegaard's texts are "really" about language, and that the purpose of indirect communication is simply to exhibit the capacity of language (= reflection)[28] for uninterrupted self-reference and interminable deferment. It would certainly be ironic to think that the truth communicated by indirect communication is a truth that can only be communicated by not being communicated at all.

That is tempting and not altogether wrong. But perhaps not good enough. Or better, a bit too ironic (and therefore not ironic at all), like the possibility, entertained and rejected by Climacus, that God might have topped his own understatement in the Incarnation by entering the world and passing through it completely unnoticed.[29] That, he suggests, would not be irony but wrath. An ironic communication, albeit incalculably indirect, is still communication—the silence *in* speech, not the silencing *of* speech.

Because it confounds sense and obstructs reference, Climacus' language may be said to undercut itself as language. But that is too facile. How can language, *being* language, undercut itself *as* language? Can language ever do more than repeat itself, even if not especially when it tries to deny itself? Is literary language a special case, an exception, or is it not rather a distillation of the "essence" of language: to question meaning by multiplying meanings and to fold the referentiality of discourse back on itself. Human language, as Climacus observes, is rooted in self-love (*PF*

27. Søren Kierkegaard, *Either/Or*, trans. David F. Swenson and Lillian Marvin Swenson (Garden City, N.Y.: Doubleday, 1959), 1:31.

28. Søren Kierkegaard, *Johannes Climacus or, De Omnibus Dubitandum Est*, trans. T. H. Croxall (Stanford: Stanford University Press, 1958), pp. 146–54.

29. *PF* 69, *PS* 52. Cf. above, n. 11.

34-35, *PS* 25). Its extravagant fascination with itself in literature is not a perversion of language but a singularly pellucid manifestation of its true nature.

Indirect communication—negative capability, the literary or aesthetic principle—is also, Climacus knew, Socrates' maieutic, a *magisterium* perfected in ignorance and ironic detachment. But Christianity is something else again: not man's communication to men but God's communication to man. The expression of God's (strictly unimaginable) love for man and the execution of his (strictly unthinkable) resolve to consummate this love in the union of Incarnation (*PF,* chap. 2, passim; *PS* 20-34).

Exceeding the normative indirection of Socrates ("this project indisputably goes further than the Socratic" [*PF* 139A, *PS* 106]), the *Philosophical Fragments* wills to be the expression of this expression and the execution of this execution. Which it can only accomplish in the mood of audacious suggestion, by asking the unaskable question:[30] is it possible that Something Else has invaded language, foisting upon it both an interpretation and a meaning, dissolving its autonomy, enslaving it to a sense and committing it to a referent—all of which, as language, it must and will be free of? Is it possible that there is Something that can make language speak what cannot be spoken? Possible. But scarcely thinkable. And surely unspeakable.

> So then perhaps it is no poem, or at any rate not one for which any human being is responsible. . . . But then my soul is filled with new wonder, even more, with the spirit of worship; for it would surely have been strange had this poem been a human production. . . . as you yourself voluntarily exclaim, we stand here before the *Miracle.* . . . the poem is so different from every human poem as not to be a poem at all, but the *Miracle.* [*PF* 44-45, *PS* 33-34]

But what is the difference between a poem and—the Miracle? That is a question hardly to be answered. Can it even be asked?

Maybe that is what Kierkegaard meant when, in presenting

---

30. Cf. above, sect. I.

himself poetically to posterity, he ascribed his work to "Providence," and described that work itself as a "teleological suspension in relation to the communication of truth."[31] That God is uniquely revealed as God in man's nothingness and need is a common theme in Kierkegaard's writings.[32] Man's weakness is God's opportunity. So also perhaps the impotence of language to lay hold on being, its necessary and voluntary self-contentment,[33] is the aperture through which the Other intrudes itself into the affairs and the discourse of men. The language of Kierkegaard's texts is not, like the language of Socratic dialogue, self-effacing. It is effaced in advance by the unspeakable which is incredibly given it to utter. More ironical even than the irony of Socrates, the *Philosophical Fragments* is ~~Kierkegaard's~~ discourse of the Other.

VI

In 1852 Kierkegaard made the following entry in his journal:

Melancholy

Somewhere in the Psalms it says of the rich man that he collects a treasure with great care and "knows not who shall inherit from him": and so too I shall leave behind me, intellectually speaking, a not so little capital; alas, and I know at the same time who will inherit from me, that figure which is so enormously distasteful to me, who up till now has always, and will continue to inherit all good things: the Docent, the professor. . . .*

31. Søren Kierkegaard, *The Point of View for My Work as an Author,* trans. Walter Lowrie (London: Oxford University Press, 1939), p. 91 and chap. 3, passim. On this whole matter, cf. Edward W. Said, *Beginnings: Intention and Method* (New York: Basic Books, 1975), pp. 73–78, 85–88.

32. Cf., e.g., the discourse, "Man's Need of God Constitutes His Highest Perfection," in Søren Kierkegaard, *Edifying Discourses, vol. 2*, trans. David F. Swenson and Lillian Marvin Swenson (Minneapolis: Augsburg Publishing House, 1962), pp. 120–60.

33. Cf. *PF* 18–21, 20 n, on the willed but inevitable nature of sin. *PS* 12–15, 14 n.

*And even if "the professor" were to come across this it would not stop him, it would not have the effect of making his conscience prick him, no, this too would be taught. And this remark again, if the professor were to come across it, would not stop him, no, this too would be taught. For the professor is longer than the tapeworm (which a woman lately got rid of and which measured, according to her husband, who gave thanks in the paper, 200 feet) longer even than that is the professor; and no man in whom there is "the professor" can be freed by another man from that tapeworm, only God can do that, if the man is willing.[34]

Anyone who writes about Kierkegaard (if he is not *all* professor) must confront the tapeworm in fear and trembling. Kierkegaard himself did not escape altogether. Who inscribed that little note in his journal and then doubled back and wrote a footnote to it? Devolutions of the tapeworm.

The image is to be taken with all gravity. Reflection, which is another name for language, is interminable, segment after segment propagating itself and prolonging itself. Without relief. Unless the head is rooted out. The principle must be extirpated. But, as Kierkegaard says, only God can do that.

Who?

---

34. I quote from *The Journals of Søren Kierkegaard*, trans. Alexander Dru (London: Oxford University Press, 1938), nos. 1268 and 1269. I have altered Dru's translation. The original may be found in *Søren Kierkegaards Papirer*, X⁴ A 628, 629.

8

"Psychological Fragments": Kierkegaard's Religious Psychology

VINCENT A. MCCARTHY

At the periphery of nineteenth-century romanticism and well in advance of twentieth-century existentialism, Søren Kierkegaard lived and thought immersed in moods. It is well known and oft-related in his *Journals* and in later biographies that Kierkegaard was cast into emotional depths by circumstances in his own life, many of which he brought upon himself.[1] How Kierkegaard reached these depths is of course not unimportant, but the principal interest in these pages is the self-examination he conducted from them. In these emotional depths, *before* the existentialists and *beyond* the romantics, he explored the self with an eye for detail and with a reflective brilliance that is only slightly marred by his lapses into metaphysics.[2] His preoccupation with and analysis of the emotional life must be understood in relation to the romantics and, as so often with Kierkegaard, as a "corrective." For just as the pseudonym Constantine Constantius set out in *Repetition* to debunk the idea that the cure for a young man's melancholy is simply to fall in love, so Kierkegaard set out more generally to show that an entire sphere of emotional life has a meaning, depth, and ultimate clarity that goes far beyond popular wisdom, poetic *Schwärmerei*, and superficial psychologies of all kinds.

---

1. Cf. Josiah Thompson, *Kierkegaard: A Critical Biography* (New York: Knopf, 1973), which successfully undercuts Kierkegaard hagiographies à la Walter Lowrie.

2. For example, in *The Concept of Anxiety* [Dread], the psychologist Vigilius Haufniensis describes the soul before birth.

The Religious Presupposition

In accomplishing his goal, he remained true to his prediction that if ever there were to be any such thing as *Danish* philosophy, it would distinguish itself from the German in not beginning with nothing.[3] For in his nonpresuppositionless philosophizing, Kierkegaard unabashedly and unembarrassedly presupposes the religious as the deepest ground of the person and as the intentionality of the important sphere of emotional life that he singled out for sustained analysis. In light of this stand, no philosophy—and no psychology—that seeks to investigate his authorship and harvest its fields can proceed in intellectual honesty without confronting that from which, he asserts, all rises. The religious is indeed for Kierkegaard a presupposition, but also a discovery—the discovery of the only sense-giving and equilibrium-restoring source for a series of emotional upheavals. The discovery and its articulation are two-sided: both conceptual and emotional or, in his own terms, dialectical and pathetic. In conscious contrast to all too many romantic poets, Kierkegaard does not engage in a celebration of the range and power of feeling but rather in the discernment of a "logic of the heart" through an examination, empirically and reflectively-speculatively, of the truth of human growth and then in a philosophical statement of the underlying elements that are necessary if emotional life is to make sense (and he was convinced, as an emotional rationalist, that it does). He also engaged in existential experimentation—personal and imaginative —in which other proposed solutions proved to be bankrupt, both in his own life and in the literary existences of aesthetic pseudonyms.

By no means did Kierkegaard consider his "discovery" original. The truth that "Our hearts are restless until they rest in Thee [O

3. In an undated entry of 1844, Kierkegaard writes in his *Journals:* "Danish philosophy—if there ever comes to be such a thing—will be different from German philosophy in that it definitely will not begin with nothing or without any presuppositions whatsoever or explain everything by mediating, because, on the contrary, it begins with the proposition that there are many things between heaven and earth which no philosophy has explained." *Journals and Papers,* trans. Howard V. Hong and Edna H. Hong (Bloomington: Indiana University Press, 1975), vol. 3, pp. 513–14 (no. 3299).

Lord]" can be found in Augustine of Hippo,[4] and of course is older as well. It is an "original" discovery for Kierkegaard only perhaps in the same sense that original sin is original: It is personal and individual and herein has its true significance.[5] Kierkegaard self-consciously inherited his religious understanding of the depths and final end of the person from certain strains in the Christian tradition, particularly from Augustine and Luther and, as he read it, from their New Testament source as well. For him the religious is not simply a frame that encloses a psychological portrait accessible to secular, nonreligious, and even antireligious explorers of the psyche who might simply discard the frame and hold onto the picture. He at least tried to make the religious an integral element in his analysis. To expand the simile of a frame, the religious is like a frame painted onto the canvas itself. He sought to articulate the religious so integrally into his thought that anyone who sought to ignore or discard the religious dimension would have to tear the whole. Whether he fully succeeded or to what extent he did succeed in making the religious an integral part of the whole are questions that deserve to be posed to Kierkegaard, and no less to would-be philosophical and psychological eclectics who seek to make off with only what suits them. Rejection he did not fear, arbitrary eclecticism he would abhor as much as any other thinker, even he who entitled works *Philosophical "Fragments"* and *"Unscientific" Postscript*. For such titles are playful and, for those who know him, finally underline rather than distract from the seriousness of his enterprise.

The Concept of Moods

What, then, is Kierkegaard about, in seriousness and jest, in an authorship that is formally a parody of much of the poetic, philosophical, and theological literature of the day? He was of course, like any classic and complex author, about a great deal and yet in the end about one principal idea. His description of himself as a religious writer—in addition to his stress on the religious as his presupposition—is the clue, should we need one.

---

4. *Confessiones,* I, ii.
5. The literal meaning of the Danish *Arvesynden* is "inherited sin."

In this paper, I confine myself to his analysis of the stormy emotional life of the potentially religious subject, his presentation of the human spirit weathering the internal storms involved in reaching Infinite Spirit. Kierkegaard restricted his psychologizing to the religious and focused on four moods in the evolution of religious subjectivity. Further, he had a concept of these moods, even if he never wrote a formal treatise on moods as such. His presentation of his concept of moods is neither simple nor straightforward, in characteristic fashion, and for this he had his deliberate reasons. Moreover, despite the extensive descriptions he provides, he never really defines a mood as such; and the four cardinal moods that he emphasizes, as well as their manner of presentation, are surprising: irony, anxiety, melancholy, and despair.

Anxiety and despair are the less problematical: each is the clear subject of a treatise by a transparent pseudonym (*The Concept of Anxiety* [Dread] by Vigilius Haufniensis and *The Sickness unto Death* by Anti-Climacus). Irony, which is initially the most surprising "mood," was the subject of Kierkegaard's Copenhagen dissertation, for which he was awarded a degree by the university and the epithet "master of irony" by the public. Irony, for Kierkegaard, was not essentially a matter of wit or a sharp tongue but a coloration of the entire personality, a tonality (Danish: *Stemning*) that characterized the way one experienced the world and oneself in the world. It is a mood of rebellion and rejection of finitude. Melancholy is longing for the Beloved, not as the young and the romantics understood it but rather as did the Christian mystics. Kierkegaard's concept of the moods of religious subjectivity contains a discernible "dialectic of moods." And his rational examination of emotional life constitutes a logic of moods, a clear and meaningful ordering of crisis and resolution in what would at first appear to be merely a chaos of emotions. Moreover, in each instance he would hold that crisis is both predictable and necessary.

"Mood" and the Moods of Religious Subjectivity

Kierkegaard is interested principally in moods related to reflection and self-consciousness, moods that intensify the experience of subjectivity and call one's identity into question. A mood for Kierkegaard is an attunement, a coloration affecting perception—minimizing, maximizing—while one is in the mood. "Being in a mood" is a way of indicating its hold. For some, such as Heidegger, one is always in a mood, always colored, attuned; and one mood gives way to another in a steady stream. One does not choose one's mood in the sense of selecting it, but for Kierkegaard as for Heidegger, once in a mood one needs to accept it and the revelation about the self effected by it.

The four moods of religious subjectivity that Kierkegaard examines have no external objects and are essentially about the self, as indicated by their intensification of subjectivity. The moods make one more conscious of oneself, of the problem of the self in two senses: the self as shattered and a burden and the self as task to be accomplished. The moods thus throw one back upon oneself and reveal the task and destiny of becoming an authentic self: whole and grounded once again in the One Possible Source who is by degrees recognized.

Moods come and go, but all four that Kierkegaard considers are tied to one fundamental existential state—that is, the shattered self in need of reconstitution; and they endure and return for as long as this state endures. The moods can, however, lie dormant, and a dialectic of moods, as Kierkegaard portrays it, only occurs in the religiously sensitive personality. This is, however, no privileged sphere; all are religiously conditioned, even if apparently to different degrees. Each of the moods is in a sense already there: its message is implicitly present in the personality until explication begins in an awakening, setting-into-motion of spirit in which the consciousness and task of religious subjectivity emerge. Accepting and going through the moods thus constitute a passageway for finite spirit advancing toward the Infinite.

The "solution" to a mood is, in choosing it (in the sense of accepting), to choose oneself in each of the four in a somewhat different way, as I shall explain. Each for Kierkegaard comes and goes, but each also builds to a crisis stage demanding resolution. However, there is no assurance that the crisis will be resolved, no assurance that one will arrive where the moods ever more clearly direct one. This is true in two senses: first, in that each step requires an act of the will that one is not compelled to make (even if one is emotionally punished for not making it); second, in that the final resolution—reconciliation of God and man, refusion of the self—results from a divine grace that, although promised, cannot be presumed. As a spiritually qualified being, one is equally free to become oneself and to destroy oneself; and Kierkegaard's writings portray characters who rather clearly will *not* go the whole way, most notably Johannes of *Either/Or*, who is thereby considered "diabolical."[6]

Hegel and Kierkegaard

Such terms as "concept," "dialectic," "crisis," "contradiction," and "necessity" (to name but a few) immediately conjure up the ghost of Hegel. Hegelian terminology abounds in Kierkegaard and, for all his rebellion against the Berlin philosopher, the Copenhagen writer remains more indebted to him than he would probably wish to acknowledge. The dialectic of moods, which we will examine in more detail below, has nothing less than a Hegelian structure, as does Kierkegaard's thought generally. Each mood has an initial state; a crisis phase in which inner opposition is brought into open contradiction and then intensified to the point of requiring resolution; and finally a resolution that is itself nothing less than a Hegelian *Aufhebung*—a cancellation and preservation.[7] Kierkegaard's psychology of moods is a detailed examination of the second phase, although attention is devoted to the first and third as well. His study of moods is in fact the study of

6. In *Purity of Heart*, Kierkegaard, in his own name, writes: "Alas, it is horrible to see a man rush toward his own destruction. It is horrible to see him dance on the rim of the abyss without any intimation of it. But this clarity about himself and about his own destruction is even more horrible. It is horrible to see a man seek comfort by hurling himself into the whirlpool of despair. But this coolness is still more horrible . . . that he should quietly choose to be a witness to his own destruction!" (trans. D. V. Steere [New York: Harper & Row, 1956], p. 65).

7. Kierkegaard has, however, *four* cardinal moods rather than the expectable Hegelian triad. There are many additional departures from and twists on Hegelian structure, of course.

inner conflict in the delicate human synthesis as it moves toward a demand for resolution that consciousness can no longer ignore.

The principal difference between Hegel and Kierkegaard is contained in the Kierkegaardian category of the "individual." For Kierkegaard, the concrete existing individual seemed to have been dissolved in the Hegelian System of philosophy.[8] His writings therefore begin with a highly individualized subject who, while surely an intellectual and philosophically inclined, is unaffected by the Hegelian world-historical absent-mindedness about being an existing subject and in fact increasingly agonizes over the meaning of his subjectivity. And although the aesthetic character Johannes is a creation of Kierkegaard's mind (and partly based on his own romantic youth), there is still no question of privileged access to him. One need not have reached the level of "absolute knowledge" in Hegelian philosophy in order to understand the pathetic and critical nature of his existence. His records—principally the "Diary of the Seducer" and the "Diapsalmata" but also the more theoretical "Rotation Method"—are available to all.[9]

Subsequent Kierkegaard works become increasingly abstract and general as the pseudonyms become increasingly transparent. Nonetheless, while in the later works the analysis is of Everyman, the universal subject, rather than the highly individualized, fan-

8. Kierkegaard has not infrequently been proved to be wrong. Indeed, he was narrow-minded, overzealous, and self-righteous in all of what he regarded as the major "occurrences" of his life. He thus precipitously broke his engagement to Regine Olsen, provoked attack by the *Corsair,* and in the process ruined the academic career of a prominent contributor, P. L. Møller, and mocked Grundtvig, whose popular socialism his own bourgeois isolation could not comprehend. Only in the instance of his broken engagement did he subsequently acknowledge error.

For philosophers, the most famous event in his largely literary existence was his attack upon Hegel. And here he may have erred as well, and with his characteristic excesses. Although his direct objects are in many cases Hegelians in Copenhagen rather than G. W. F. Hegel himself, Kierkegaard proves underinformed about Hegel's philosophy time and again—or at least does not indicate that he has taken other interpretative possibilities into account.

9. That is, once they have been sprung loose from the writing-table where Victor Eremita, "editor" of *Either/Or,* originally "found" them.

tastic subject of *Either/Or,* the emphasis remains (with its limitations) upon the *individual* who must individually realize the universally open and proper destiny of Christian subjectivity. In contrast, the aesthete Johannes possesses only a false and deceptive individuality, which then gradually unmasks itself. And the true, religious individuality promised at the stage of the grace beyond sin-consciousness in *Sickness unto Death* is no less genuine in being available to Everyman. It is never a collective destiny. The individual becomes himself through personal deed. He is not, à la Hegel, united into identity with the Infinite. For Kierkegaard, the divine-human relationship is decidedly vertical, a relationship of subjects who remain distinct, in contrast to the horizontal divine-human encounter and merger in Hegel's monism.[10]

The main point in the Hegel-Kierkegaard comparison relevant to the topic of this paper is made in the opening pages of *Either/ Or,* which disputes the Hegelian contention that the outer is the inner and the inner the outer. Kierkegaard did not need to think of himself as standing Hegel on his feet (Hegel had described speculation as walking on one's head). He sought rather to turn Hegel's method not inside-out but *outside-in:* to describe a phenomenology of finite spirit not in the race or social group, nor in the broader culture, but in the inner life of the existing subject. This he did self-consciously against a Hegel whose intellectual accomplishment he respected—not as absolute knowledge but rather as a thought-experiment of a high order, and as such a form of intellectual romanticism.

10. Much more could be said of the Hegel-Kierkegaard relationship, of the Hegelian backdrop to much of Kierkegaard's authorship, and much more of course has been written about it elsewhere. One cannot and should not ignore it; but one equally ought not to be seduced by it (any more than by Kierkegaard's biography). It is intrinsically interesting and exercises a legitimate fascination. But the result of attention to a Hegelian background ought not to be the obscuring of a Kierkegaardian foreground, if it is one's intention to write about *Kierkegaard.* (Writing about *Hegel* through a Kierkegaard-Hegel comparison is perfectly legitimate but simply a different exercise.) Here again it must be conceded that Kierkegaard contributes to the problem, but always sets his "fragments of philosophy" in relief against—and as relief from—the Hegelian System.

Diagnosing a Moody Aesthete

Kierkegaard's analysis of moods begins before his "formal authorship" (which he describes in *The Point of View for My Work as an Author*) in his dissertation, *The Concept of Irony with Constant Reference to Socrates*. There he engages in a criticism of romantic and Hegelian irony, and he continues in more concentrated form in the examination of aesthetic existence in the formal and pseudonymous authorship. The dissertation criticizes romantics (and Hegel, whose System he regarded as intellectual romanticism) on intellectual points, while the aesthetic authorship criticizes the bankruptcy of a lived-out romantic existence. But the two lines merge in the aesthete Johannes of *Either/Or,* who is an intellectual aesthete, and also in the young Johannes Climacus of the unpublished "De omnibus dubitandum est."

Johannes of *Either/Or*[11] is a formidable and fascinating character, an individualist and would-be individual whose existence is rooted in imagination and who in an awakening consciousness of the religious defies it and the true individuality it promises because it is not his own creation. Kierkegaard's aesthete (like Kierkegaard himself) is in fact burdened with self-consciousness. He can neither "let himself go" nor quite contain himself. No sooner does a possibility occur to him than his fantasy spins out every conceivable variation, which he then compares and judges. In the process, he robs himself of the spontaneity of action; he wears himself out in this fashion. He both loves it and hates it; but more significantly still, he cannot stop it.

He is an *intellectual* aesthete: his are the pleasures of thought, of fantasy, of the detailed plan of action. As seducer his pleasure consists in developing the *idea* of seduction, which is crowned by the successful execution of the idea. The idea is more important than the physical conquest, and the latter is almost an afterthought (except that it is a necessary aspect of the idea). Moreover, it is his intellectuality that makes the seducer so diabolical in

11. Following a clue given by Victor Eremita, I hold Johannes to be the anonymous author of all the papers of part 1 of *Either/Or.*

the "Diary of the Seducer," not the number of maidens. Don Juan needed 1,003 conquests;[12] Johannes boasts of only one and feels he compares very well. The same intellectuality renders him so pitiful in the "Diapsalmata," which although formally opening *Either/Or* really record the results of the intellectual aestheticism depicted there.

Kierkegaard's subsumption of the intellectual into the aesthetic stage is an important point in his writing. Under what other existential category might it be placed? Little of it is moral, and it would certainly not claim for itself the title religious.[13] His major point against Enlightenment philosophy, romanticism, and Idealism is that an exclusively intellectual life is existentially bankrupt. The roller-coaster moods of the aesthete are witness to this.

But Kierkegaard does not merely depict an intellectual romantic who is a prisoner of moods, who is ironic and melancholy, anxious and despairing, in our usual senses of these words and in the special sense he will emphasize. He scrutinizes the emotional life of his intellectual aesthete as others in his time did not and thereby takes emotional life with the utmost seriousness, as the unfolding development of spirit on the individual level.

What is the solution for the aesthete of *Either/Or*? Not the bourgeois ethical humanism of part 2, as becomes clear in a rereading of Johannes's papers after the judge's criticisms in the letters of part 2. For part 1 successfully anticipates many of the good judge's objections and sees through to the limitations of the alternative (that is, ethical humanism) proposed by Judge William even before the judge poses it. Thus *Either/Or* constitutes an existential neither/nor, requiring a third option and, true to its Hegelian thought structure, also a both/and, since elements of the aesthetic and of the ethical will be preserved in the religious.

The sole solution Kierkegaard holds out for Johannes and for

12. "The immediate Don Juan must seduce 1,003; the reflective need only seduce one, and what interests us is how he did it." *Either/Or*, trans. David F. Swenson and Lillian Marvin Swenson (New York: Doubleday, Anchor Books, 1959), part 1, p. 107.

13. Of course, moral and religious people can also be intellectual and aesthetic as well.

every aesthete—the religious—emerges gradually from the aesthetic writings but is declared openly along the way in parallel religious discourses that Kierkegaard published under his own name. The solution for this crisis of reflection is not "absolute knowledge" in the manner of Hegel but, more modestly, knowledge of the self in a God-relationship.

The aesthete already has an inkling of the religious, but certainly not the religious as represented by the Danish state church, nor by systematic theology, which even in out-of-the-way Copenhagen had been infected with the intellectual aestheticism of Hegelian philosophical theology (the chief symbol being Martensen, who as professor was attacked in Kierkegaard's dissertation and as bishop was prominently included in the "attack upon Christendom"). Nor is the religious comprised of pietistic sentimentality about Jesus, even if, as we shall see, something of pietistic sin-consciousness remains in the treatise on despair. The religious for Kierkegaard means, in the end, contemporaneousness with the Jesus of the New Testament, in the ongoing and developing encounter of the individual finite spirit with the Infinite (terminology one may view as straight out of Hegel, but the relationship surely not).

The process in which this takes place is traced in the analysis of the aesthete Johannes—in *Either/Or*, the treatise on melancholy—and in the more general treatises on anxiety and despair, as well as in the dissertation itself. Moving from *Either/Or* to the formal treatises, one may even "flesh out" the moods of Johannes and locate him in Kierkegaard's scheme.[14]

Irony: The Mood of Rebellion against Finitude[15]

Irony is the first crisis-mood in an aesthetic existence on the verge of dissolution—that is, an existence lived on the level of

14. This I have done at greater length in *The Phenomenology of Moods in Kierkegaard* (The Hague: Martinus Nijhoff, 1978), chap. 5.

15. Irony is mentioned as a mood in *The Concept of Irony* in a discussion of Solger's attempt at a philosophical grasp of irony. There irony is termed "that mood wherein contradictions annihilate themselves," p. 334.

pleasure (sensual and intellectual) and centered exclusively in oneself. As the pseudonym Johannes Climacus remarks:

> Irony is an existential determination, and nothing is more ridiculous than to suppose that it consists in the use of certain phraseology.... Whoever has essential irony has it all day long, not bound to any specific form, because it is the infinite within him. [*Postscript*, p. 450]

Irony represents a decisive *prise de conscience* about the world (finitude) and about oneself in the world. It begins in that first moment of reflection in which one realizes that one is unsatisfied, uncompleted by the world. Kierkagaard thus speaks of it as raising one out of immediate (nonreflective) existence and, having raised one, leaving one in midair (*Irony*, p. 85 n.). The ironist is suspended in the air, like the coffin of Mohammed, between two magnets—in this case, the magnets of finitude and infinitude.

One ironizes, according to Kierkegaard, because the world has lost its validity (*Irony*, p. 276). The implicit promise of the world to satisfy man's higher needs is experienced as broken and, in reflection, is increasingly recognized as unfulfillable. Here Kierkegaard means in particular the needs of man as a spiritually qualified being. Kierkegaard's insight is psychological but also metaphysical—based on an understanding of the person as tied to and ultimately grounded in a higher Spirit, that is, God. Disappointment breeds resentment, and the ironist turns increasingly against the world and his fellows, and sometimes against himself.

Kierkegaard's dissertation first discusses the more usual associations of irony as a tool of discourse, which he does not deny but rather views as only a surface phenomenon. Thus the rebel against finitude sometimes employs rhetorical irony: saying the opposite of what he means but at a deeper level reflecting the difference between reality and appearance; sometimes he indulges in the private irony of letting others appear as fools in their illusions, as he watches from some superior and unshared viewpoint. In the first instance he plays on the fact that everything is not as it appears or sounds; in the second he engages in exploding the cherished illusions of others.

Kierkegaard draws a neat line between the ironist and the satirist, which we may find less than convincing. His view is that the satirist is a reformer at heart, seeking to correct the foibles of mankind (whether in the gentler Horatian mode or in the harsher Juvenalian). But his point in the contrast is that the ironist, at this stage in his development, is unethical: he has no serious concern for others. His goal in engaging in ironic discourse is a kind of one-upmanship, the self-satisfaction of an ailing and solitary self taking some brief pleasure in the enduring illusions of others. In this view, the ironist is still tied to the aesthetic even if already at its boundaries. Kierkegaard also distinguishes between the ironist and the prophet and holds that the prophet, even if disclaiming some present state of affairs, does not break with his contemporaries but stays among them and calls them to a higher and common future. (Kierkegaard does not mention a prominent biblical exception to his conception of the prophet—the reluctant prophet Jonah, who was hardly disposed to bring Yahweh's message of reform and pardon to his long-standing enemy in Nineveh). The neat division does not really hold, but we grasp Kierkegaard's point: the ironist is here self-centered and careless of a world whose illusions he has rejected.

When Kierkegaard's dissertation turns to the deeper manifestations of irony in the new ironist's existence, he breaks new ground in the concept of irony. And here he indicates both positive and negative aspects of its negating power.

On the positive side, Kierkegaard recognizes the rebellion of irony as representing the first moments of genuine subjectivity, of the break with the masses and the emergence of an individual. He terms irony an incitement to subjectivity, and the ironist himself he calls a prophecy of and abbreviation for a complete personality (*Irony*, p. 177). He even goes so far as to say that no authentic human life, no life worthy of being called human, is possible without irony.[16] Here he means not the tool irony, which only a few can wield, but ironic consciousness, which is accessible to all.

16. *Irony*, p. 338. This is also thesis XV of the dissertation itself.

Irony is negativity itself—"infinite absolute negativity," as he terms it—and it will be no surprise to anyone familiar with Hegelian dialectic that it will have negative aspects that will require something beyond irony. (The expectation arises from the Hegelian underpinnings of the dissertation, indeed, the Hegelian structure in which irony is considered under the rubrics of possible, actual, and necessary. Hence movement into negative moments and beyond are fully in order.)

Irony as negativity means quite simply that it *only* negates. Herein lies its contribution to subjectivity—freeing from the hold of finitude in a nonreflective existence—but also its limitation. For irony does not provide content to the existence that it has severed from the world. The ironist is cut off from the world, or so he experiences himself in what is really only but another illusion. He no longer looks to the world for the sustenance of his spiritual life, yet he still requires sustenance. He becomes alienated from others. Even a relationship to other ironic subjects proves illusory since irony, while it can be seductive and an incitement to love,[17] cannot provide the positive bond that establishes a relationship, the positive third element that makes love or friendship possible. In Kierkegaard's view, the German romantics of the late eighteenth and early nineteenth centuries illustrate the dangers of irony. For, cut off from the finite, they seek new moorings in the infinite. Kierkegaard would be the first to stress the Infinite that alone can ground subjectivity but rejects the false infinity that is approached only in and through imagination. The danger of irony is that it succumbs to the illusion that it can accomplish what it now desires. The ironist, having broken with the finite, seeks to soar to the infinite. One might term the infinity to which he would soar a "bad infinity" à la Hegel—an infinity that does not contain the finite within it. The solution for the ironist amounts to a kind of "good finitude" along the same Hegelian model—a reacceptance of a finitude in which the Infinite is recognized as present.

17. So Kierkegaard views it in the famous relationship between the sage Socrates and the adventurer Alcibiades. Cf. *Irony*, pp. 213 ff.

Irony breaks other illusions but must catch itself before it plunges into an empty infinity of fantasy. For having realized the unworthiness of former objects of desire, it may seek to satisfy itself through the creation—and destruction—of imaginative objects of desire.

Without genuine content, without continuity, and without perspective, the ironist by degrees moves into a crisis in his rebellion against finitude: he has rejected the world but cannot reach the Infinite, and certainly not an Infinite outside of the finite. He lives "hypothetically and subjunctively"; he lapses under the sway of moods and feelings (*Irony*, pp. 300–01). And the only unity in the discontinuity that is his life is the "hungry satiety" of boredom.[18]

His very reflection that at first freed him now entraps him, as he finds it impossible to act spontaneously. He is always the spectator-actor (*Irony*, p. 300), watching from out of the tiny window of the isolated ego every action, which often enough he has even thought out in advance (as in the case of Johannes of *Either/Or*).

Incapable of satisfying the deeper spiritual needs of subjectivity, the life of irony finally leads to despair.[19] Since we have been tracing a Hegelian movement here, we may expect resolution and degrees of resolution as well. Indeed, the Hegelian triadic movement of (1) universal initial state, (2) particularization and movement into opposition, and finally (3) resolution-reconciliation-individualization can be discerned here and one may well assign phases of the ironic existence to different Hegelian moments—even if, in imitation of Hegel himself, one may seem to be stretching things a bit in this instance in order to press the disorganized stuff of existence into neat conceptual slots.

One may thus schematize the life of irony as follows: an initial moment of immersion in a finitude which in and of itself cannot

18. *Irony*, p. 302. Kierkegaard goes on, pseudonymously, to a witty, ironic analysis of boredom in the "Rotation Method" of *Either/Or*, part 1.

19. *Irony*, p. 286. This is despair in its usual sense. Only mastered irony leads on to despair as sin-consciousness.

satisfy the infinite longing of the human spirit; a moment of opposition between the finite self and the finite world[20] that culminates in rejection of the world and in the requirement of reconciliation; finally, a moment of reconciliation and resolution that resolves the crisis of the rebellious mood of irony.

Reconciliation with finitude takes place only after the finite subject, in an increasing self-consciousness, moves on to acquaintance with the Infinite—that is, to discovery of the presence of the divine life of Infinite Spirit within individual human spirit. Here one chooses oneself in one's eternal validity, based on a relationship to the divine.[21]

The first choice of self (the second choice of self will be discussed in the outline of the mood of despair) constitutes the final positivity after the negativity of irony and also constitutes passing beyond the boundaries of aesthetic categories to the ethico-religious. In addition, it constitutes a "mastered irony": an irony in which one is freed from finitude but also is able to live in finitude and to act in the finite world once again (in contrast to the ironic poet, who only dreams)—a world now enriched by the consciousness of the infinite. One does not, however, come to a mastered irony before passing through other crisis moods and their ever-more-explicit revelation of the religious depths of the self.

Anxiety: The Mood of Possibility

The second critical mood of the internally dissolving aesthetic life is anxiety. Since its "material cause" is at base human possibility, it belongs to every sphere of life and not exclusively to the aesthetic. For Kierkegaard, however, there is a special anxiety crisis in the aesthetic that leads to the surmounting of the asethetic itself. Human being—for Kierkegaard a synthesis of body, mind, and spirit—always has possibility. And having possibility is precisely that which is experienced in the mood of anxiety. But since

20. An opposition of the finite to the Infinite is presupposed.
21. This—to try to clarify Kierkegaard's paradoxical terminology—I would term the first act of despair. This is the despair to which Judge William advises the aesthete Johannes.

possibility is unactualized, Kierkegaard and subsequent existentialist writers term it the "nothing" of anxiety. The experience of possibility finally means the experience of one essential possibility, and its actualization constitutes crossing over into the ethico-religious. Moreover, the resolution of the essential anxiety crisis is also for Kierkegaard the resolution of the negativity of irony—that is, the choice of the self in relation to the Infinite. The seriousness of the mood is reflected in the alarm and fascination that attend it and that constitute the ambiguous aspect of the experience. Kierkegaard speaks of it as the "sympathetic antipathy" and "antipathetic sympathy" of anxiety.

Kierkegaard's 1844 treatise on anxiety, published under the thinly pseudonymous name Vigilius Haufniensis, "Watchman of Copenhagen," was such a serious undertaking that he departed from his custom of publishing accompanying edifying discourses and instead sought to balance it with the witty (and as yet untranslated) *Prefaces.* The work on anxiety is subtitled "a psychological deliberation oriented in the direction of the problem of original sin." It begins with sin and will end with sin but first seeks the proper mood for dealing with sin. This, its author notes, must not be the mood of metaphysics, that is, indifference, nor the mood of psychology, that is, curiosity (*Dread* [*Anxiety*], p. 14). For the point of the work is not to *think* about sin or merely to observe it but to discern the psychological process by which finite spirit moves according to an inner dynamism toward recovering itself from sin. When sin is talked about, Haufniensis remarks, the mood tells whether one has the right concept. Seriousness is the mood for discussing sin, and this leads to the mood of anxiety in which the exit from sin can begin.

The work begins with the sin of Adam and attempts to interpret the theological teaching on original sin in such a way that Adam keeps a special role in the human race and in the history of sin but without releasing every other man from the responsibility of his own fall into sin.[22] Original sin as "sinning in Adam" comes to

22. Adam is the first to experience anxiety and the first to sin and also the first to bring the curious quantity "objective anxiety" into the world. This category is

mean sinning *as* Adam. *Why* one sins is not really explained and remains a mystery (as it also does in Kant's treatment of the fall[23]). *How* one sins leads Kierkegaard-Haufniensis into the speculative re-creation of the first state, of Adam and of Everyman, before sin: how it must have been, if man falls and is to be considered responsible for the fall, and therefore how it was. This leads to a consideration of what we might term "primal anxiety," in which Kierkegaard tries to think that twinkling-of-an-eye in which sleeping spirit, already immersed in the nothing of anxiety by virtue of innocence-ignorance, awakens and swoons in the dizzying moment of possibility from which it then arises to find itself in sin.[24] The treatise then moves on to the heart of the matter: anxiety in the sinner and anxiety that paves the way for overcoming sin.

Kierkegaard-Haufniensis is essentially concerned with the possibility of continuing in sin or else of overcoming it, an emphasis reflected in the fact that approximately one-fourth of the treatise is devoted to this, under the category "anxiety for the good." Here he examines the attempt to flee from the good and from the consciousness of oneself as sinner—a flight that he terms demoniacal.[25]

---

not the only dubious point in the work. In addition, one might cite the speculative re-creation of the fall and the assertion of the culmination of anxiety for a second time in women at the moment of childbirth. Modern feminists will also take offense at the underlying notion that men are more spiritual than women, the latter being more sensual.

23. Kierkegaard gets no further in finding a satisfactory explanation for the passage from innocence to sin than did Kant in part 1 of *Religion within the Limits of Reason Alone* (1793) (trans. Theodore M. Greene and Hoyt H. Hudson, New York: Harper Torchbooks, 1960 [orig. pub. La Salle, Ill: Open Court, 1934]).

24. In his interpretation of the biblical account of the Fall, Kierkegaard-Haufniensis sees the prohibition not to eat of the fruit as awakening anxiety, for it awakens the possibility of freedom (p. 47). Kierkegaard seeks to make an important point against Hegel here. According to Kierkegaard, innocence is a state sufficient unto itself and does not require perfection in a dialectical movement. For Hegel, ignorance requires fall, that is, knowledge of good and evil. Cf. Hegel, *Lectures on the Philosophy of Religion* (1821–31), part 3 ("The Absolute Religion," in vol. 3 of translation), trans. E. B. Speirs and J. B. Sanderson (1895) (New York: Humanities Press, 1962), pp. 48 ff.

25. The parallel category—"anxiety for the evil"—would be the inauthentic

The decisive and religiously qualified anxiety crisis revolves around the essential possibility confronting the fallen individual. Sin is not overcome in one single step, but the shattering experience and recovery of possibility in anxiety represents a decisive break from its hold. Passing into and through anxiety, and thus in some sense overcoming it by accepting its revelation of religious possibility, occurs in the first choice of self as a self in relationship to God. But since one is fallen, the choice of self also means taking on the consciousness that the relationship is at present one of separation and that one is alone responsible for this. (In the higher crisis of despair, one reaches the distressing consciousness that one is unable to reconstitute the original divine-human unity as it existed before fall.)[26]

So long as a subject lives he has possibilities. Hence anxiety is never annihilated (*Dread*, p. 104). More Hegel-like, it is *aufgehoben:* canceled/preserved (p. 86). Choice of the self in God-relationship is the actualization of possibility, a kind of giving positive content to the "nothing" of anxiety. But further possibility remains and thus anxiety with it. Anxiety is most decisively— but still not completely—overcome in the mood of despair, with which Kierkegaard links anxiety in several places.[27]

If we should wish to see Hegelian triadic movement here (but with the qualification that for Kierkegaard there is no *necessity* of moving from innocence to fall), it would be as follows. Primordial state: innocence as ignorance. Particularization and opposition: fall and the opposition of the finite to the Infinite within, culminating in the wrenching experience of one's essential religious possibility. Resolution: the first choice of the self.

Kierkegaard-Haufniensis' upbuilding teaching in *The Concept*

---

attempt, through fake remorse, to escape from sin-consciousness and the attendant pain through some bargain-priced salvation.

26. Kierkegaard, like Hegel, speaks of taking on responsibility for the fall. Unlike Hegel, however, he does not regard the fall as necessary. More unlike Hegel still, he does not regard rising from a fallen state as a natural possibility. Self-recovery is only partial, before the moment of free grace.

27. It is another paradox of his terminology that the cure for anxiety, that is, actualizing possibility, is termed "despair." Here it is conceived in the same sense as in *Either/Or:* choice of the self in relationship to the Eternal.

of Anxiety culminates in chapter 5: "Anxiety as a Saving Experience by Means of Faith." The emphasis is upon both saving experience and faith. For only faith properly identifies the possibility that will restore the fallen self—that is, a relationship, as repentant sinner, to the God who appeared in time. It "saves" insofar as it delivers one from the finite over to the Infinite, in the *prise de conscience* of a God-relationship. The experience of anxiety is also held to be the final purging from the finitude from which the ironist was already in flight but which he can only imaginatively escape. There is no leaving finitude. Instead, anxiety brings the revelation of the possibility of an authentic finitude restored to relationship with the Infinite. It is the break with the old, the first step into the new and the positivity sought.

"Religious Melancholy": The Mood of Longing for the Infinite

"Religious melancholy" (*Tungsind*) is already a second moment of melancholy. It is the melancholy of a subject become reflective in the wake of the failure of all finite objects to satisfy an unquenchable longing. *Melancholi,* the first moment and etymologically the same word we use for all forms of melancholy, is (merely) the longing of poets and young men, the sweet and seductive pain of not possessing an object of desire. *Tungsind* (German: *Schwermut*), which I here loosely render as "religious melancholy," is an advanced case of the same spiritual malady. For it is indeed as a spiritual condition that Kierkegaard regards it: the search and longing of an evolving finite human spirit for a worthy and attainable object of desire. In the second and reflective moment of melancholy, the possible object of desire is becoming increasingly and unavoidably clear to the subject's consciousness. This occurs for Kierkegaard's several melancholic aesthetes in a "process of elimination" of finite objects until they are left only with the possibility of the Infinite itself.

Tungsind is a reflective and more critical melancholy. Etymologically it means "heavy-spirited" and refers to the increasingly heavy burden of a subjectivity no longer nourished by the finite and as yet not positively linked to the Infinite. In Kierkegaard's aesthetes, it is also a melancholy of gloom, reserve, and empty isolation.[28]

Kierkegaard depicts *Tungsind* as the natural development of *Melancholi* and would thereby imply that any melancholy cured by romantic love is not the genuine article. This is his clear meaning in *Repetition,* for example.

Kierkegaard analyzes melancholy in three works. *Either/Or,* part 1, is the presentation of an engaging melancholic; part 2 is the analysis of his melancholy by an older, married friend, who embodies the ethical and has essentially overcome melancholy. The aesthete of part 1 is well on his way to becoming reflective about his melancholy and knows that his attempt to live in aesthetic categories—sensual and intellectual—cannot succeed. But he refuses, "demoniacally" Haufniensis might add, to make the act of will required—that is, to affirm himself in a relationship to the Infinite. One of the reasons for his defiant stance seems to be a pride offended by the idea of "salvation" from some source other than himself. The theologian might say that he simply refuses to accept the fact of his "creaturehood," that he would be his own god and creator or perish in the attempt rather than fulfill some spiritual destiny he himself had not ordained. His only real choice is to accept his God-given spiritual destiny or to refuse it. Both refusal and non-choice are choices against spirit, and the chaos and eruptions in the aesthete's inner life are interpreted by Judge William in part 2 as spirit's revenge: "The spirit will not let itself be mocked, it revenges itself upon you, it binds you with the chain of melancholy [*Tungsind*]" (p. 208). However, the judge also tries to console the suffering aesthete with the positivity of melancholy: it indicates the movement of finite spirit toward the Infinite so that what appears as present bad fortune may appear someday in retrospect as good fortune (p. 194)—if only the aesthete will advance as inner dynamism presses him.

Repetition, by the aesthetic psychologist Constantine Constantius, is a self-proclaimed psychological examination of a young man whose melancholy has not been cured by romantic love.

28. Literally "shut-upness" (*Indesluttethed*).

"Such a melancholy [*Melancholi*] has never before presented itself in my practice" (*Repetition,* p. 38), remarks the surprised psychologist, and he ultimately withdraws when he begins to see that the religious is the base of the problem. He has reached the limits of his competence, as he puts it. Constantine and the young man (whom Constantine later admits is a poetic fiction) simultaneously discover the religious nature of melancholy, the latter through reflection, the former through observation (and both adding conjecture, since the religious is not reached by either reflection or observation).

The young man, described as at the age when maturity of spirit announces itself (p. 36), was melancholy, has fallen in love, and comes to his friend-psychologist more melancholy than ever. His is *Melancholi.* But prompted to reflection by his romance and the crisis of an engagement he feels he cannot carry through to marriage, he is well on his way to *Tungsind.* The young girl was not the object of his longing after all. She is not the ideal and is unlikely to take consolation in being called his "muse" (p. 44). She is—more unflattering still—an Aristotelian efficient cause of his melancholy, bringing it to the point of crisis and the demand for resolution.

Stages on Life's Way contains another version of a broken romance and presentation of a melancholy at the stage of *Tungsind* in Quidam's Diary ("Guilty?/Not Guilty?"), where in alternating morning and evening entries the melancholy young man by day recreates the break-up of his engagement one year ago and by night agonizes over a lingering guilt.[29]

Quidam, the diarist (who later turns out to be a poetic creation of Frater Taciturnus), begins his entries in *Tungsind* and recognizes it as his very nature from the very first page (*Stages,* p. 198). When his engagement breaks up, he echoes the struggle of the young Augustinus recorded in the *Confessions* when he writes, "And are there not as it were two natures striving within me?" (p.

29. It hardly needs to be said that both *Repetition* and "Guilty?/Not Guilty?" are highly autobiographical, but it does need to be emphasized that Kierkegaard's point is not indulgence of his own undeniable susceptibility to melancholy but rather an analysis of the mood.

205). He reflects in a midnight entry, "The eternal, a God-relationship, relationship to ideals, was what moved my soul, but such a middling thing I could not understand" (p. 214). By degrees he recognizes his root problem as the religious, as the need to come to terms with its pressing manifestation. One of the reasons for the rupture is that the young girl (the absent Quaedam) is not sensitive to the religious ("she has no eye for the religious" [p. 222]). His last hope is to reconcile the union *by stirring the religious in her* and thereby effect a positive third element that can hold the relationship together.

If he recognizes the religious, he is, however, not yet reconciled with it and candidly observes: "I am not actually a religious individual. I am only a properly and completely formed possibility of such a thing" (p. 242). His relationship in the end shatters: "I was melancholy . . . I required an ideality under the weight of which I sank. . . . Only religiously can I now understand myself before God" (p. 322).

Frater Taciturnus confirms the religious analysis of this second lover's melancholy:

> His reserve is essentially a form of melancholy [*Tungsind*] and again this melancholy in his case is the condensed possibility which must be gone through within the experience of a crisis if he is to become clear to himself in the experience of the religious. [p. 388]

This *Tungsind*, unlike that of poets, artists, and thinkers, Taciturnus identifies as religious: "So the melancholy of this lay figure of mine is a crisis anticipatory of the religious experience" (p. 389).

Religious melancholy is the moment of crisis when the separation of the finite from the Infinite reaches a point of unendurable severity. The starting-point and presupposition of *Tungsind* is the religious (p. 343), and the religious is the sole resolution (p. 345). What this "third moment"—religious resolution in a restored God-relationship—would be like is never described either by the aesthetes or by Kierkegaard himself. The analysis of melancholy, as of the other moods, revolves around crisis in existences at-

tempted under nonreligious categories. *Tungsind* also reveals that
the resolution to irony and anxiety—the first choice of the self in a
God-relationship recognized as separation resulting from human
fall—is ultimately not sufficient, that nothing less than reunion
can satisfy the longing of the human heart.

Despair: The Mood of Sin-Consciousness

Sin-consciousness is the second crisis moment of the mood of
despair, the second crisis of a shattered self seeking reconstitution. In the resolution of this mood, at its second and higher
phase, God is assigned an indispensable role in refusing the self.
The first moment of despair is the choice of self in relationship to
the Eternal, the taking consciousness of a God-relationship but, as
noted above, a relationship of separation. The second moment is
still one of separation, but at the point at which finite spirit recognizes its need for reunion with the Infinite and wills this, at the
same time agonizing in the consciousness of inability to reestab-
lish what it requires.

Despair is in a true sense also a mood of possibility—the highest
natural possibility available to man—sin-consciousness. And sin-
consciousness brings with it consciousness of a yet higher possibility beyond the reach of the natural. As a mood of higher possibility, the second moment of despair is an intensified form of anxiety. Kierkegaard's treatises on anxiety and despair are allied. *The
Sickness unto Death* (1849), by the pseudonym Anti-Climacus, is in
part a continuation of the 1844 treatise by Vigilius Haufniensis,
The Concept of Anxiety. While their styles are technically different,
their principal concern is sin and related psychological states. *The
Sickness unto Death* proceeds with the same seriousness as the work
on anxiety and turns that seriousness, in part 2, to a consideration
of despair as continuation in sin. Like *The Concept of Anxiety,* it is
profoundly and self-consciously existential, not an example of
"indifferent learning" (*Sickness,* p. 142). The difference between
the psychological pseudonyms is that Anti-Climacus is a *religious*
author. He writes from the perspective of a Christian religious

understanding of the self and completes the analysis of overcoming sin that Haufniensis only began.

The state of not being the self Kierkegaard terms "despair." In his use of the Danish *Fortvivlelse,* he plays upon the root *Tvivl* ("doubt"). *Fortvivlelse* (German: *Verzweiflung*) is an intensification of the split—the twoness—indicated by *Tvivl* (German: *Zweifel*), but in an existential sense.[30]

Kierkegaard not only plays on the etymology of the word but uses it in various senses as well. When Judge William urges despair upon the aesthete Johannes as the cure for despair, he clearly has two different senses in mind. Despair is for Kierkegaard both a state and an act. As a state, it is the condition of disequilibrium within the human synthesis comprised of infinite and finite, eternal and temporal, possibility (freedom) and necessity. The synthesis, he notes, is not yet actual. Kierkegaard begins with the observation of human disequilibrium, in rather Hegelian fashion analyzes the person into antithetical components requiring synthesis, and posits synthesis as the natural state from which one is alienated and as the destined state. Although synthesis may be regarded as the natural state, it was not the *original* state. For although there was unity with God before fall into sin, the synthesis was not actual. The synthesis is thus a higher self than the original, unawakened self described in *The Concept of Anxiety.* Consciousness and reflection, in Kierkegaard as in Hegel, really mean a higher self. "Reintegration" is not literally such—it is rather integration into an originally destined state, not one that had been actualized. Unlike Hegel, however, Kierkegaard would hold that spirit could have awakened without a fall. How this would have happened he does not even speculate about. But this puts him in line with traditional Christian teaching on the subject, and he would go the whole way with the notion that the fall indirectly effected a higher relationship to God than the one originally intended, since the fall brought about the Christ-event.

30. Kierkegaard also notes, in the posthumously published *De omnibus dubitandum est* (written 1842–43; English translation by T. H. Croxall [London: A. C. Black, 1958]), that the life of Cartesian doubt (*Tvivl*) leads to despair (*Fortvivlelse*). The wordplay is lost in English.

As an act, and to repeat what has been indicated above, despair first means choice of the self in relationship to the Eternal (guilt-consciousness) and then sin-consciousness as the fuller grasping of the human condition. The elements of the synthesis are not observed but rather arrived at speculatively and dialectically. And nowhere does Kierkegaard offer for observation or speculative description either an unfallen self or a reconstituted self.[31] The forms of despair are arrived at by reflecting upon the elements of the synthesis and are the despair of infinitude, the despair of finitude, the despair of possibility, and the despair of necessity. Two more basic forms are arrived at: the despair of willing to be oneself (in the sense of a self of one's own creation) and the despair of willing to be rid of oneself. But all forms of despair, and the root reason for the disequilibrium among the elements of the synthesis, are a misrelationship to the Constituting Power that grounds the synthesis. Man is spirit and inescapably in relationship to eternal spirit, whether it be a relationship of separation or of unity. There is no severing oneself completely from the Eternal: "But the eternal he cannot get rid of, no, not to all eternity; he cannot cast it from him once for all, nothing is more impossible" (*Sickness,* p. 150).

The issue in despair is staying in sin or overcoming it. And, according to Kierkegaard, only the religious psychologist will see this. The elements of the synthesis will not come to equilibrium without a readjustment of the relationship to the Constituting Power—who is not a Watchmaker God, who creates and lets creation run its course, or even a Watch-repairman God, who must intervene once to repair a faulty mechanism. For Kierkegaard, while there are special moments of divine action, the Divine must be present and active at every moment, and an *ongoing* relationship to the Constituting Power becomes the key.

Of course, no one is forced to take on this relationship, and Kierkegaard portrays aesthetic characters who will not, in de-

31. Even the religious pseudonym Anti-Climacus does not explicitly cite Christ as the human example of perfect synthesis and relationship to the Constituting Power. In contrast, both Kant and Hegel cite Christ as the perfect example of being well pleasing to God and as consciousness of personally actualized, divine-human unity, respectively.

fiance and in self-destruction. The despair of defiance even seeks to prove from its misery the wretchedness of all existence:

> Revolting against the whole of existence, it thinks it has hold of a proof against it, against its goodness. This proof the despairer thinks he himself is, and that is what he wills to be. Therefore he wills to be rid of himself, himself with his torment, in order with this torment to protest against the whole of existence. [*Sickness,* p. 207]

Despair understood as sin-consciousness situates Kierkegaard's thinking within a Christian, Lutheran, and even somewhat Pietist framework. For the mood of sin-consciousness is a mood of helplessness in sin before the Divine, in the anxious expectation of forgiveness. But because this mood of helplessness is not a passive mood of weakness but rather a crisis moment attained only after an arduous effort of self-recovery, it does not fit into the Pietist mold. It therefore invites theological interpretations as to the degree of human contribution.[32] Is human inability to attain reunion with the Constituting Power, and thereby to restore equilibrium to the human synthesis, merely a fact swept away in some lightning-swift grace of forgiveness appearing on cue when the proper consciousness has been attained, or is it a moment to be suffered through? Clearly the latter is Kierkegaard's sense. The mood of sin-consciousness is an existential moment brought to an end by a *free* grace.

Worthy of note here is that Kierkegaard does not engage in an analysis of possible states of relative equilibrium. The religious psychologist Anti-Climacus is interested only in the total cure, not in the temporary alleviation of disturbances. And he thinks that so long as the total cure is not attained, the sickness of the spirit will break forth again.

Concluding Remarks

With the revelation-proclamation of the need of grace, Kierkegaard's religious psychology abruptly ends. His psychology—

32. It also invites theological arguments about Pelagianism and semi-Pelagianism.

or perhaps more correctly put, his "philosophical anthropology"—is rich and provocative. It advances toward a definition of the modern self, with unmistakable metaphysical underpinnings and an undisguised religious presupposition. It is truly self-conscious, but it is by no means complete.

Whether regarded as philosophy or psychology, it remains a part of the nineteenth century in its language, in its thought structure, and in its method. It not only presupposes the religious but also presupposes G. W. F. Hegel, without whom it never would have attained its form. Kierkegaard taunts Hegel's System, but Hegel survives to haunt Kierkegaard's fragments. One might even ask oneself how Kierkegaard might have described the self if Hegel were not always there to be criticized and contradicted posthumously.

Yet Kierkegaard would seek to transcend his century and intellectual context. To the extent that he succeeds in reformulating a timeless wisdom, he makes his positive contribution to modern self-understanding. He seeks at once to be contemporary with the Jesus of the New Testament and to urge such contemporaneousness upon the reader. This must be a spiritual Jesus, rooted in history, and not the spiritualized, desensualized Jesus of Hegel's *Philosophy of Religion* (1821–31). What contemporaneousness means when concretized neither Anti-Climacus' subsequent *Training in Christianity* nor Kierkegaard's *Edifying Discourses* fully reveal to us. The positive side of the religious life is never described psychologically—not even metaphysically. "Grace," "forgiveness," and "reconciliation" are but hints.

Kierkegaard's psychological fragments can never be normative, for they are self-consciously incomplete. They intend to be a corrective, as does his authorship generally, and he must be conceded some measure of success here. He is not systematic in his treatment of emotional life, even of its religious dimension. Although Hegel brought systematizing into bad repute for a time, one must still regret the incompleteness and nonsystematic nature of Kierkegaard's enterprise. He never engages in a fuller philosophical exploration of human nature and emotions as did Hume. And while his avowed interest in the moods selected for sustained attention is resolution, he explores only the crisis. Emotions of resolution, such as peace and bliss, are not analyzed or described or portrayed but merely inferred. This may finally make his presentation less than convincing for secular empiricists, less than desirable perhaps even for religious empiricists who defend an ultimate silence about the "unspeakable bliss" of mystical union in a yet higher stage.

Kierkegaard's individual, for all the relief he provides from the Hegelian sweep of world history, for all his merits and all his importance, remains a bourgeois Christian self of nineteenth-century Protestant Copenhagen. Kierkegaard's famous definition of the self at the opening of *The Sickness unto Death* ("The self is a relationship which relates itself to its own self . . .") has been faulted time and again for its lack of a social dimension, and it cannot be excused simply by invoking the intention of corrective. In a philosophy ostensibly concerned with authentic subjectivity, there is not nearly enough on the category of intersubjectivity, even if there are hints and suggestions. And for a philosophy which affirms against Hegel that the outer is not the inner and the inner not the outer, there is little on the subject as actor in the world. Hegel is far ahead of him in this respect.

Kierkegaard's category of the religious is also narrow and limited, even if self-consciously. While invoking Christianity, he limits himself to a very narrow understanding of this particular world religion and exhibits little grasp of others.[33] Both Hegel and the Enlightenment are apparently better read in this regard. Hegel's curious philosophy of the history of religions is in some senses more complete. Kierkegaard evidences no appreciation of how the task of religious subjectivity might be carried out in religious traditions not tied to the historical Jesus, nor to what extent it might be carried out in them. Nor will the good pagan Socrates suffice as a universal example of non-Christian religiousness. Kierkegaard's distinction between "religiousness A" and "religiousness B" and the affirmation of personal religious comple-

33. He thereby misses, for example, the *four* stages of life in Hindu thought (student, householder, forest-dweller, ascetic).

tion only in the latter—Christianity—does not silence or dismiss the Buddhist's claim that he can attain religious bliss in the timeless Nirvana revealed by another historical figure. Nor does Kierkegaard exhibit a concrete appreciation of how far the humanist might get, even if he gives us a humanist in the character of Judge William.

His authorship restricts itself to an analysis of antireligious subjects within the culture of the absolute religion. He analyzes but also pleads a case—for Christianity in an age of secular momentum. He opposed Hegel's gratuitous "salvation" of Christianity in a secularized religion under a priesthood of philosophers, and his polemical concern, in this instance as in others, ruled out a broader consideration of religion.

His teaching, while rich and suggestive, is finally a very hard one. Those alienated from the tradition and its Christ or else totally unfamiliar with them are not his intended audience. His religious presupposition is intended as a challenge and affront to secularists who have been exposed to the tradition and its Teacher but who would seek to transcend them.

One may or may not be able to overcome the religious and Kierkegaard's defiantly narrow statement of it. What he does, however, make difficult is altogether circumventing them. He wishes to reinsert into philosophical discourse, and allied psychology, the *scandalon* of Christianity. In the process, he makes it nigh impossible to move secularly and eclectically through his own thought without tripping up against the stumbling-block of the religious, so carefully placed in the center of the road.

REFERENCES

Kierkegaard, S.

    Journals and Papers [1834–55]. Translated by H. and E. Hong. Bloomington: Indiana University Press, 1975.

    The Concept of Irony [1841]. Translated by L. M. Capel. Bloomington: Indiana University Press, 1968.

    Either/Or [1843]. Translated by D. and L. Swenson with revisions by H. A. Johnson. New York: Doubleday, Anchor Books, 1959.

Repetition [1843]. Translated by W. Lowrie. Princeton, N.J.: Princeton University Press, 1941.

The Concept of Dread [Anxiety] [1844]. Translated by W. Lowrie. Princeton, N.J.: Princeton University Press, 1957.

Stages on Life's Way [1845]. Translated by W. Lowrie. New York: Schocken Books, 1967.

Concluding Unscientific Postscript [1846]. Translated by D. Swenson and W. Lowrie. Princeton, N.J.: Princeton University Press, 1941.

Purity of Heart [1847]. Translated by D. V. Steere. New York: Harper & Row, 1956.

The Sickness unto Death [1849]. Translated by W. Lowrie. Garden City, N.Y.: Doubleday, 1954.

9

Subjectivity in Psychoanalysis

W. W. MEISSNER

The Problematic

The problem of subjectivity in psychoanalysis is closely related to the problem of the nature of psychoanalysis as a science. The intention of psychoanalysis as a science is to provide an account of human behavior and experience in basically objective terms. The problem arises from the fact that analysts deal with individual patients and their inner psychic experience. The material that patients provide in the analytic process has the immediacy of personal experience and derives from the world of inner significance, meaning, and motive that reflects the world of the patient's inner subjective experience. What methodology, then, makes it possible for a science, which bases itself on subjectively derived inner experience in large measure, to become an objective science of human behavior? Nearly half a century ago, Hartmann (1927) discussed this tension in the analytic methodology in terms of the contrast between understanding and explanation. Understanding has to do with the interpretive grasp of the connection between meaning structures or signs. Explanation refers to the scientific discovery of causal sequence and the construction of hypotheses.

The discussions that have evolved out of this internal difficulty in psychoanalytic methodology have focused on the issue of whether psychoanalysis is a natural science or a humanistic psychology. A second aspect of the discussion has focused on the question of the role of the personal agent in the therapeutic technique and the theoretical understanding of psychoanalysis. One important offshoot of the debate between the natural science and humanistic views of psychoanalysis has been the discussion of the extent to which psychoanalysis may be more closely akin to history as an intellectual discipline than to the more objective physical sciences (Novey, 1968).

My purpose in the present discussion is to explore various aspects of this problematic from the point of view of the development of psychoanalytic thinking, particularly as related to the evolving critique of metapsychology as the basic psychoanalytic theory. We can then call on Kierkegaard for consultation, in the hope that his own struggles with the tension between system and subjectivity, particularly focused in his formulations about the individual, will offer some basis for a renewed approach. Finally, we will return to the issue of subjectivity in psychoanalytic theory, particularly in reference to the emerging and evolving conceptualization of the self in psychoanalysis, and attempt some integration of the approach to subjectivity with the concept of the self.

Psychoanalytic Approaches to the Problem of Subjectivity

At the beginning of the psychoanalytic enterprise, subjectivity was not a matter of concern. Freud opted more or less definitively for a natural science account of mental phenomena. At the very beginning of his abortive "Project for a Scientific Psychology" (1950 [1895]), Freud makes an unabashed and unequivocal commitment:

> The intention is to furnish a psychology that shall be a natural science: that is, to represent psychical processes as quantitatively determinate states of specifiable material particles, thus making those processes perspicuous and free from contradiction. [p. 295]

The elusive complexity of the task and the limitations of available neurological knowledge left Freud feeling frustrated and defeated after his feverish attempt to provide such an objective and quantitative account.

The disappointment forced Freud to turn to a more explicit

psychology. That shift in Freud's thinking from the physiological to the psychological was given an added impetus by the abandonment of his seduction hypothesis. In his early years Freud had gradually formulated the hypothesis that at the root of every neurosis there lies an actual infantile trauma. On the basis of repeated accounts by his patients, he hypothesized that the early trauma was characteristically sexual in nature. In spite of convincing evidence in support of this hypothesis, Freud began to have doubts and finally, apparently as a result of his own self-analysis, in which he found suggestions of such infantile trauma, came to realize that his assumption regarding infantile sexual seduction might be invalid.

The insight was momentous and provided a critical turning point in the history of the development of psychoanalytic thought. If the apparent memories of infantile seduction recovered by the patients were not memories of real events, then, Freud argued, these memories must be the products of internal instinctual forces that used the relationship with the parents as a vehicle for expressing infantile sexual wishes. The way was open for an exploration of the internal world of psychic experience, a world of meanings, symbolic expressions, significances, fantasies, and affects. The psychoanalytic inquiry correspondingly took a significant step in the direction of the lived immediacy of intrapsychic experience. The emphasis fell on subjectively derived aspects of intrapsychic experience. Subjectivity was not an area of analytic concern, but it remained present and active as the assumed or taken-for-granted originative source of intrapsychic activity.

Nor was there any serious or systematic attempt to conceptualize it. Insofar as any attempt at formulation was made, the agent within the psychic apparatus was thought of as a sort of observing ego. But it remained an unthematized aspect of psychic functioning. Nevertheless, Freud's account of both defense and consciousness ultimately depended on the operation of this unnamed and unexplained agency. In both cases there seemed to be a form of infinite regress that postulated an unending series of ego states. At the heart of his scientifically determined and mechanistically functioning system, Freud was forced to leave an island of vitalism. The unnamed ego that somehow stood at the subjective pole of all internal experience was able somehow to sense the danger and to set into action mobilization of defenses against it or was able to perceive the indications of quality in a wide variety of conscious experience; yet the ego itself remained a sort of primary willer and ultimate knower—a center of personal agency and awareness that operated within the theory and yet could not be reduced to the physicalistic terms of the psychic machinery it served. It was the "ghost in the machine" (Ryle, 1949).

It is not that Freud was without a theory of consciousness. In the *Interpretation of Dreams* Freud distinguished between the concept of the conscious-preconscious system (*Cs.-Pcs.*) and consciousness as subjective experience. The *Cs.-Pcs.* was the equivalent of the ego for his topographic theory and would evolve in the later tripartite theory into the structural ego. Freud also postulated an apparatus of consciousness, distinct from both the subjective experience and the system *Cs.-Pcs.*, whose function was to account for the phenomenon of subjective conscious experience. The attributes of this functional apparatus of consciousness have been detailed by Rapaport (1959, 1960) and pertain to the nature of attention cathexis and the manner in which its distribution as part of the energy system in the *Cs.-Pcs.* gives rise to conscious experience. However, behind the interplay of cathectic processes there remained the observing, guiding, sensing, and perceiving agency, somehow silent and unobserved yet palpably present, inhabiting the subjective pole of human experience.

In the later years of his career, Freud found good reason to completely overhaul his model of the operation of the mind. The existence of unconscious defenses made it necessary to revise the theory of the agency of repression, which could no longer be regarded as coextensive with the *Cs.-Pcs.* system. The tripartite structural ego, therefore, embraces both conscious and unconscious functions, but one of the major ego functions is that of consciousness. Here again, however, subjectivity itself escapes exploration but remains a residual unanalyzed and unsystematized element within the theory. The tendency to regard consciousness as a specific function of the structural ego reinforces the systematic tendency to regard the ego as the source of and location of self-determining agency and initiative and the locus of subjective experience.

The direction that had been set by Freud's natural science option was followed up by Heinz Hartmann, particularly in the powerful elaboration of an ego psychology. In considering the tension between understanding of inner subject-related states and the objective explanatory account of the natural science perspective, Hartmann (1927) commented:

> But we must recall that at the outset of our investigation into the scientific status of psychoanalysis we came to the conclusion that no scientific psychology is capable of preserving in its concepts the lived immediacy of its primary material, and that any psychology has to sacrifice to the scientific goal the illusion of that "deeper penetration" into its subject which belongs to immediate experience. [p. 402]

What was at issue was the relationship of the more subjective categories of understanding, intentionality, purpose, and will to the presumed causal sequences that were more properly the object of scientific methodology. Hartmann, as a good psychoanalyst, was unwilling to surrender the subjective rooting of the scientific psychoanalytic account, but he saw no room for the subjective experimental dimension in psychoanalytic theory. He tried to strike a satisfactory balance, which in itself underlies and reflects the inherent tension within scientific methodology:

> Many understandable connections (including the "as-if" understandable connections) are . . . actually causal connections. We must not forget that the emergence of a voluntary action from an act of will is the paradigm not only of the understanding connection but also of the causal relationship. The concept of causality, however . . . has freed itself from its origin in the experience of causality. This subjective experience no longer is a valid criterion of causal connections.

Understanding connections are, as hypotheses, in many ways indispensable, but their validity must in every case be established empirically. No psychology of the more complex aspects of the mind can fully dispense with understanding. But as long as it is a science, it must not use understanding without having established the limits of its reliability. To ascertain these limits and thereby to determine the sphere within which understanding and causal connections coincide is one of the essential tasks of psychoanalysis. [p. 403]

The paradigm of the emergence of voluntary action from an act of will served as a guiding theme for Hartmann's later work. Action was the function of the ego:

Normal action in all of its varieties, even instinctual or emotional action, is formed by the ego. But between action and the ego there exist manifold relationships. In action we have an intention toward a goal; and the motor and other phenomena used to reach this goal are controlled and organized accordingly. [1947, p. 39]

The trend toward increasing subjectivity, defined here in terms of the initiatives of agency, was formulated in terms of degrees of increasing internalization. Freud's later theory of anxiety as a danger signal for the mobilization of defenses was a useful example. The signal provides the means for mastering inner danger before it can be translated into external danger. Action that is both motivationally and operationally organized can be brought into play and is gradually substituted for the reactive impulse to motor discharge. Trial activity, for example, in the case of thinking, can be mobilized in the service of mastery or problem-solving and may then be gradually internalized. The gradual internalization of various forms of action, moreover, both in the ego and superego, contributes to a growing independence from the outside world in such a way that processes of inner regulation come to replace processes of external reaction and/or regulation (Hartmann, 1947).

The action paradigm led Hartmann's thinking in the direction of his powerful and immensely liberating ideas of the conflict-free sphere of ego functioning, ego autonomy, and the shift of emphasis in the understanding of ego potential from an emphasis on defense to that of adaptation. The initiative had been offered by Freud in his epochal transformation of the understanding of anxiety in *Inhibitions, Symptoms and Anxiety* (1926). This theoretical shift and the linking of the principle of action with ego functioning tended to support the concept of the ego as the seat of intention, purpose, will, intentionality, and subjectivity.

The analysis of the paradigm of voluntary action was extended in the systematizing work of Rapaport (1961). The tension between activity and passivity became a central element in his metapsychological thinking, and the essence of activity came to reflect the capacity for control, regulation, and synthesis by an integral and cohesively functioning ego. The model of passivity included (a) the helpless-passive experience of tension, and (b) the passive-gratifying tension discharge. Correspondingly, the model of activity came to embrace (a) the defense against and/or control of drive tension doing away with passive helplessness in the face of drive demands, and (b) the ego-controlled discharge of tension, through ego apparatuses by detour processes aiming to find the drive object in reality. The link of activity with ego autonomy was made explicit and specific:

> The development of activity . . . appears to be coterminous with the developing autonomy of the ego. Activity appears as the measuring rod of the extent to which the ego as an autonomous agency enters the clash of drive demand and reality and transforms it into intrapsychic conflict. Ego autonomy, the roots of the subjective experience of volition, ability to delay discharge and to undertake detour actions toward the drive object, and activity are somehow closely related. [p. 541]

The interplay and the polarization of aspects of passivity and activity play themselves out at all levels of mental organization and even on the highest levels of conceptual experience. Rapaport concluded:

... where structure controls drive we find thought phenomena which may be characterized dynamically as activity and may even be accompanied by a subjective experience of activity; where drive imposes itself upon structure we find thought phenomena bearing the dynamic—and perhaps even the subjective experience—earmarks of passivity. [p. 563]

The last decade or so of development in psychoanalytic thinking has seen a retrenchment from the apogee of metapsychological systematization provided by the elaboration and dominance of ego psychology by Hartmann and his collaborators Kris and Lowenstein and by the metapsychological constructions of Rapaport. There has ensued over the intervening years a well-orchestrated attack upon the natural science suppositions of psychoanalytic metapsychology. In 1966, Home argued that Freud's discovery that the symptom in psychoneurosis has meaning equivalently took the study of neurosis out of the realm of science and transformed it into a humanistic discipline, insofar as meaning does not derive from causes as such but from the creative activity of an experiencing and meaning-giving subject. The argument essentially deals with the role of subjectivity in psychoanalysis and in psychoanalytic theory. Insofar as a natural science methodology eliminates subjectivity, its logic and method become radically different from the humanistic disciplines, though the methodology of the humanistic approach is no less respectably rational or disciplined. Home writes:

> To psychoanalysis the difference may be best known directly as the difference between "interpretation" and "explanation." Or again it is expressed in the canons of scientific method which demand that a clear distinction always be maintained between observation and inference, whereas in a humanistic study a clear distinction is demanded only in respect of who is saying what. Or yet again in the fact that science asks the question how does a thing occur and receives an answer in terms of causes, whereas a humanistic study asks

the question why and receives an answer in terms of reasons. [pp. 43-44]

We are back then at the dichotomy between understanding and explanation that Hartmann had addressed over a half century ago. Hartmann's decisive option had then been to support and reinforce the natural science bent in Freud's thinking, so that he chose scientific explanation over understanding. Home, however, takes the opposite tack and opts for understanding in preference to explanation. Instead of the explanation through causes, the emphasis is shifted to the role of understanding through empathy and identification. Home writes:

> When we identify with an object we feel what it would be like to be that object. This gives us an *understanding* of the object and particularly of how it is feeling and therefore of how it will behave. The accuracy of the information we derive from an act of identification will depend on the accuracy of our perception, on our capacity to criticize our transference and our ability to identify only within the limits of what is actually identical. Within those limits, cognition through identification gives us accurate information and information which can be obtained in no other way. [p. 44]

The argument was taken up and carried forward by Guntrip (1969, 1971), who argued that the basing of psychoanalytic understanding on an instinctual theory that was biologically rooted and based on natural science explanations was a distortion of psychoanalytic methodology. Rather, the true psychodynamic science rested on a more authentic understanding of inner experience and its related meanings and on the relationship of the experienced subject to significant objects. For Guntrip, psychic phenomena are recognized by an inner subjective process that is related to an immediate personal experience. He wrote:

> We know that our thoughts and feelings do not have any necessary objective counterpart in the outer world, but they have a reality of their own, *psychic reality*. This direct im-

mediate knowledge of psychic reality is quite different from our sensory experience of the outer world. Our knowledge of our thoughts and feelings is our experience of ourselves as "subjects." We can mentally know ourselves in this manner without any intermediary method or technique of investigation. There is nothing else *at all* that we can know in this direct manner.... [1969, p. 370]

Thus, the psychoanalytic study of human behavior bases itself on the knowledge of subjective reality as opposed to the exclusively objective emphasis of natural science. Consequently, there is posed a genuinely new scientific problem that cannot yield to the classical methods of scientific investigation and theorizing.

Guntrip (1969) then turned his attack against Hartmann and ego psychology. Hartmann's ego, composed of structures, processes, and functions, is designated as the "system-ego" and is opposed to a more truly psychodynamic concept of "personal ego." Guntrip argues that "Hartmann's 'system-ego' with autonomous power (as against the id) to adapt and adjust to outer reality, does not give us a 'person' with capacities for spontaneous self-expression and creative originality, not simply adapting to external reality but producing from internal reality" (p. 399). The ultimate charge against Hartmann and his followers is that the natural science account of the structural organization and function of the ego is essentially divorced from and irrelevant to the understanding of the difficult and important dynamic problems of experiencing and relating to significant objects and gives no direct or immediate assistance to dealing with therapeutic problems. The psychodynamic essence, for Guntrip, has to do with persons' inner experience giving meaning and symbolic significance to their relationships to important life objects. The account provided by Hartmann and classical psychoanalysis abstracts, depersonalizes, and mechanizes the dynamic aspects of the patient's inner world (Guntrip, 1969, pp. 405–06).

The criticism of the natural science modality in psychoanalytic theorizing since then has found its most articulate and developed advocacy in the recent work of Roy Schafer (1976). Schafer argues that the natural science model operates by inferring entities, structures, processes, and other properties and qualities as means for making intelligible the observable regularities in the external data of the object of investigation. In psychoanalysis, this approach produces a complex set of explanatory constructs for a wide range of behavior. Schafer's words forcefully sharpen the issues:

> The terms of Freudian metapsychology are those of natural science. Freud, Hartmann, and others deliberately used the language of forces, energies, functions, structure, apparatus, and principles to establish and develop psychoanalysis along the lines of a physicalistic psychobiology.
>
> It is inconsistent with this type of scientific language to speak of intentions, meanings, reasons, or subjective experience. Even though in ... the psychoanalytic situation, psychoanalysts deal essentially with reasons, emphases, choices, and the like, as metapsychologists they have traditionally made it their objective to translate these subjective contents and these actions into the language of functions, energies, and so forth. In this way they have attempted to formulate explanations of action in the mode ... of natural science explanation. They have suppressed the intentionalistic, active mode.... And, in keeping with the assumption of thoroughgoing determinism, the word *choice* has been effectively excluded from the metapsychological vocabulary. Action, if it is not used in the sense of acting-out, is understood merely as motoric activity with respect to the so-called world. [p. 103]

One of the striking paradoxes in Freud's work is that regardless of his insistence on a natural science mode of thinking, he did not adhere rigidly to that approach, but rather spontaneously and unabashedly tended to anthropomorphize it. In other words, in discussing various aspects of psychic structure or topographic systems or even instinctual drives and derivatives, he tended to dramatize them as though they were expressing purposes, and as if they had the capacity for creating meaning, positing choices, and engaging in deliberate and voluntary action. Schafer takes issue with this practice, pointing out that it is as though Freud were speaking of separate minds within the mind or of homunculi working within the psychic apparatus.

Freud's failure to follow the natural science method consistently and his resort to anthropomorphism tend to prove an important point: psychoanalysis cannot do without the person as agent. The interpreting analyst in the analytic situation does not address himself to a set of structures, capacities, or functions; rather, he addresses himself to an individual person as a human being. Similarly, it is not the ego as structure or organization of functions that enters into a therapeutic alliance, but rather the integral personality. The gap between the person on the one side and the natural science apparatus on the other is unavoidable and unbridgeable.

Schafer then trains his guns on the staggering accomplishments of Hartmann and Rapaport, precisely because he finds in their elaboration of ego psychology the best exemplar of the application of a natural science methodology. Even the exemplar fails to meet its objective and inevitably slips into contradiction. Schafer summarizes his critique of Hartmann's contribution in the following terms:

> Broadly viewed, however, the problems arise from Hartmann's commitment to the natural science approach to conceptualization. This approach excludes meaning from the center of psychoanalytic theory. It deals with meaning only by changing it into something else (functions, energies, "principles", etc.). But meaning (and intention) is the same as "psychic reality"—that which is at the center of clinical psychoanalytic work. Consequently, a radical split between the mode of theorizing and the mode of investigation is a major consequence of adhering to the natural science model. Hartmann's emphasis . . . is shown to lead in certain instances to behavioristic, as opposed to truly psychoanalytic formulations. It also retains the anthropomorphism it is in-

tended to expunge from metapsychology. And finally it is inadequate *on its own terms* for rendering the complexity of clinical understanding and thus to support claims of exact explanation. [pp. 100–01]

It is of interest that Schafer takes up his counterproposal to a natural science metapsychology from very nearly the same point as Hartmann. He makes the paradigm of action the heart of his construction, but unlike Hartmann, who chose to emphasize the conditions and the energic-structural causes of action, Schafer turns to an analysis of action based on the notion of the person as the initiating agent, the intentional source of all human activity. The key concept is that of action:

> By action I do not mean voluntary physical deeds only. In my sense, action is human behavior that has a point; it is meaningful human activity; it is intentional or goal-directed performances by people; it is doing things for reasons. There is nothing the psychoanalytic interpretation can deal with that is not action as here defined. For example, to think of something is to do an action; to see or remember something is to do an action; to be silent or otherwise inactive is as much an action as to say something or to walk somewhere. It is one kind of action to say something and another to think it and not say it. [p. 139]

Consequently, in the action-language approach there is no appeal to causes. Rather, explanation is accomplished in terms of specific intentions, reasons, purposes, and other aspects of goal-directed action. Thus, the language of action has no room for the adjectival-substantive mode of existence, since that implies the existence of entities or structures within the organism which may account for observable behavior or activity. In the action-language approach one does not speak of unconscious drives, since such language implies that drives exist which have certain properties that qualify their mode of being. The action language, therefore, is articulated in terms of actions and the modes of

action, that is to say, by the use of verbs (action-words) and ad-
verbs. It is this revised language that Schafer claims as the native
tongue of psychoanalysis.

It is apparent that the points of view and theoretical orientations span the full range from a natural science orientation that
seeks to translate almost all aspects of human experience and
psychic functioning into terms of energies, forces, functions, processes, and structures, to an equally radical if quite opposite orientation that seeks to jettison the metapsychological contraption
and to start all over again from the basic observations of the
psychoanalytic situation, basing its humanistic conceptualizations
on the intentionality, purpose, and meaning derived from immediate experience and explained by a personal agent acting for
specific motives and reasons and seeking to fulfill specifiable
goals.

If the attack on metapsychology and the alternate proposals
advanced by these critics[1] have accomplished anything, they have
certainly brought home to us the realization that psychoanalysis
cannot survive and becomes relatively empty and meaningless
without including the meaningful aspects of immediate subjective
experience.

There are also important currents in psychoanalytic thinking
that lie much closer to the phenomenology of clinical experience.
Undoubtedly, the leading contribution in this respect has been
the work of Donald Winnicott, the English pediatrician turned
psychoanalyst, whose genial contributions toward focusing on aspects of subjectivity within the psychoanalytic experience are well
known.

Winnicott takes as his point of departure the infant's early developmental experience, in which he emerges from a relatively
inchoate state of merged interaction with the mother to a
gradually articulated experience of objects outside of himself. As
the result of his experience in interaction with the mothering

1. Including Apfelbaum (1965, 1966), Holt (1965, 1972, 1975), and Klein
(1976).

figure, the child's ego changes from an unintegrated state to a gradually more structured integration, which makes it possible for him to begin to experience anxiety and the possibility of disintegration. In normal, healthy development the infant retains some capacity for reexperiencing unintegrated states, but his capacity depends on the continuity of reliable care by the mother or on the build-up of the infant's memories of the mother's care.

In articulating the transition from subjective experience to objectively perceived experience, Winnicott has made his most powerful and influential argument. The model for his analysis of this important shift in the child's infantile experience is provided by the common experience of transitional objects in infancy. In Winnicott's view, such transitional objects become the child's first "not-me" possession. He comments:

> I have introduced the terms "transitional objects" and "transitional phenomena" for designation of the intermediate area of experience, between the thumb and the teddy bear, between the oral erotism and the true object-relationship, between primary creative activity and projection of what has already been introjected, between primary unawareness of indebtedness and the acknowledgement of indebtedness. [1971, p. 2]

Both the subjective and the objective aspects of experience contribute to this intermediate area. To Winnicott's mind, "It is an area that is not challenged, because no claim is made on its behalf except that it shall exist as a resting-place for the individual engaged in the perpetual human task of keeping inner and outer reality separate yet interrelated" (p. 2). Further:

> I am therefore studying the substance of *illusion*, that which is allowed to the infant, and which in adult life is inherent in art and religion and yet becomes the hallmark of madness when an adult puts too powerful a claim on the credulity of others, forcing them to acknowledge a sharing of illusion that is not their own. We can share a respect for *illusory experience*,

and if we wish we may collect together and form a group on the basis of the similarity of our illusory experiences. This is a natural root of grouping among human beings. [p. 3]

It remains to determine the ways and extent to which subjective and objective phenomena interact and interplay within the analytic situation. We will return to this subject later, but at this point it seems useful to point out that the analytic process creates, in Winnicott's terms, an area of illusory experience within which the elements of subjectivity and objectivity of both analyst and analysand are intermeshed in a unique and creative human experience.

Kierkegaard and Subjectivity

We have come to a point in our inquiry at which it seems useful and judicious to call for expert consultation. The tension between psychoanalytic viewpoints is clear and dramatic enough, but we are left in a quandary as to how these divergent perspectives can, in any meaningful sense, be integrated. We are left with only the acute perplexity of realizing that we cannot do without each of them—that the subjective alone loses its scientific relevance and validity, while an objective account devoid of subjective reference and meaning becomes abstract, mechanical, and irrelevant to human concerns and intentions. Let us see, then, what Kierkegaard has to offer in our dilemma.

Kierkegaard decisively declared the relevance of subjectivity over against the claims of objective systematic thinking. In the context of his reaction against the sweeping systematic rationalizations of the Hegelian system, he laid the ground for the claims of individuality. Without dispelling or devaluing the necessity of objective scientific accounts, Kierkegaard was exquisitely sensitive to the risks and limitations in an exclusively objective approach. The tendency of such "abstract thought" or "objective reflection" was to move away from the personal, intentional subject toward a statement of human nature in terms of impersonal laws and determined facts. When human nature is studied by methods of objective reflection alone, it is reduced to terms of the same laws and determining conditions that prevail in nature. Such an approach is valid enough until it makes the claim of being the only valid way of understanding human nature. To Kierkegaard's mind, such a claim evacuates all that is essential and basic in man's nature.

In the face of the exclusivity of such an objective claim, Kierkegaard sought to find room for another approach, another kind of truth about man. He regarded the truths of objective science as "hypothetical" or "approximate." The method of natural science is hypothetical insofar as it fails to give an adequate account of the human knower who must think and act within the structural processes of the objective account. The same method is also approximate, insofar as it never attains a real understanding of man in his own proper mode of being, particularly as a subject exercising existence in his own right. Beyond the realm of objective reflection there lie essential questions about the meaning of existence, the nature of man, and the uses of freedom, which cannot be addressed by scientific methods and fall more properly within the purview of what Kierkegaard calls "subjective reflection" or "existential thinking."

I must here introduce a note of caution in the attempt to utilize Kierkegaard in the service of understanding some aspects of psychoanalysis. It must be remembered that Kierkegaard is fundamentally a philosophical and religious thinker. However, we are not concerned here with the philosophical or religious implications of his formulations, but rather with the implications of his thought for an understanding of the psychoanalytic situation and process. Consequently, we must here proceed by a step-by-step translation of Kierkegaard's ideas, continually refocusing them toward the more immediate context of our present concern.

This will become particularly critical when we are discussing Kierkegaard's ideas about faith and despair, where the implications have far-reaching spiritual and religious applications. The refocusing of such ideas will involve not simply a disregard of those implications but a refashioning of them by analogy to the demands and concerns of a psychoanalytic inquiry. For Kierkegaard, subjectivity implies an inwardness or existential attitude of the individual psyche. The Augustinian implications of this position have been previously noted (Collins, 1953), in that Kierkegaard gives this notion of the *homo interior* a specifically religious connotation, such that humanly significant truth gained through inwardness and subjectivity is primarily an ethico-religious truth. In this sense, man's subjectivity implies a personal, inward embrace of morality and religious life, an aspect of the reality of human nature that is not open to scientific inspection. As we shall see, the culmination of Kierkegaard's understanding of subjectivity and individual reality is joined in his concept of faith.

In addition, Kierkegaard's writings are the distillation of the inner torment of his own soul. There is nothing calm, distanced, or "objective" about his thinking. Rather, it boils over from the inner turmoil of his own subjectivity, his own inner conflict and torment, and issues in a view of man that reflects his own existential condition—namely, that of an isolated individual, alone and solitary, struggling less with the forces around him than with those within himself, and with his God.

In the face of the reductive claims of objectivity, Kierkegaard proclaimed a bold and fundamental thesis—truth is subjectivity. He shifts the ground of the inquiry from a concern with the object of apprehension, the *what* of thinking, to the nature of the subject's relationship to what he thinks, the *how*. This shifts the emphasis to a kind of relationship that allows us to say that the individual in this relationship to an object has a certain form of truth, even though that object may turn out to be a deception or untruth. It is this more decidedly ethical and personal kind of truth that Kierkegaard has in mind when he joins it to subjectivity. As he writes:

> Objectively we consider only the matter at issue, subjectively we have regard to the subject and his subjectivity; and behold, precisely this subjectivity is the matter at issue. This must constantly be borne in mind, namely, that the subjective problem is not something about an objective issue, but is the subjectivity itself. For since the problem in question poses a

decision, and since all decisiveness as shown above, inheres in subjectivity it is essential that every trace of an objective issue should be eliminated. If any such trace remains, it is once a sign that the subject seeks to shirk something of the pain and crisis of the decision; that is, he seeks to make the problem to some degree objective. [1846, p. 115]

There is something quite specific and special about being a subject. Kierkegaard notes that there is also something special about becoming a lover or even a hero: "And yet, being a lover, a hero, and so forth, is precisely a prerogative of subjectivity; for one does not become a hero or a lover objectively" (1846, p. 117). The same can be said of religious devoutness: devoutness inheres in subjectivity and no one ever becomes devout objectively. The relevance to psychoanalysis is immediate and evident: the effort of psychoanalysis is to enable the individual to be a subject; one does not become an individual, one does not become a subject, objectively.

Kierkegaard goes on to discuss the nature of subjective truth in the following terms:

> When the question of truth is raised in an objective manner, reflection is directed objectively to the truth, as an object to which the knower is related. Reflection is not focused upon the relationship, however, but upon the question of whether it is the truth to which the knower is related. If only the object to which he is related is the truth, the subject is accounted to be in the truth. When the question of the truth is raised subjectively, reflection is directed subjectively to the nature of the individual's relationship: if only the mode of this relationship is in the truth, the individual is in the truth, even if he should happen to be thus related to what is not true. [1846, p. 178]

As an example, he takes the knowledge of God. Objectively, the question is whether the object of knowledge is, in fact, the true God. But subjectively, the question has more to do with whether the nature of the individual's knowledge implies a relationship to something in such a way that his relationship is a God-relationship. The emphasis here is less on what is known than on the relationship of the individual cognitively and personally to that which is known. Within the psychoanalytic context, it can be said that what is of greater import to the subject analysand is not what is known but how it is known. The actual content of what is discovered through the psychoanalytic inquiry in terms of the historical account of the patient's life experience is not unimportant but can be regarded as less important than the way in which it is known, the relationship the subject adopts toward it in the course of his psychoanalytic inquiry.

Kierkegaard does not abandon the realm of objectivity, but rather envisions the role of subjective truth as taking its point of departure from the junction at which objective uncertainty arises. It is as though the process of understanding had reached a fork in the road at which objective knowledge must be placed in abeyance. At such a point there is objective uncertainty, but it is precisely this point that increases the tension of subjective inwardness. The truth, then, takes on a special meaning that can be defined in the following terms: "An objective uncertainty held fast in an appropriation-process of the most passionate inwardness in the truth, the highest truth attainable for an existing individual. . . . The truth is precisely the venture which chooses an objective uncertainty with the passion of the infinite" (1846, p. 182).

When truth is thus subjectively grasped, the objective truth becomes paradoxical. Thus:

> The paradoxical character of the truth is its objective uncertainty; this uncertainty is an expression for the passionate inwardness, and this passion is precisely the truth. So far the Socratic principle. The eternal and essential truth, the truth which has an essential relationship to an existing individual because it pertains essentially to existence (all other knowledge being from the Socratic point of view accidental, its scope and degree a matter of indifference), is a paradox. But the eternal and essential truth is by no means in itself a paradox; it becomes paradoxical by virute of its relationship

to an existing individual. The Socratic ignorance is the expression for the objective uncertainty; the inwardness of the existing individual is the truth. [1846, p. 183]

If we shift back to the psychoanalytic frame of reference, the issues of objective uncertainty and subjective inwardness become immediately relevant. If we envision the psychoanalytic inquiry as a process through which the subject seeks the truth about himself, that is to say, a true understanding of himself that allows him in some definitive way to come to know, acknowledge, and accept himself and his way of existing (in Kierkegaard's terms, choosing himself), then the objective inquiry has a limited scope and validity. The historical account is itself limited by the vicissitudes of the patient's memory and by the fact that the recapturing of that account is always conditioned by the patient's subjective awareness and the need to construct the account in terms of certain inner significances that he constantly attributes to the experienced events.

Thus, there are no psychoanalytic "facts" that are not ultimately embedded in a context of meaning and relevance which bears an immediate relationship to the patient's subjectivity. There is a constant tension between the meaning of the events in themselves and the meaning attributed to them in the patient's mind. The ultimate explanation, then, does not lie so much in the determining causal effect of given factual sequences and their resultant effects in the patient's experience as in the meaningful construction given to such events and their integration in a pattern of relevance within the patient's experience. In a sense, the patient constructs a meaning out of his experience and it is this constructed meaning that serves as the basis for the sense of self to which he must ultimately commit himself.

The commitment must take place in relation to the residual objective uncertainty, which can never be totally eliminated or absolved. This aspect is given poignant expression by Kierkegaard:

The thing is to understand myself, to see what God really wishes me to do; the thing is to find a truth which is true to me, to find the idea for which I can live and die. What would be the use of discovering so-called objective truth, or working through all the systems of philosophy and of being able, if required, to review them all and show up the inconsistencies within each system; what good would it do me to be able to develop a theory of the state and combine all the details into a single whole, and so construct a world in which I did not live, but only held up to the view of others; what good would it do me to be able to explain the meaning of Christianity if it had no deeper significance for me and for my life; what good would it do me if truth stood before me, cold and naked, not caring whether I recognized her or not, and producing in me a shudder of fear rather than a trusting devotion? [1834-55, p. 15]

We are exceedingly close at this juncture to what psychoanalysis has come to refer to as "insight." As is well recognized, insight is not a matter of formulation, or a matter of cognitional or notional assent to causal explanations or to the relevance between events and experience. Insight rather is a subjectively and emotionally grasped realization and actualization within one's own experience of a basic truth about oneself. The norms of psychoanalytic insight, therefore, are identical to the claims of Kierkegaard's subjectivity and inwardness. One could almost take Kierkegaard's words and put them in the mouth of the analysand who has come to the end of a successful psychoanalytic inquiry.

> One must know oneself before knowing anything else. It is only after a man has thus understood himself inwardly and has thus seen his way, that life acquires peace and significance. . . .
> And so I stand once again at the point where I must begin my life in a different way. I shall now try to fix a calm gaze upon myself and begin to act in earnest; for only thus shall I be able, like the child calling itself "I" within its first conscious action, to call myself "I" in any deeper sense. [1834-55, p. 17]

Thus, for Kierkegaard existential truth is practical, never completed, and basically paradoxical. It is concerned with human

actions and self-development as opposed to the making or transformation of external objects. It is concerned with individual
human existence rather than with general laws and impersonal
processes. Its ultimate aim is the cultivation of the self, especially
in its free relationships with other human selves, and in Kierkegaard's view, ultimately with God. For the human subject this
remains unfinished business since man must be regarded not as a
completed reality but rather as evolving in a continuing and
dynamic process of becoming and striving. It is less a body of
truth than the manner in which the subject applies this truth to
himself with particular concern for the implications for his inner
life. Human life is a continuing process of adaptation, changing
circumstances, losses, and unremitting striving. The analytic process, like life itself, is open-ended and unending. What it achieves
is not so much a static and finished product as the activation of a
process, an inquiry, a dynamic and personal methodology, which
allows the individual to choose and unendingly to continue to
choose his self, his life, his way of being and existing. Like existential thought itself, it is practical, unfinished, and paradoxical.

One of the most fundamental dimensions of Kierkegaard's
thinking, which took on added importance in his later writings
particularly, is his notion of the individual—for him specifically
the sense of man as an individual before God. For Kierkegaard,
for man to be a human being means that he must also be an
existing individual. There are two ways in which man can be such
an individual, and this becomes a fundamental option, a basic
either/or in Kierkegaard's thinking. *Either* he can forget that he is
such an existing individual, and so becomes a comic figure, since
man must exist whether he wills it or not. *Or* he can focus his
entire energy on the realization of the fact that he is such an
existing individual. The primary concern, then, is not what it
means to be human in some general or abstract sense, for this
would be an objective consideration, but rather "what it means
that you and I and he are human beings, each one for himself"
(1846, p. 109).

Central to the notion of the individual and subjectivity is the
question of ethical choice. What is of primary importance for

Kierkegaard is not the object of choice but the manner of choice. Ethical choice is absolute, that is, the choice is made in some unlimited way so that the individual assumes complete responsibility for it. As Kierkegaard puts it in the second part of *Either/Or*: "If you will understand me aright, I should like to say that in making a choice, it is not so much a question of choosing the right as of the energy, the earnestness, the pathos with which one chooses. Thereby the personality announces its inner infinity, and thereby, in turn, the personality is consolidated" (part 2, p. 171). Such an act of choosing is unavoidably an expression of the ethical.

The only absolute either/or is the choice between good and evil, and that is an ethical choice. Ethical choice is opposed to aesthetic choice, which Kierkegaard describes as either entirely immediate or as losing itself in the multifarious. In Kierkegaard's words:

> It is, therefore, not so much a question of choosing between willing the good *or* the evil, as of choosing to will, but by this in turn the good and the evil are posited. He who chooses the ethical chooses the good, but here the good is entirely abstract, only its being posited, and hence it does not follow by any means that the chooser cannot in turn choose the evil, in spite of the fact that he chose the good. Here you see again how important it is that a choice be made, and the crucial thing is not deliberation, but the baptism of the will which lifts up the choice into the ethical. [1843a, part 2, p. 173]

Thus, it is precisely through the medium of ethical choice that the individual becomes an individual and becomes detached from the crowd, so that he becomes aware of himself as a vital personal center of responsibility and selfhood.

Kierkegaard undoubtedly saw the risk in his emphasis on subjectivity and individuality, particularly the danger of self-isolation and of withdrawal from human society. The *Journals* contain frequent references and cautions regarding the overextension of his thesis. His own vocation he described as analogous to that of the spy in an enemy territory, or to the sentry on the lonely battlefield—both circumstances that amplify the need for inner resourcefulness and emphasize the individual. He reviled the appeal to public opinion and mass movements as criteria of truth among his contemporaries. He was troubled by the tendency to adopt a herd mentality, as the result of social forces that led toward egalitarian ideals and the engulfment of the individual in the political mass, whether that be the democratic majority, the race, the class, the nation, or even humanity itself.

Although the specter of the mass man is a threat to human existence and value, Kierkegaard insisted that every man in the crowd has the power within himself to become an individual, a true and authentic self. Thus, his *Christian Discourses* are addressed to individuals, that is, to every human being precisely as an individual. For him the summons of Christianity to mankind was for each and every human being to become an individual, to posit that fundamental ethical choice which led inexorably to becoming an individual and to realize in its fullness his own subjective selfhood.

The culmination point of existential truth and the highest act of man's individual subjectivity took place for Kierkegaard in the act and assent of faith. For him, faith was man's supreme passion and his most meaningful act of existence. It is an act in which man engages his entire self in a temporal and historical process that is at the same time a synthesis of the temporal and eternal and an act in which the believer becomes identified with Christ. Fundamentally, faith implies an act of the will, a fundamental choice in which man both makes a radical expression of his subjectivity and posits himself in his choosing to will the infinite. Because it was the ultimate expression of individuality and subjective truth, the act of faith was for Kierkegaard a kind of Archimedean point upon which he could base his philosophical stand and which would allow him to break out of the constraints and limits of systematic thinking, particularly as presented by the dialectic idealism of Hegel.

The paradox is that faith does all this by virtue of the absurd, and not by virtue of human understanding. The paradox of faith is cast in terms of the contrast between the knight of faith and the knight of infinite resignation. The knight of infinite resignation is

like the ancient Stoic or the modern romantic hero who re-
nounces everything in life without any glimmer of hope of get-
ting it back. He, therefore, denies himself the finite, the world
and everything in it, and lives in the infinite. The knight of faith,
however, also undergoes an infinite resignation but at the same
time believes by virute of the absurd that he will gain it back in the
end. His life encompasses the double movement of infinite resignation while living in the finite.

The model of the knight of faith was Abraham, whose profound faith and obedience to God's command to slay his son Isaac
is the subject of Kierkegaard's powerful discourse on faith, *Fear
and Trembling*. The first movement in Abraham's faith was the
infinite resignation, but the movements of faith lie beyond infinite
resignation. Of the knight of faith Kierkegaard writes:

> And yet, and yet I could become furious over it—for envy, if
> for no other reason—because the man has made and in every
> instant is making the movements of infinity. With infinite
> resignation he has drained the cup of life's profound sad-
> ness, he knows the bliss of the infinite, he senses the pain of
> renouncing everything, the dearest things he possesses in the
> world, and yet finiteness tastes to him just as good as to one
> who never knew anything higher.... And yet, and yet the
> whole earthly form he exhibits is a new creation by virtue of
> the absurd. He resigned everything infinitely, and then he
> grasped everything again by virtue of the absurd. [1843b, p.
> 51]

Thus, faith in a fundamental way participates in a paradox,

> that the individual as the particular is higher than the univer-
> sal, is justified over against it, is not subordinate but
> superior—yet in such a way, be it observed, that it is the
> particular individual who, after he has been subordinated as
> the particular to the universal, now through the universal
> becomes the individual who as the particular is superior to
> the individual, *inasmuch as the individual as the particular stands
> in an absolute relation to the absolute*. This position cannot be

mediated, for all mediation comes about precisely by virtue
of the universal; it is and remains to all eternity a paradox,
inaccessible to thought. And yet faith is this paradox....
[1843b, p. 66]

Thus, in faith there is a suspension and a transcending of the
ethical as universal. The story of Abraham contains what Kierkegaard calls a "teleological suspension of the ethical," a suspension of the basic principle that a father should love his son and not
kill him. The difference between Abraham and the tragic hero is
that the tragic hero remains within the ethical. The tragic conflict
is between one expression of an ethical *telos* and another.

In going beyond the realm of the ethical entirely, Abraham did
so in terms of a higher *telos*. There is no way in which Abraham's
action can be brought into relation with the universal; it is a purely
personal and individual action. Kierkegaard sums up the story of
Abraham as follows:

> As the individual, [Abraham] became higher than the uni-
> versal: this is the paradox which does not permit of media-
> tion. It is just as inexplicable how he got into it as it is inexpli-
> cable how he remained in it. If such is not the position of
> Abraham, then he is not even a tragic hero, but a murderer.
> To want to continue to call him the father of faith, to talk of
> this to people who do not concern themselves with anything
> but words, is thoughtless. A man can become a tragic hero by
> his own powers—but not a knight of faith. When a man en-
> ters upon the way, in a certain sense the hard way of the tragic
> hero, many will be able to give him counsel; to him who
> follows the narrow way of faith no one can give counsel, him
> no one can understand. Faith is a miracle, and yet no man is
> excluded from it; for that in which all human life is unified is
> passion, and faith is a passion. [1843b, p. 77]

In driving a wedge between the finite and the infinite, between
infinite resignation and faith, between the universal and the individual, and between the ethical and faith, Kierkegaard sets up a
radical, perhaps too radical, dissociation of faith from any form of

reason or rational assent (Edwards, 1971). Faith is rooted in a radical subjectivity that is suspicious of any intellectual processing or motives in connection with faith. He writes:

> In this way Christianity protests every form of objectivity; it desires that the subject should be infinitely concerned about himself. It is subjectivity that Christianity is concerned with, and it is only in subjectivity that its truth exists, if it exists at all; objectively, Christianity has absolutely no existence. If its truth happens to be in only a single subject, it exists in him alone; and there is a greater Christian joy in heaven over this one individual than over universal history and the system, which as objective entities are incommensurable with that which is Christian. [1846, p. 116]

The task of becoming a subject is arduous in the extreme, since it must work against so many ingrained resistances in human nature and in society. It runs against the admired wisdom of the age that the task of the subject is increasingly to divest himself of his subjectivity so that he may become more and more objective. Philosophy teaches that the way is to become objective, while Christianity teaches that the way is to become subjective, that is, to become a subject in truth.

But it must be remembered that faith asserts itself only in virtue of the absurd. With this, logic and objective inquiry cannot grapple:

> Suppose a man who wishes to acquire faith; let the comedy begin. He wishes to have faith, but he wishes also to safeguard himself by means of an objective inquiry and its approximation-process. What happens? With the help of the approximation-project the absurd becomes something different: it becomes probable, it becomes increasingly probable, it becomes extremely and emphatically probable. Now he is ready to believe it, and he ventures to claim for himself that he does not believe as shoemakers and tailors and simple folk believe, but only after long deliberation. Now he is ready to believe it; and lo, now it has become precisely impossible

to believe it. Anything that is almost probable, or probable, or extremely and emphatically probable, is something he can almost know, or as good as know, or extremely and emphatically almost *know*—but it is impossible to *believe*. For the absurd it is the object of faith and the only object that can be believed. [1846, p. 189]

Kierkegaard distills this sentiment and perspective on faith into one synthetic statement:

Subjectively, what it is to become a Christian is defined thus:
The decision lies in the subject. The appropriation is the paradoxical inwardness which is specifically different from all other inwardness. The thing of being a Christian is not determined by the *what* of Christianity but by the *how* of the Christian. This *how* can only correspond with one thing, the absolute paradox. There is therefore no vague talk to the effect that being a Christian is to accept, and to accept, and to accept quite differently, to appropriate, to believe, to appropriate by faith quite differently (all of them purely rhetorical and fictitious definitions); but to *believe* is specifically different from all other appropriation and inwardness. *Faith is the objective uncertainty along with the repulsion of the absurd held fast in the passion of inwardness, which precisely is inwardness potentiated to the highest degree.* This formula fits only the believer, no one else, not a lover, not an enthusiast, not a thinker, but simply and solely the believer who is related to the absolute paradox. [1846, p. 540]

One of the most powerful aspects of Kierkegaard's argument regarding subjectivity and existential truth comes in his analysis of despair, which he sees as the radical converse of faith. The man who is in despair is essentially double-minded, that is, having two wills such that he is unable to will one thing: specifically, he is unable to will to be himself. In *The Sickness unto Death,* Kierkegaard writes:

A despairing man wants despairingly to be himself. But if he despairingly wants to be himself, he will not want to get rid of himself. Yes, so it seems; but if one inspects more closely, one perceives that after all the contradiction is the same. That self which he despairingly wills to be is a self which he is not (for to will to be that self which one truly is is indeed the opposite of despair); what he really wills is to tear his self away from the Power which constituted it. But notwithstanding . . . all the efforts of despair, that Power is the stronger, and it compels him to be the self he does not will to be. But for all that he wills to be rid of himself, to be rid of the self which he is, in order to be the self he himself has chanced to choose. To be *self* as he wills to be would be his delight (though in another sense it would be equally despair), but to be compelled to be *self* as he does not will to be is his torment, namely, that he cannot get rid of himself. [1849, p. 153]

The immediate man is immersed in the earthly and the finite; he has no infinite consciousness of the self or of the nature or fact of despair. His despair is passive. Kierkegaard says of him:

The *immediate* man (insofar as immediacy is to be found without any reflection) is merely soulishly determined, his self or he himself is a something included along with "the other" in the compass of the temporal and the worldly, and it has only an illusory appearance of possessing in it something eternal. Thus, the self coheres immediately with "the other", wishing, desiring, enjoying, etc., but passively. [1849, p. 184]

Such a man has no self and does not become a self but lives on only in the immediacy of his experience. He lives by acquiring some little understanding of life, by learning to imitate others around him, seeing how they live their lives, and by mimicry he too manages to live after a fashion. Kierkegaard focuses this form of despair specifically in terms of a pathology of the self: "When immediacy despairs, it possesses not even enough self to wish or to dream that it had become what it did not become. The immediate man helps himself in a different way: he wishes to be another" (1849, p. 186).

When the immediate man may be assumed to have some degree of self-reflection, there may be some degree of consciousness of himself and of his despair: but the despair is essentially a despair of weakness and passivity. It remains a form of not wanting to be oneself. His degree of self-reflection allows him to become aware of himself as essentially different from his environment and from the external aspects of it. But he finds himself without perfection, and this difficulty frightens him away. He is left with the despair of weakness, of passive suffering of the self that he can only do his best to defend.

Man may also despair about the eternal or about himself: "This despair represents quite an advance. If the former was the *despair of weakness,* this is *despair over his weakness,* although it still remains . . .'despair of weakness'. . . . The despairer understands that it is weakness to take the earthly so much to heart. . . . But then, instead of veering sharply away from despair to faith, humbling himself before God for his weakness, he is more deeply absorbed in despair and despairs over his weakness" (1849, p. 195).

Ultimately, there is despair over himself, for despair about the eternal is impossible without some concept of self. Along with this greater consciousness, there is a greater knowledge of what despair is, that it is a loss of the eternal and oneself.

Beyond this despair of weakness, Kierkegaard places a further form of despair, which becomes conscious of the reason why it does not want to be itself; this is the despair of willing despairingly to be oneself—namely defiance.

> defiance . . . really is despair by the aid of the eternal, the despairing abuse of the eternal in the self to the point of being despairingly determined to be oneself. But just because it is despair by the aid of the eternal, it lies in a sense very close to the true, and just because it lies very close to the true, it is infinitely remote. The despair which is a passage way to faith is also by the aid of the eternal: by the aid of the eternal the self has courage to lose itself in order to gain itself. Here on the contrary it is not willing to begin by losing itself, but wills to be itself. [1849, p. 201]

This despair is conscious of itself since it does not come from something external as a form of suffering but comes directly from the self. This willing of oneself in despair requires a consciousness of what Kierkegaard calls the infinite self:

> By the aid of this infinite form the self despairingly wills to dispose of itself or to create itself, to make itself the self it wills to be, distinguishing in the concrete self what it will and what it will not accept. The man's concrete self, or his concretion, has in fact necessity and limitations, it is this perfectly definite thing, with these faculties, dispositions, etc. But by the aid of the infinite form, the negative self, he wills first to undertake to refashion the whole thing, in order to get out of it in this way a self such as he wants to have, produced by the aid of the infinite form of the negative self—and it is thus he wills to be himself. [1849, pp. 201–02]

But such a self can never become any more than it is in itself, hence in its despairing efforts to will to be itself it ends up by becoming, in fact, no self—a hypothetical self.

The despair that wills desperately to be itself is not willing to hope. Such a sufferer becomes offended at the whole of existence and in spite of his suffering he wills not to be himself without it, for as Kierkegaard notes, this would be to move in the direction of resignation. And so he defiantly wills the whole of his existence, wills himself as suffering, almost defying his torment. To hope in the possibility of help, let alone to seek help by virtue of the absurd, by virtue of the fact that for God all things are possible— that he will not do. The more consciously this sufferer determines in despair to be himself, all the more does his despair become demoniac.

Subjectivity and Self in Psychoanalysis

The attempt to integrate Kierkegaard's contribution requires some translation into more specifically psychoanalytical terms— both clinical and theoretical.

Kierkegaard's unique formulations come very close to describing a phenomenology of clinical conditions that is readily recognizable from a psychoanalytic perspective. The analysis of despair, for example, yields readily to a translation into more clinical terms. At the core of despair lies the inability to will oneself. The clinician can recognize here a core disturbance that is found, with variations on the theme, throughout the whole spectrum of psychopathology. The inability to will oneself in an honest and authentic and responsible manner lies at the core of most neurotic difficulties—regardless of the patterns of symptomatology and defensive organization that arise as a secondary reaction to this core deficit. In the light of my own theoretical orientation, I translate this difficulty into the terms derived from the vocabulary of internalization.

The human psyche takes shape and undergoes development through the progressive organization and integration of internalizations that derive in important ways from the experience of objects in the individual's human environment (Meissner, 1979).

The sense of self, the sense of what and who one is in oneself, arises out of the amalgamation and integration of the introjections and identifications consequent to such interaction. When the introjections acquired over the course of one's developmental history are relatively harmonious and positively tinged, they give rise to a relatively unconflicted and positive sense of self, which can serve as the basis for a harmonious and well-functioning internal psychic integration and for the capacity for healthy adaptation to one's environment and nonneurotic personality adjustment. However, when these configurations arise out of situations of conflict, tension, or other forms of dysphoria or disharmony in the relationships with significant objects, the introjective organization reflects instinctual imbalances and the forms of pathogenic defensive organization correlative to these. Phenomenologically, such an individual develops a sense of self characterized by feelings of inadequacy, vulnerability, worthlessness, extreme sensitivity and pride, grandiosity, excessive and exquisite dependency, hostility and rage, shame, and so forth. Part of the work of psychoanalysis—perhaps the most significant part—is to undo and to revise the component elements of this composite sense of self, so that the individual can surrender the pathogenic self-organization that lies at the root of his symptomatology and his other psychological difficulties and replace it with something more authentically his own (Meissner, 1978).

The work of analysis entails the stripping away of aspects of this pathological organization, tracing their origins in the individual's life experience, unearthing the usually hidden and unconscious motivations that preserve and reinforce them, and enabling the individual little by little to abandon his attachment to them and to fulfill some of his developmental potentialities for new, healthier, and more adaptive configuration. But the man of despair who wills this pathogenic configuration and clings to it in the face of the efforts of his therapist to pull him away from it can will only the self that he sees and senses; it is his misfortune that that self is not himself.

Kierkegaard's description of this condition is also reminiscent of some familiar schizoid variants in the clinical situation. The schizoid dilemma is essentially one between the intense need for objects and an equally intense fear of engulfment by objects, of being swallowed up and consumed by them (Burnham, Gladstone, and Gibson, 1969). Such patients complain of feeling isolated and cut off, shut out, strange; they complain of an inner emptiness, of a life that seems futile, meaningless, leading nowhere and accomplishing nothing. The schizoid person cannot effectively choose his own self as involved with and related to objects. External relationships are affectively empty and characterized by emotional withdrawal. The individual draws behind a defensive shell into a hidden inner world so that his unconscious sense of himself is emptied of any vital feeling and capacity for involvement and so seems to have become unreal. His attitude to the world around him is one of noninvolvement and mere observation, without any feeling, attachment, or participation.

Two prominent variants of the schizoid condition are the false-self organization, originally described by Winnicott (1960), and the as-if personality, defined originally by Helene Deutsch (1942). In the false-self variant there is a turning away from interpersonal relationships out of a need to preserve the sense of inner autonomy and individuation. Deutsch's account of the "as-if" personality focuses on an apparent impoverishment of emotional relationships. These patients seem lacking in wholeness or genuineness, and yet their lives move along as if they were somehow complete.

Similarly, Kierkegaard's immediate man, who manages to live a sort of life based on compliance and mimicry, is left in the condition of despair. Clinically, the issues involved in the spectrum of alternatives can be recognized as basically narcissistic. Such a despairing individual is unwilling to choose himself because he is unwilling to accept his weaknesses, imperfections, shortcomings, inadequacies, and limitations. He holds out for something better, something nobler, something more ideal, something closer to the perfection he envisions and desires for himself.

One extreme defensive posture in this context of narcissistic entitlement and adherence is defined by Kierkegaard in terms of defiance, that is, the will to be oneself despairingly. In clinical terms, we can recognize this as akin to the paranoid disorders. The paranoid patient, in a sense, stakes a defiant claim in his own individuality, specialness, and difference. Here the self defiantly proclaims itself to be what it wills to be and rejects, often hostilely and destructively, what it cannot accept within itself. Rather, it retreats to a sense of self embedded in grandiosity and often sets up against the rest of the world in embattled hostility. Such a man cannot accept his true self at all but must substitute for it a fiction, a hypothetical self, a self such as he wills it to be but not as he is.

When we ask what is entailed in the choosing of one's self, Kierkegaard's answer is in terms of resignation followed by a gaining back of what has been lost, by virtue of the absurd. This can be translated into a psychoanalytic perspective in terms of the dynamics of narcissism. The analytic process, in order to reach its goal, must entail a resignation that entails all of those elements which have been embedded in the pathogenic sense of self. We can immediately recognize what the momentousness of such a requirement may be. The individual has spent a lifetime shaping and constructing the self-organization that has become the core of his experience of himself. How does one come to a point at which it becomes possible to resign oneself, to detach oneself from it, to give it up? After all, we are talking about one's self, that which is closest, most precious, most identified with our sense of who and what we are. The very idea of resigning oneself is threatening in the extreme, more threatening than the idea of resigning any possession or quality that we can regard as extrinsic to ourselves. But it is precisely this resignation that is required in order for the analytic resolution to take place.

Moreover, from a dynamic point of view, the resignation of the self is all the more difficult because it has become the locus of intense narcissistic investments. This may seem paradoxical, since we are talking about individuals in whom the pathogenic sense of self has become the source of so many psychological difficulties, conflicts, anxieties, and other painful dysphoric affects. One would think that such a patient would be only too eager to surrender this source of pathogenic dismay. But it is not so. The patient mobilizes powerful resistances to surrendering this precious sense of himself because it is his self, it is the only self he has ever known, the only self he has ever had. Literally, for him to resign it is to resign himself.

The situation, it seems to me, is something analogous to that described by Kierkegaard in terms of the infinite resignation leading to faith. The second moment of the process is the choosing of oneself by virtue of the absurd and by this choosing to gain back everything that has been lost, and more. The analytic process, then, must hold a mirror up to the subject, showing him what is contained and involved in his pathogenic self, the self that he has chosen but that is not himself. The individual must be able to resign that self, particularly because of the narcissistic investments it entails.

The dynamics of narcissism display themselves in two decisive and polarized directions: one gives rise to a sense of specialness, entitlement, grandiosity, being different from and somehow superior to one's fellow men; the other gives rise to a sense of shame, inferiority, worthlessness, and inadequacy. These dimensions of the narcissistic self-portrait tend to accompany each other in an inextricable and irrevocable bond. In clinical terms, if one sees the aspects of narcissistic inferiority in a patient's self-demeanor, as is frequently the case in depressed patients, one

knows that behind the depressive facade, with its feelings of de-
valuation and loss of self-esteem, there lurk the elements of narcissistic superiority with the accompanying sense of entitlement,
specialness, and the wish to be treated in some extraordinary and
acknowledging way.

The art and the science of psychoanalysis are dedicated to the
task of finding a way, in terms of generalizable principles and
theory and in terms of the inner struggle in every psychoanalysis,
to make possible the patient's fundamental choice in virtue of the
unknown, in virtue of the absurd. When the patient can make this
choice, can choose himself in the face of the objective uncertainties of what and who he is in himself, then all is regained, and
more than all. For in this very choice the patient gains himself, a
self that he has never before possessed, a self that he has in many
ways never known to exist. Ultimately and irreducibly, that choice
is an expression of the individual's subjectivity; it is his assertion
and grasp of a subjective truth that is himself.

The psychoanalytic process, viewed in this perspective, is essentially a dialectic of subjectivity. The analytic situation, and particularly the relationship between analyst and analysand, provides a
matrix within which elements of the subjective and the objective
mingle on both sides of the analytic equation. In the analytic
"space" (Green, 1975) that is constructed between them, there
evolves an area of illusion (Winnicott, 1971) in which the
dynamics of the analytic interaction are played out. This aspect of
the subjective realm of experience of each participant is contributed by projections that derive from the organization of their
respective introjects (Meissner, 1978).

The area of illusion becomes the testing ground for the patient's subjective truth. Within this area the transference and
countertransference develop through the interweaving of reciprocal projections and introjections. By revivifying and reexperiencing in the transference matrix the vicissitudes of object
relationships that derive from various levels of his developmental
experience, the patient comes to reexperience aspects of his own
subjectivity in their vital interplay with both the objectivity of a
highly invested object and that object's own respective subjectiv-

ity. Through the experience of this transferential "illusion" the analysand comes to recognize the dimensions of his own subjectivity and gradually, often in a painstaking and piecemeal fashion, to acknowledge the parts of that subjective experience which belong essentially to another rather than himself. By this process of recognition he begins to realize that the self he has always affirmed as his own may be inauthentic, falsely and defensively motivated, and may have little to do with that which ultimately is authentically his own.

One way of interpreting the analytic dialogue is as a continual winnowing process by which the false components of the analysand's apparent self, and the motivations behind them, are gradually isolated, defined, analyzed, and ultimately—in Kierkegaardian terms—resigned. Once the residues of infantile fixation, dependence, and omnipotence are stripped away and recognized, the analysand is left with a vacuum that ultimately only he can fill. His transference to the analyst, his trust in and dependence on the analyst, the capacity for meaningful alliance in collaboration with the analyst, serve him as a strong sustaining force to undergo the bitter and difficult work of disengaging the pathogenic aspects of his own self and gradually resigning them.

But at some point the basic choice, which Kierkegaard described so vividly—the choice of himself, with all of the disappointment, disillusionment, inperfection, and limitation of reality—must unalterably be made. I say *must* because it is an intrinsic demand of the analytic process itself; but at the same time the choice can be avoided or short-circuited in myriad ways that have an infinite capacity to deceive both the analysand and his analyst. Although the analytic dialectic leads inexorably in the direction of a clarification of one's own subjectivity, in its imperfect resolution, the process can—and often does—yield only a partial resignation and a partial grasping of one's own subjectivity. One possible outcome of this kind is an acceptance of an ideal of analytic perfection that rests ultimately on compliance with the analyst's expectations and is therefore substitute and false but that nonetheless provides a workable identity and sense of subjective truth for the analysand.

In the beginning of this essay the problem of subjectivity was posed primarily from a theoretical perspective. In the debate between the objective and subjective adherents within psychoanalysis, I have taken the position here that is intermediate and consequently open to ambiguity. I think the argument over subjectivity cannot avoid the telling conclusion that psychoanalysis cannot do without the inclusion of individual subjectivity within its scope. The question is whether or not there is room for such subjectivity within its scientific account of itself. For the Hartmann school, the data of subjectivity and of meaningful content within psychoanalysis were regarded as nontheoretical, that is, as part of the empirical substratum with which analysts worked and out of which it compounded its theories. The contemporary argument, however, reaches further, since it demonstrates not only the operation of subjective factors within the analytic process but places a further demand that these elements be given theoretical recognition.

The argument as it developed historically lacked a concept or set of concepts that might have effectively mediated the polar contentions. The debate over subjectivity, as I have traced it above, labors under a theoretical framework, or "paradigm" in Kuhn's (1970) terms, that did not reach beyond the merely functional, mechanical, and structural account provided by a systematized ego psychology. In such a theory, there was no place for the personal agent, the meaning-giving, meaning-taking, interpreting, and intentional source of individual responsibility and action. I would like to take the argument a step further by saying that a properly elaborated concept of the self may provide the overriding conceptual framework so that the elements of the objective structuralized account may take their appropriate place alongside the more subjective concerns we have been discussing.

From this point of view, it seems that the notion of the self lends itself readily and appropriately as the locus of subjectivity. As Hartmann pointed out, the self is the appropriate notion that stands in proper opposition to the object and the objective. Consequently, the linking of self-awareness and self-activity with the notion of subjectivity seems an easy next step. Clearly, the self as so delineated must stand in opposition to the structural apparatus that has been the substance of classical psychoanalytic metapsychology. But that opposition need not be and I do not think is exclusive. Rather, it seems reasonable to regard the self at a minimum as a supraordinate psychic organization that embraces as objective components and subsystems the traditional tripartite entities of the structural theory—id, ego, and superego. Thus, the frame of reference provided by the structural entities is specifically that of intra- or intersystemic conflict and/or integration. The theoretical frame of reference provided by the self, however, not only entertains these subsystems as participating entities but provides a more meaningful frame of reference for their theoretical integration and for their conjoint functioning in terms of the operations of the self vis-à-vis objects and the external environment.

The conceptualization of the self in systemic terms as a supraordinate organization within which the individual psychic agencies carry out their appropriate functions can be specified in terms of the following points:

(1) The self as theoretical construct provides a focus for formulating and understanding the complex integrations of processes that involve combinations of functions of the respective psychic agencies. This would have specific reference to such activities as affects, in which all of the psychic systems seem to be in one way or another represented, the superego-ego integration reflected in the formation of value systems, and interactions involving fantasy production, drive-motor integration, cognitive-affective processes, and so forth. There is room here for a considerable reworking and refocusing of traditional psychoanalytic ways of looking at psychic phenomena. Particularly important is the whole area of the understanding of internalizations and their role in development and psychic structure formation, especially the commerce between introjections and projections as they play themselves out in the self-other interaction of interpersonal relationships.

(2) The self-concept as a supraordinate organization provides a

more specific and less ambiguous frame of reference for the articulation of self-object interrelationships and interactions, including the complex area of object relations themselves. It should be noted that the important theoretical underpinnings for our understanding of the therapeutic alliance cannot simply rest on an ego-psychological basis, as has been the case to date. Rather, the therapeutic alliance, analogous to but decidedly different from the phenomenon of transference, involves important classes of interaction between subject and object that need to be specifically delineated and understood in those terms.

(3) The emergence of a self-concept provides a locus in the theory for articulating the experience of a personal self, either as grasped introspectively and reflexively or as experienced as the originating source of personal activity. As numerous criticisms have indicated, the conceptual apparatus having to do with the functions of id, ego, and superego cannot provide an adequate account of this sense of personal agency. However, the full understanding of the experience of selfhood involves various aspects of the integrated functions of these respective psychic agencies, and something more. The something more has to do specifically with the subjectivity of the personal agent, the dimension of human experience so exquisitely addressed by Kierkegaard.

One way of dealing with the integration of the classical structural entities and the phenomenology of the self has been to view them as complementary accounts of the analytical data. The model of complementarity, however, following the classic wave-particle complementarity of light physics, implies that the same phenomena are being viewed from two theoretical perspectives that remain in some degree exclusive—a fundamental theoretical either/or in Kierkegaard's terms. Thus, an adequate account of the reality becomes impossible because of the divergence of observational approach or of measurement techniques. However, in psychoanalysis the situation is somewhat different. Here the method of observation or measurement remains the same, but what we are dealing with are essentially different phenomena or different aspects of the organization and functioning of the human psyche. The phenomena addressed by a structural, conflict-related, drive-defense model are not the same as those addressed in a self-perspective.

For example, the classical paradigm focuses on aspects of the analytic transference experience that are different from those focused on by the self-psychology paradigm. In the classical paradigm, transference has more to do with the libidinal and/or aggressive impulses directed toward significant objects and the resultant conflicts. The locus of the conflict, therefore, is primarily intrapsychic and intersystemic. In transference from the perspective of the self, however, the issues of difficulties in the relationship between self and object, the emergence of issues of trust and dependence, and the narcissistic issues related to self and object valuation are considerably more predominant (Kohut, 1971). Clinical experience suggests that not all of these aspects will come into focus to the same degree in every patient. The more classically neurotic patients may be quite adequately conceptualized for purposes of therapy in terms of the classical model, while patients in whom narcissistic, object-relational, and self-organizational problems play a more significant part in the pathology will bring the self-related aspects of the transference into much clearer focus.

The important contribution that Kierkegaard makes to this internal psychoanalytic dialectic is the understanding that there is a dimension of the analytic experience and a kind of analytic truth that can be regarded strictly in subjective terms. Thus, the *what* of psychoanalytic understanding must be combined with the *how* of the analysand's comprehension and choice related to that content. The analytic process reaches a culmination not merely when the objective account reaches a level of clarity and reasonable reconstruction, but rather when that objective account comes to meet the realm of subjectivity and subjective truth and becomes a truth for the subject in a meaningful and embracing way. It is at that point that there is the potentiality for meaningful existential choice and commitment. That choice and the subjective truth in question represent ultimately a knowing choice of oneself in the face of objective uncertainties, ambiguities, and imperfections and can be seen as the process of resignation, which then issues in a willing of oneself specifically in virtue of the unknown, the indeterminate, and the uncertain. This, it seems to me, is none other than Kierkegaard's formula—to will one's self in virtue of the absurd.

REFERENCES

Apfelbaum, B. "Ego Psychology, Psychic Energy, and the Hazards of Quantitative Explanation in Psychoanalytic Theory." *International Journal of Psycho-Analysis* 46 (1965): 168-81.

———. "On Ego Psychology: A Critique of the Structural Approach to Psychoanalytic Theory." *International Journal of Psycho-Analysis* 47 (1966): 451-75.

Bretall, R., ed. *A Kierkegaard Anthology*. Princeton, N.J.: Princeton University Press, 1946.

Burnham, D. L.; Gladstone, A. I.; and Gibson, R. W. *Schizophrenia and the Need-Fear Dilemma*. New York: International Universities Press, 1969.

Collins, J. *The Mind of Kierkegaard*. Chicago: Henry Regnery, 1953.

Deutsch, H. "Some Forms of Emotional Disturbance and Their Relationship to Schizophrenia" [1942]. In *Neuroses and Character Types*. New York: International Universities Press, 1965.

Edwards, P. "Kierkegaard and the 'Truth' of Christianity." *Philosophy* 46 (1971): 89-108.

Freud, S.

The Origins of Psychoanalysis: Letters, Drafts and Notes to Wilhelm Fliess (1887-1902). New York: Basic Books, 1954.

Standard Edition of the Complete Psychological Works. London: Hogarth, 1953-74.

The Interpretation of Dreams (1900), vol. 4.

"Mourning and Melancholia" (1917), vol. 14.

The Ego and the Id (1923), vol. 19.

Inhibitions, Symptoms and Anxiety (1926), vol. 20.

"Project for a Scientific Psychology" (1950 [1895]), vol. 1.

Green, A. "The Analyst, Symbolization and Absence in the Analytic Setting (On Changes in Analytic Practice and Analytic Experience)." *International Journal of Psycho-Analysis* 56 (1975): 1-22.

Guntrip, H. *Schizoid Phenomena, Object Relations and the Self*. New York: International Universities Press, 1969.

_____. *Psychoanalytic Theory, Therapy and the Self.* New York: Basic Books, 1971.

Hartmann, H. "Understanding and Explanation" (1927). "On Rational and Irrational Action" (1947). In *Essays on Ego Psychology.* New York: International Universities Press, 1964.

_____. *Ego Psychology and the Problem of Adaptation* [1939]. New York: International Universities Press, 1958.

Holt, R. R. "A Review of Freud's Biological Assumptions and Their Influence on His Theories." In N. S. Greenfield and W. C. Lewis, eds., *Psychoanalysis and Current Biological Thought.* Madison: University of Wisconsin Press, 1965.

_____. "Freud's Mechanistic and Humanistic Images of Man." In R. R. Holt and E. Peterfreund, eds., *Psychoanalysis and Contemporary Science,* vol. 1. New York: Macmillan, 1972.

_____. "The Past and the Future of Ego Psychology." *Psychoanalytic Quarterly* 44 (1975): 550–76.

Home, H. J. "The Concept of Mind." *International Journal of Psycho-Analysis* 47 (1966): 43–49.

Kierkegaard, S.
  The Journals of Søren Kierkegaard [1834–55]. Edited by A. Dru. New York: Oxford University Press, 1938.
  Either/Or [1843a]. New York: Doubleday, 1959.
  Fear and Trembling and The Sickness unto Death [1843b, 1849]. Translated by W. Lowrie. New York: Doubleday, 1954.
  Concluding Unscientific Postscript [1846]. Princeton, N.J.: Princeton University Press, 1941.

Klein, G. S. *Essentials of Psychoanalytic Theory.* New York: International Universities Press, 1976.

Kohut, H. *The Analysis of the Self.* New York: International Universities Press, 1971.

Kuhn, T. S. *The Structure of Scientific Revolutions.* Chicago: University of Chicago Press, 1970.

Meissner, W. W. *The Paranoid Process.* New York: Jason Aronson, 1978.

_____. "Internalization and Object Relations." *Journal of the American Psychoanalytic Association* 27 (1979): 345–60.

Novey, S. *The Second Look: The Reconstruction of Personal History in Psychiatry and Psychoanalysis.* Baltimore: Johns Hopkins University Press, 1968.

Rapaport, D. "The Theory of Attention Cathexis" [1959]. "On the Psychoanalytic Theory of Motivation" [1960]. "Some Metapsychological Considerations Concerning Activity and Passivity" [1961]. In *The Collected Papers of David Rapaport.* Edited by M. M. Gill. New York: Basic Books, 1967.

Ryle, G. *The Concept of Mind* [1949]. New York: Barnes and Noble, 1965.

Schafer, R. *A New Language for Psychoanalysis.* New Haven: Yale University Press, 1976.

Winnicott, D. W. "Ego Distortion in Terms of True and False Self" [1960]. In *The Maturational Process and the Facilitating Environment.* New York: International Universities Press, 1965.

―――. *Playing and Reality.* New York: Basic Books, 1971.

10

Two Encounters with Kierkegaard:
Kierkegaard and Evil
Doing Philosophy after Kierkegaard

PAUL RICOEUR

Part I: Kierkegaard and Evil

The task of celebrating Kierkegaard, who had no pity for ministers and professors, may call forth derision. Can we talk about Kierkegaard without excluding either him or ourselves? We are here to face this ridicule as honestly and modestly as possible. After all, we must also confront Kierkegaard's sarcasm. It is still the best way of honoring him. In any case, it is better to run this risk than to prove him correct out of good manners or through convention.

I propose two very different encounters with Kierkegaard. In the first, we shall attempt to listen and to understand by simply putting before ourselves a few texts upon which we shall concentrate as narrow and intense attention as possible. These texts are taken from two writings, *The Concept of Dread*, which dates from 1844, and *The Sickness unto Death*, published five years later, in 1849. I want to extract from these two essays Kierkegaard's thought concerning evil by means of as rigorous an exegesis as

"Kierkegaard et le mal" and "Philosophie après Kierkegaard," *Revue de Théologie et de Philosophie* 13 (1963): 292–302, 303–16. Translated by David Pellauer. These two essays, along with an essay by Gabriel Widmer on "Kierkegaard et le Christ," were originally presented under the auspices of the Theology Faculty of the University of Geneva and the Marie Gretler Foundation on the occasion of the 150th anniversary of Kierkegaard's birth. They are here combined and slightly altered to fit the format of this volume. Reprinted by permission.

possible. It is through this *explication de texte* that we run the biggest risk of excluding ourselves. In the second encounter, I will try to explicate and apply the precept taught by Karl Jaspers more than forty years ago. Our task, he said, we who are not the exception, is to think in the face of the exception. Thus, we will attempt not to exclude Kierkegaard by posing the question, How is it possible to do philosophy after Kierkegaard?

Why are we stopping with these two texts and why the question of evil?

Let us consider the question of evil first. There is scarcely any need to emphasize that evil is the critical point for all philosophical thought. If it comprehends evil, this is its greatest success. Yet evil understood is no longer evil. It has stopped being absurd, scandalous, beyond right and reason. Yet if philosophy does not comprehend evil, then it is no longer philosophy—at least if philosophy ought to comprehend everything and set itself up as a system with nothing outside itself. In the great debate between Kierkegaard and the system—which is to say, Hegel—the question of evil represents a touchstone beyond compare. This debate will lead us to our second problem, can we do philosophy after Kierkegaard? In view of this question regarding a vote of confidence in philosophy, it is important to understand how Kierkegaard himself thought in the face of the irrational, the absurd. For he did not proclaim; he thought.

There is another reason for talking about evil. It is not only the touchstone for philosophy, it is also the occasion to take by surprise the quality of Kierkegaard's Christianity; I mean his Christianity of the Cross more than of Easter or of Pentecost. But above all, I want to attempt to show how Kierkegaard speaks and thinks about evil; that is, about what is most opposed to the system.

I shall begin with the following brief comment. Neither of these two books constitutes, in any way, a journal or a confession. You will find no trace in these two writings of the terrible confession his father made to him about that day in his youth, when, shepherding his sheep on the Jutland heath, he climbed up on a rock and cursed God. Or anything about the precipitous marriage of the widower father to his servant mistress, or of all the deaths that struck the paternal home, as if in punishment for the earlier blasphemy, or of Søren's melancholy, or of the splinter in his flesh. We would be wasting our time if we took the short way of psychoanalytic biography and if we looked in these complicated and argumentative writings for the direct transposition of an emotional life weighed down by torments and remorse. This direct way, from the life to the work, is absolutely forbidden to us. Not that a psychoanalysis of Kierkegaard, or at least a fragmentary psychoanalytic approach, is impossible, but rather we must resolutely take the inverse way to him—that is, start with the exegesis of texts and perhaps return from them to the life, for there is more in these texts than the biographical odds and ends we might collect.

Thus, let us turn directly to the texts. These two treatises have in common that they are built upon the basis of two feelings or moods, more precisely, two negative feelings or moods whose object remains indeterminate: dread (or anxiety) and despair. Anxiety about what? Despair about what? Yet it is from these two that we must begin, for if we adopt as our starting point what we already know about evil, we will miss precisely what these two moods can teach us. To begin from known evil is to begin from a purely moral definition of guilt, as the transgressing of a law or as an infraction. On the contrary, the question is to discover a quality and a dimension of "sin" that only these profound emotions, ordinarily linked to melancholy or fear, can announce. Because the determination of evil occurs entirely within the orbit of these two moods, the resulting "concept" of evil is profoundly different in each treatise. The analysis of anxiety leads to a concept of sin as event or upheaval. Anxiety itself is a sort of slipping, of fascination wherein evil is circumscribed, approached from back and front. To the contrary, the *Treatise on Despair*—another name for *The Sickness unto Death*—takes place in the midst of sin, no longer as a leap, but as a state: despair is, if we may put it this way, the evil of evil, the sin of sin.

Let us successively consider these two approaches. To finish, we shall try to understand their conjunction.

The first is deliberately anti-Hegelian: leap, upheaval, event, are opposed to mediation, synthesis, reconciliation. In this way, too, the equivocal mixing of the ethical and the logical is broken off: "In logic this is too much, in ethics too little; it fits nowhere if it has to fit both places" (*The Sickness unto Death,* p. 13). But who then will speak justly about sin? The metaphysician? He is both too disinterested and too comprehensive. The moralist? He believes too much in man's effort and not enough in his misery. The preacher? Well, perhaps, for he addresses himself to the isolated individual, one to one. But do not let him be a Hegelian minister! The dogmatician too, though he only explains sin by presupposing it: "The concept of sin does not properly belong in any science; only the second ethics"—the one that follows dogmatics and that knows the real and sin without "metaphysical frivolity or psychological concupiscence" (p. 18)—"can deal with its apparition but not with its origin" (p. 19). And yet it is as a psychologist that Kierkegaard is going to speak. To isolate the act's radical leap, the psychologist outlines its possibility, thereby in a way approaching the discontinuity of upheaval through the continuity of a sliding or slippage.

The paradox here is that of a beginning. How does sin come into the world? By a leap that presupposes itself in temptation. This is the "concept of anxiety": a psychology as close as possible to the event, a psychology that clings to the event as an advent, a psychology of the *durée* wherein innocence loses itself, is already lost, where it seesaws, totters, and falls. But we do not know innocence. We only know its loss. Innocence is something that "only comes into existence by the very fact that it is annulled, comes into existence as that which was before it was annulled and now is annulled" (p. 33). Hence I only know innocence as lost. I only know the leap of sin in its transition. This is something that is in between innocence that is lost and a leap that proceeds itself in anxiety.

What can be said about anxiety per se? It is the birth of spirit, of that spirit the Bible calls discerning of good and evil. But spirit is still a kind of dreaming. It is no longer innocence, nor yet good and evil. About what then does spirit dream? About nothing. Nothing at all. This nothing gives birth to anxiety. It is why "dread

is freedom's reality as possibility for possibility" (p. 38).
Nothing—possibility—freedom . . . One sees that ambiguity—the
word is Kierkegaard's—is more enigmatic than the already too
ethical "concupiscence." A "sympathetic antipathy and an antipathetic sympathy," the subtle Kierkegaard prefers to say (p.
38). And he calls this ambiguity dialectical, but psychological, not
logical. We will return to this point in our second encounter: "Just
as the relation of dread to its object, to something which is nothing
(language in this instance also is pregnant: it speaks of being in
dread of nothing), is altogether ambiguous, so will the transition
here from innocence to guilt be correspondingly so dialectical
that the explanation is and must be psychological" (p. 39).

Will someone say that it is prohibition that awakens desire? Yet
innocence does not understand prohibition. This is an explanation after the fact. We should rather say that prohibition is the
word—the "enigmatic word"—that crystallizes anxiety. The decree alarms Adam because it awakens in him the possibility of
freedom. Nothingness becomes the "possibility of the possibility
of being able to do something." This is what Adam loves and what
he flees.

We should not say that Kierkegaard delights in the irrational.
He analyzes, he dissects, he abounds in words. He is the dialecti-
cian of the antidialectic. And this paradoxical dialectic culminates
in the representation of human beings as a synthesis of soul and
body, united in this third term: spirit—spirit that dreams about
nothing, spirit that projects the possible. Spirit is the "hostile
power" that constantly disturbs this relation, which, however,
only exists through it. On the other hand, it is a "friendly power,"
which desires to constitute exactly this relation: "What then is
man's relation to this ambiguous power? How is spirit related to
itself and to its situation? It is related as dread" (pp. 39–40).

Hence psychology comes too soon or too late. It recognizes
either the anxiety of before, which leads to the qualitative leap—
the anxiety of dreaming, of nothing—or the anxiety of afterward,
which augments evil—the anxiety of reflection, about something,
become in a way nature insofar as it henceforth has a "body." This
is why anxiety permeates sex: not that it comes with it but because

it comes to it. The anxiety of dreaming becomes flesh and extends an "inexplicable deep melancholy" over everything. It would be a mistake here to look for some kind of puritanical repugnance to sexuality. Before Max Scheler, Kierkegaard understood that anxiety does not come from sex but descends from the spirit into sexuality, from dreaming into the flesh. It is because man is disturbed in spirit that he is ashamed in his flesh. The spirit is uneasy in modesty and frightened over assuming sexual differentiation. Thus sin enters the world, becomes a world, and increases quantitatively.

Yet we do not know better what sin is through subsequent anxiety than through prior anxiety. It remains anxiety, closely circumscribed, yet empty at its center: "No science can explain how. Psychology comes nearest to doing so and explains the last step in the approximation, which is freedom's apparition before itself in the dread of possibility, or in the nothingness of possibility, or in the nothing of dread" (p. 69).

The Sickness unto Death, or *Treatise on Despair,* is also a psychological essay. More precisely, according to its subtitle, it is "A Christian Psychological Exposition for Edification and Awakening." Consequently, this treatise associates psychology, in the sense of *The Concept of Dread,* with edification in the sense of the *Edifying Discourses.* We have spoken already of the difference that separates these two treatises: the first speaks of evil as an event, a leap; the second speaks of it as a state of affairs. The substitution of despair for anxiety expresses this shift: anxiety tends toward . . . , despair resides in. . . . Anxiety "ex-ists"; despair "in-sists." What does this shift signify? It is impossible to understand *The Sickness unto Death* without referring back to an earlier essay, *Fear and Trembling,* which situates the meaning of faith and sin beyond the sphere of the ethical. Sin is not the contrary of virtue but of faith, which is a theological category. Faith is a way of being face to face with God, before God. This liaison is elaborated in *Fear and Trembling,* not by means of an abstract discussion about theological concepts, but by way of an *exegesis.* The new concepts are deciphered by means of the interpretation of a story, the story of Abraham. The *meaning* of the sacrificing of Isaac decides the meaning of the concepts of law and faith. Sacrificing Isaac would be a crime according to the moral law. According to faith, it is an act of obedience. To obey God, Abraham had to suspend the ethical. He had to become the knight of faith who moves forward alone, beyond the security of the universal law, or, as Kierkegaard puts it, of the universal. Hence *Fear and Trembling* opens a new dimension of anxiety, which proceeds from the contradiction between ethics and faith. Abraham is the symbol of this new species of anxiety linked to the theological suspension of the ethical.

The concept of despair belongs to the same nonethical but religious sphere as does Abraham's faith. Despair is the negative version of Abraham's faith. This is why Kierkegaard does not first say what sin is, then what despair is; instead he constructs and discovers sin in despair as its religious signification. From there on, sin is no longer a leap but a stagnant stage, a persisting mode of being.

Second consequence: the question is no longer, How did it enter into the world?—through anxiety; but, How is it possible to escape? Despair is thus comparable to one of the "stages on life's way" that Kierkegaard explores in another work. It is a sickness, a sickness one dies of without dying. It is the sickness "unto death," in the way that injustice, according to Plato, in book 10 of *The Republic,* is a living death and the paradoxical proof of immortality. Despair, according to Kierkegaard, is a greater evil than injustice according to Plato, which still refers to the ethical sphere. Yet because it is more grave, it is closer to recovery.

Now, how can we speak of despair? Structural analysis of *The Sickness unto Death* should bring us closer to our problem: What is Kierkegaard's mode of thinking? How is it possible to do philosophy after Kierkegaard? What is remarkable, is that Kierkegaard constructs the concept of despair. A quick look at the table of contents of this treatise reveals a tangle of titles and subtitles. The plan is even curiously didactic. The first part demonstrates this: "The Sickness Unto Death Is Despair." Its possibility, actuality, universality, and forms are carefully distinguished. Its forms are even elaborated in a rather systematic manner, from the point of view of a "lack of finitude" and a "lack of infinitude," from a "lack

of possibility"—which is to say of imagination and dreaming—
and a "lack of necessity"—which is to say of submitting to our tasks
and general duties in this world. The same balancing is renewed
with the appearance of new distinctions. The most subtle one is
presented as follows: "Despair viewed under the aspect of consciousness," wherein it knows itself or does not know itself.
Therefore, there is a despair over "not willing to be oneself" and
over "willing to be oneself."

Then the second part, entitled "Despair Is Sin," elaborates all
the characteristics of sin according to the model of despair and
leads to the conclusion that "sin is not a negation but a position." I
will stop with this conclusion, which I will oppose to the nothingness of anxiety.

But first I want to interrogate the strange structure of this
treatise. It is impossible not to be impressed by the heavy and
laborious aspect of its construction, which resembles an interminable and awkward dissertation. What does it signify? We are confronted by a sort of grimacing simulacre of Hegelian discourse.
Yet this simulacre is at the same time the means of saving its
discourse from absurdity. It is didactic because it cannot be dialectic. In other words, it replaces a three-term dialectic by a cut-off
dialectic, by an unresolved two-term dialectic. A dialectic without
mediation—this is the Kierkegaardian paradox. *Either* too much
possibility *or* too much actuality. *Either* too much finitude *or* too
much infinitude. *Either* one wants to be oneself *or* one does not
want to be oneself. What is more, since each pair of contrary terms
offers no resolution, it is not possible to construct the following
paradox on the one that precedes it. The chain of paradoxes is
itself a broken chain—hence the didactic framework, which is
substituted for the immanent structure of a true dialectic. The
rupture that threatens this discourse must constantly be conjured
away or compensated for by an excess of conceptuality and
rhetorical hability. From this, finally, comes the strange contrast
that it is the most irrational term—despair—that sets into movement the largest mass of conceptual analyses. In my second encounter, we shall begin from this strange situation: a hyperintel-
lectualism linked to a fundamental irrationalism.

Let us examine this somewhat forbidding construction a bit more closely. The kernel about which the great antinomies of despair are constructed is a definition of the self that *The Concept of Dread* prepared us for when it spoke of spirit as the third term—the spoilsport—in the tranquil relation between soul and body. This definition in its disconcerting abstraction runs as follows: the human self is "a relation which relates itself to its own self, and in relating itself to its own self relates itself to another" (*The Sickness unto Death,* p. 146). Whether out of derision or loving vexation (we will discuss which later), this definition bears the mark of the Hegelian dialectic. But as a difference from Hegel, this relation that relates itself to itself is more a problem than an answer, more a task than a structure. For what is given in despair is what Kierkegaard calls the "disrelation." This priority of the disrelation throughout the subsequent analysis rests on the structure's relation as an impossible task: the possibility of despair resides in the possibility of a disrelation—that is, in the fragility of the relation that relates itself to its own self, as the expression "and in relating itself to its own self relates itself to another" signifies. For this relation, to constitute oneself is to unmake oneself.

We can already understand what force this union of mood and analysis can give to the Kierkegaardian rhetoric of pathos. Despair exists—or as I have tried to say, insists—in the figures of disrelation. Consequently, everything will be more complicated than in *The Concept of Dread*. Dread or anxiety was fascinated by the nothingness of pure possibility; despair "is the disrelationship in a relation which relates itself to itself. But the synthesis is not the disrelationship, it is merely the possibility, or, in the synthesis is latent the possibility of the disrelationship. . . . Whence then comes despair? From the relation wherein the synthesis relates itself to itself, in that God who made man a relationship lets this go as it were out of His hand, that is, in the fact that the relation relates itself to itself" (pp. 148–49). The latter remark allows us to further our explication of the strange expression about a relation that "in relating itself to its own self relates itself to another." In this abandonment, it is *related* to itself as to *another.* Dereliction is the reflective aspect of this abandonment by

God, who lets go of the relation as though it escaped his grasp. Kierkegaard, prior to existentialism, discovered this identity of reflection and dereliction.

From here on, all of Kierkegaard's art consists in applying his psychological subtlety to the numerous possibilities offered by the dissociating of this relation that relates itself to its own self in relating itself to another. Kierkegaard's literary, psychological, philosophical, and theological genius seems to me to lie in this half-abstract, half-concrete way of presenting these artificially constructed possibilities, of making the *opéra fabuleux* of despairing states of the soul correspond to this conceptual game. The reader's astonishment, unease, admiration, and irritation depend on this incessant oscillating between the most pointed imaginary experimentation and the most artificial conceptual dialectic. Here are some examples: Man, we are told, is a synthesis of infinitude and finitude, of possibility and necessity. Despair springs up as soon as the will to become infinite is felt or experienced as a lack of finitude, and vice versa. This interplay between opposed concepts is fed by an extraordinary power to create human types, among whom we recognize the hero of fantastic possibilities, the Don Juan of the aesthetic stage, the seducer of the "Journal of a Seducer," Goethe's Faust, and also the poet of the religious stage, the explorer of the open according to Rilke; in brief, the imagination, the crucible of every process of infinitization. The self is reflection, says Kierkegaard, and imagination is the possibility of all reflection. This is why the loss of a place to stand, the endless distance from oneself, is felt or experienced as a loss, as despair. The abstract paradox becomes a concrete one: the "either/or" of the infinite and the finite is the "either/or" that confronts the seducer and, on his level, the hero who does his duty, depicted through the traits of Judge William. The lack of infinity, the narrowness of a mediocre life, the loss of a horizon, are very concrete possibilities, as anyone will discover who feels his own existence as that of a pebble on the shore or one number lost in the crowd.

Yet it is perhaps the last dialectic that clarifies all the others. The worst despair is "the despair that is unaware of being despair." The ordinary person is desperate, is in despair, but does not know it. Thus it is because despair may be unconscious that it has to be discovered, even constructed. The dialectic of the unconscious and the conscious unfolds inside of despair as if within the heart of an ontic possibility, of a mode of being. Consciousness does not constitute despair. Despair exists, or, as I have said, insists. This is why even consciousness attaches itself to despair. The great despair, despair over oneself, the despair of willing despairingly to be oneself, which Kierkegaard calls defiance, represents the final degree of "the constant heightening of the power of despair." Here, more than anywhere else, this possibility may only be tried out in imagination: "This sort of despair is seldom seen in the world, such figures generally are met only in the works of poets, that is to say, of real poets, who always lend their characters this 'demoniac' ideality (taking this word in the purely Greek sense)" (*The Sickness unto Death,* p. 206). In real life, this supreme despair can only be approached in the most spiritual despair, the despair that no longer has to do with some earthly loss, the despair of not wanting to be helped.

We may now confront *The Concept of Dread* and *The Sickness unto Death* on the point of sin, so circumscribed by two opposed approaches.

The two treatises agree that sin is not an ethical reality but a religious one. Sin is "before God." But while *The Concept of Dread* remains outside of this determination of sin as "before God," *The Sickness unto Death* stands within its heart. *The Concept of Dread* stays purely psychological; *The Sickness unto Death* "edifies and awakens," according to its subtitle. While anxiety was a movement toward . . . , despair is sin. To say this is no longer psychology: "There here may be introduced, as the most dialectical borderline between despair and sin, what one might call a poetic existence in the direction of the religious . . ." (p. 208, trans. altered).

This "poetic existence in the direction of the religious" has nothing to do with a mystical effusion. It is, says Kierkegaard, "prodigiously dialectical, and is in an impenetrable dialectical confusion as to how far it is conscious of being sin" (p. 208). Everything that will be said from here on belongs to this reduplication of the dialectic when it passes from psychology to poetic existence in the direction of the religious. First, psychology designates sin through the experience of vertigo as a fall, then it designates it as a lack, consequently as "nothing." For poetic existence, sin is a state, a condition, a mode of being; further, it is a *position*.

Let us consider these new dimensions that could not appear in *The Concept of Dread,* first because this treatise stays purely psychological, next because it approaches sin as a leap.

That sin is a *state* is revealed by despair itself. We cannot say that anxiety *is* sin, we can say that despair *is*. In this way, the concept of sin is definitively transported from the ethical sphere of transgression into the religious sphere of unfaith. We may even say, from the sphere where sin is flesh to the sphere where it is spirit. It is the power of weakness and the weakness of defiance. Hence sin is no longer the contrary of virtue but of faith. It is an ontic human possibility, and not just a moral category according to a Kantian ethics or an intellectual defect comparable to ignorance according to the Socratic concept of evil. In other words, sin is our ordinary mode of being before God. It is existence itself as dereliction.

But we come to the final difference between *The Concept of Dread* and *The Sickness unto Death* when we say that "sin is not a negation but a position." This thesis—which Kierkegaard takes to be the orthodox Christian interpretation of sin—is directed against all speculative philosophy. To comprehend evil philosophically is to reduce it to a pure negation: weakness as a lack of force, sensuality as a lack of spirituality, ignorance as a lack of knowledge, finitude as a lack of totality. Hegel identified comprehension with negation or, better, with the negation of negation. It is here that Kierkegaard opposes his most vigorous protest against philosophy—that is, against Hegelian philosophy. If to comprehend is to overcome, that is, to pass beyond negation, then sin is one negation among others and repentance one mediation among others. In this way, negation and the negation of negation both become purely logical processes.

But, if we only comprehend when we negate negation, what do we *say* and *understand* when we say sin is a position! Here is Kierkegaard's response: "I am merely keeping a steady hold upon the

Christian dogma that sin is a position—not, however, as though it could be comprehended, but as a paradox which must be believed" (*The Sickness unto Death*, p. 229).

"A paradox which must be believed." With these words, Kierkegaard poses the question of a genre of language suitable to poetic existence. It is language that must destroy what it says, a language that contradicts itself. In this way, Kierkegaard transfers the aim of negative theology to anthropology when it attempts to say, through the voice of contradiction, that God is a position—beyond being, beyond determinations. To believe and not understand. Of course, Kierkegaard does not refer to negative theology, or to the Kantian abolition of knowledge in favor of belief, but to Socratic ignorance.

In the second encounter, we shall begin from this baffling situation of philosophical discourse: a cunning elucidation of anxiety and of despair, an antidialectical dialectic aiming at a kind of Socratic ignorance, in service of "A Christian Psychological Exposition for Edification and Awakening."

It is within *this* situation of philosophical discourse that the question arises, How can we do philosophy *after* Kierkegaard?

Part II: Doing Philosophy after Kierkegaard

Once Kierkegaard began to be known in Germany, thanks to Gottsched's courageous translation, which seemed a lost wager, then in France, thanks to Tisseau's admirable translations and Jean Wahl's famous *Etudes Kierkegaardiennes,* the Danish thinker quickly was endowed with the twofold function of protesting and arousing us. How do things stand today, thirty or forty years after this breakthrough into European philosophical and theological literature?

We should admit that we are less clear today regarding the philosophical significance of Kierkegaard. A protesting thinker? Against what? With a single voice, we all repeat with Kierkegaard himself: against the system, against Hegel, against German idealism. A rousing thinker? About what? The Kierkegaard craze invites us to reply about existentialism. These are the two preliminary pieces of evidence that I would like to try to call into doubt in order to give a rough outline of a second reading whose groundwork I have laid in the first encounter. This reading may be able to give a new future to Kierkegaard's work, now that the first reading has exhausted its possibilities.

Let us begin with our initial doubt: Is Kierkegaard the father of existentialism? With the passing of several decades, this classification has become nothing more than a trompe l'oeil, perhaps the cleverest way of taming him by cataloging him in a known genre. We are better prepared today to recognize that this family of philosophies does not exist. With the same stroke, we are ready to free Kierkegaard from it. We used to see in him the ancestor of a family wherein Gabriel Marcel, Karl Jaspers, Martin Heidegger, and Jean-Paul Sartre were cousins. Today, the breaking apart of this group, if it ever existed elsewhere than in our handbooks, is evident. Existentialism as a form of philosophy common to them all does not exist, be it in its principal theses, its method, or even its fundamental problems. Gabriel Marcel preferred to be called Neosocratic. Jaspers emphasized his solidarity with classical philosophy. Heidegger's fundamental ontology broke away toward a meditative, archaizing, and poetic thinking. As for Sartre, he considers his own existentialism to be an ideology that needs to be reinterpreted within the framework of Marxism. The latter two extreme cases are the sign that it is less enlightening today than it way thirty years ago to take existentialism as a key for a penetrating interpretation of Kierkegaard.

The first reading is strengthened by our reading of *The Concept of Dread* and *The Sickness unto Death*. There we found a thinker who transposes living experience into a trenchant dialectic, who abstractly imagines the stages, more constructed than lived, of existence and who elaborates them by means of a broken-off dialectic: finite-infinite, possible-actual, unconscious-conscious, and so forth. We came to suspect that this broken-off dialectic may have more affinity with its own best enemy—Hegel—than with its presumptive heirs.

Yet this suspicion is immediately blocked by an apparently stronger conviction. We know that Kierkegaard was anti-

Hegelian. He says so. Perhaps he says nothing else. Moreover, we know that he inaugurates a new era of thought, coming after German idealism: the era of postphilosophy. We also take it for granted that philosophy reached its end with Hegel, that philosophical discourse is complete in and through him, and that after Hegel, something else appears, which is no longer discourse. This interpretation of modern thought is encouraged by Marx's, Nietzsche's, and Kierkegaard's attacks against idealism. The protest of the unique individual before God, European nihilism and the transformation of values, the realization of philosophy as revolutionary praxis, these three tendencies of modern thought are supposed to represent the end of philosophy, understood as total discourse, and the beginning of postphilosophy.

But is this associating of Kierkegaard with Nietzsche and Marx any more enlightening than his incorporation into so-called existentialism? I am not sure that this concept of the end of philosophy is really any clearer than that of "existentialism." My doubt is twofold. Who brings philosophy to a close? Hegel? Is this certain? As for the postphilosophy trilogy, is it really external to and foreign to German idealism?

Yes, who brings philosophy to a close? We may admit that Kant, Fichte, Schelling, and Hegel form a unique sequence that reaches its peak in Hegel's *Encyclopedia*. Yet this presupposition is already a Hegelian interpretation of German idealism. We are forgetting that Schelling buried Hegel and, I dare to say, from afar. We are also neglecting the whole unexplored riches of Fichte and the later Schelling. Above all, we are mistaken about Hegel himself. Perhaps, after all, we are the victims of the bad readings Kierkegaard and Marx made of him. A new reading of Kierkegaard is without a doubt bound up with a new reading of Fichte and Schelling—and Hegel.

But I want to push further my doubt concerning the very concept of the completion of Western philosophy and to suggest that the self-annointed postphilosophies belong to the philosophical era of German idealism. Heidegger has fairly convincingly shown that Nietzsche accomplished one of the vows of Western philosophy. If that philosophy is animated by the magnification of subjectivity, by the accomplishing of the *subjectum* as subject, Nietzsche completes this philosophical search by Western thought. If we say, on the contrary, with Marx this time, that philosophy has until now "only contemplated the world without changing it," Kierkegaard and Nietzsche still belong to the philosophies of discourse. For Nietzsche, in his turn, Marx was still devoted to the ideals of the crowd, to the mythology of science—"our last religion"—the last offshoot of Christianity and Platonism. And for a reader of Kierkegaard, Marx is still a Hegelian, but for wholly other reasons. To the extent that the dialectic of history is still a logic of reality, Marx represents the triumph of generality and the very accomplishment of the Hegelian postulate that the real is rational and the rational real.

If I have played off Schelling against Hegel, Hegel against himself, and Nietzsche, Kierkegaard, and Marx against one another, it was only to render doubtful the very idea of the completion or end of Western philosophy and to free the reading of Kierkegaard from this schematism and this prejudice. We are now ready for the question, How may we do philosophy after Kierkegaard? We are no longer required to separate his destiny from that of German idealism or to make him one tributary of existentialism.

My reply consists of three degrees. I want first of all to set aside the properly irrational aspects of Kierkegaard. Then I want to consider his contribution to a critique of existentiell possibilities. Finally, I want to put this critique into relation with the ideal of philosophical discourse as a system.

"THE EXCEPTION"

There is one aspect of Kierkegaard that cannot be continued by either the philosopher or the theologian. This part is his uncommunicable existence. But there is a part that can be continued, because it belongs to philosophical argumentation, reflection, and speculation. This part is represented by his pseudonyms. We cannot do philosophy after Kierkegaard the existing individual, but we can, perhaps, after his pseudonyms, insofar as they belong to the same philosophical sphere as does German idealism.

Let us consider the first face of this paradox. On the one hand, Kierkegaard keeps himself outside of philosophy and theology. The question that confronts us here is that of genius as the non-philosophical source of philosophy. I grant that the field of this genius extends widely. It covers not only the real—and unknown—Kierkegaard, but also the mythical Kierkegaard created by his writings. Everyone grants that the story of his actual existence constitutes something unique in the history of thought: the Copenhagen dandy, the strange fiancé of Regine, the bachelor thorn in the flesh, the unsupportable critic of Bishop Mynster, the *Corsair's* sad victim, the dying man in the public hospital—none of these personages can be repeated or even correctly understood. But what existence can?

Yet the case of Kierkegaard is still more singular. No one has succeeded as he has in transposing his own biography into a kind of personal myth. Through his identification with Abraham, Job, Ahasuerus, and other fantastic personages, he has elaborated a sort of fictive personality that completely covers over and conceals his actual existence. His poetic existence is no more situated within the framework or the landscape of ordinary communication than is that of a character in a novel, or, better, than is that of some extreme character from a Shakespearean tragedy. What is offered to and refused to philosophical comprehension is a character or personage created by his works. It is an author, the child of his works, an existing individual who disrealized himself and thus removed himself from the grasp of every known discipline. For he does not even belong to his own "stages on life's way." He was not enough Don Juan or enough a seducer to be aesthetic. He did not succeed in being an ethical person since he had no profession to gain his wages, was neither a husband nor a father, and excluded himself from the ethical program depicted by Judge William. His family was correct: "How could he not be melancholic when he is using up his fortune in such a fashion!"

Was he religious in the sense he spoke of? The Christianity he depicted was so extreme that no one could practice it. The subjective thinker before God, the pure contemporary of Christ, crucified with him, without any church, tradition, or cultus, is outside of history. "I am the poet of the religious," he said. I think we must take him at his word. But what does this mean? We do not know. Kierkegaard is somewhere, in the intervals of his stages, between them, in the passages, like some abbreviation of the aesthetic and the religious stages that would leap over the ethical one. So he escapes the alternative that he himself posed in *Either/Or*. Kierkegaard cannot be found following his own categories. We would need to conceive of the extraordinary coincidence of irony, melancholy, purity of heart, and corrosive rhetoric, add to it a bit of buffoonery, then finally crown it all with the identity of the aesthetic, the religious, and the martyr.

Yes, Kierkegaard is an "exception." We must not only repeat this but also deepen our conviction. That is, we must read Kierkegaard, then let him be what he is where he is—outside of philosophy and outside of theology. I mean what I say: let him be what he is. There is no good in correcting, refuting, or completing him. Ah, says someone. If he had a little more sense of forgiveness and a little less of guilt; a little more of collective guilt and a little more sense of the Church! Ah, says another. If he had a little more sense of community, of dialogue! Ah, says a third, who adds, If he had a little more sense of history, a little more respect for the crowd and affection for people! Ah, says the last. If he had a little more simplicity, clarity, coherence! Which of us, philosophers, politicians, or theologians, have not muttered against Kierkegaard in this sense? You feel how ridiculous and vain it is. Do you correct Othello or Cordelia? Or the Bourgeois Gentilhomme? Nietzsche said, "One does not refute a sound." What one does not refute in Kierkegaard is the existing individual—the real existing individual, the author of the works—and the mythical existing individual, the child of his works. One does not refute Kierkegaard. One reads him, meditates on him, and then does one's job, "his gaze fixed on the exception."

What does it mean for the philosopher to do his job with his eyes fixed on the exception? I think that first of all it is to rediscover the intimate relation of all philosophy and all philosophical labor with nonphilosophy. Kierkegaard the exception, the rhetorical-religious genius, the martyr dandy, does not constitute a unique situation. Philosophy always has something to do with nonphilosophy, because philosophy has no object of its own. It reflects upon experience, upon all experience, upon the whole of experience—scientific, ethical, aesthetic, religious. Philosophy's *sources* lie outside it. I speak of its sources, not its starting point. Philosophy is responsible for its starting point, its method, its achievement. Philosophy looks for its point of departure— concerning which Pierre Thévenaz said convincing and decisive things: Philosophy has its starting point before it. But, if it looks for its starting point, it receives its sources. It lays out its starting point. It does not lay out its sources, namely, what replenishes and instructs it from below (*en sous-oeuvre*). This is how I understand Karl Jaspers' saying, "We are not the exception. We have to do philosophy with our gaze fixed on the exception."

Kierkegaard, as an aesthetical-rhetorical-religious genius, is one of these sources, but so are Stirner, Kafka, and Nietzsche, although Nietzsche must also be treated as a philosophical genius. This characterizes him completely as little as it does Kierkegaard, but I am thinking here of the Nietzsche of Sils-Maria who resigned his chair at Basel, the solitary man of Engadine, the author of the aphorisms, the Nietzsche invented by Zarathustra, the Nietzsche who was the interlocuter of Dionysius and the Crucified, the Nietzsche come to grief in madness, similar in this regard to Kierkegaard, the bishop's insulter and the martyr. I will say, therefore, that philosophy debates with Kierkegaard as with every nonphilosophical genius. Its proper task remains to seek the principle or ground, the order of coherence, the signification of truth and reality. Its task is reflective and speculative.

This is my first response. But each of you will sense that this manner of recognizing Kierkegaard's aesthetical-religious genius is also a manner of exiling him from philosophy. Each of you senses that Kierkegaard is not—or not only—the non-philosopher. Kierkegaard embarrasses us because he stands in relation to philosophy, outside and inside at the same time.

THE CRITIQUE OF EXISTENTIELL POSSIBILITIES

Kierkegaard thrust himself into the interior of both philosophy and Christian dogmatics. This makes our relation to him more uncomfortable and more unbearable. This is what we now have to take into account, not his geniality—be it real or fictive, biographical or mythical, that of his *Journal* and that of the poetic transposition of his lived experience—but his argumentation. We have already been led to this inverse side of the Kierkegaardian question by the enigma of his pseudonyms. If Kierkegaard stands outside of philosophy, Constantin Constantius, Johannes de Silentio, and Vigilius Haufniensis—alleged names of Søren Kierkegaard—are philosophical authors. The problem of the pseudonyms is that of indirect communication. And indirect communication, in turn, rests on its own mode of argumentation.

We cannot, therefore, limit ourselves to recognizing the exception in Kierkegaard, then give him his leave under the pretext that he is the genial exception. He himself requires that he be one of us through his fierce force of argumentation. We are once again confronted with a question that we earlier left unanswered. Kierkegaard, we said, not only argues, he elaborates concepts— the *concepts* of anxiety, despair, sin, position. He does not even just limit himself to building up concepts. On the very terrain of Hegelian dialectic, he constructs an antidialectic, made up of unresolved oppositions that he calls paradoxes. Now a paradox is still a logical structure, the one that is suitable for the type of demonstration required by the problematic of the existing individual, the individual before God. Here we need to consider Kierkegaard's most extraordinary work, the *Concluding Unscientific Postscript to the Philosophical Fragments*. There, a whole network of concepts is unfolded: eternity and the instant, the individual, the existing individual, choice, the unique, subjectivity, being before God, the absurd. This is no longer nonphilosophy. It is hyperphilosophy, to the point of caricature and derision. Yet it is at this level, that of the categories of the existing individual, that the decisive problem is posed, the problem of the logic of Kierkegaardian discourse.

This problem may not be approached head-on without a total reevaluation of the relations between Kierkegaard and German idealism. The second reading of Kierkegaard is necessarily also a second reading of German idealism. But this reading first requires our dismantling the apparent logic of the sequence "from Kant to Hegel," to recall the title of Kroner's great book. I shall present a few suggestions with regard to this second reading.

In one sense, Kierkegaard already belongs to that general movement in German philosophy after 1840 that we call "the return to Kant." The sentence I cited earlier, in my first encounter with Kierkegaard—"the paradox requires faith, not understanding"—invincibly leads back to Kant's famous saying that "I had to abolish knowledge to make room for faith." The field of comparison must be widened even further. The philosophical function of paradox for Kierkegaard borders on the philosophical function of limit for Kant. We may even say that Kierkegaard's broken-off dialectic has some affinity with the Kantian dialectic understood as a critique of illusion. In both cases, it is by means of a broken discourse that the essential can be said. Thus, there is something in Kierkegaard that cannot be said without a Kantian background, and there is something in Kant that gets its meaning only by means of the Kierkegaardian struggle with paradox.

I admit that this confrontation with Kant is less satisfying than any of the others we are going to consider. It is just within a philosophical perspective where the only alternative would be between Kant and Hegel that this alliance thrusts itself upon us. In the last analysis, Kierkegaard is not a critical thinker in the Kantian sense of the term. Questions about conditions of possibility do not interest him, at least as an epistemological problem. But may we not say that his categories of existence constitute a new genre of critique, that of a *critique of existence,* and that they concern the possibility of *speaking* about existence?

To be an existing individual is in no way a mystical experience condemned to silence. Kierkegaard is not an intuitionist. He is a reflective thinker. To establish a deeper kinship between Kierkegaard and Kant, we must overcome a second opposition that precisely concerns the structure of reflection. Kantian reflection obeys a precise model founded on dissociating at the very heart of experience between the a priori and the a posteriori. This formalism perhaps does have a meaning and a function within the field of physical experience. I will not discuss this point here, but its transposition from the domain of physics to that of ethics is perhaps the key to all the failures of Kant's practical philosophy. This practical philosophy is constructed on the model of the theoretical philosophy and brings the critical problem of action to the formalizing of the imperative. Hence, may we not say that the Kierkegaardian concepts of existence constitute a response to problems of practical reason that Kant led into an impasse? The categories of existence are to ethics what the categories of objectivity are to physics. They are the *conditions of possibility of an experience,* not physical experience or an experience parallel to physical experience but a fundamental experience that is *the realization of our desire and our effort to be.*

Now, this liberation of practical reason from the yoke of formalism leads us from Kant to Fichte. As I said at the beginning, Fichte and Schelling are the most misunderstood thinkers of this period and also the ones who are most often purloined. Everything that is strong and valuable in modern philosophy and that does not come from Kant or Hegel has been begotten by Fichte or Schelling. I am convinced that giving more and better attention to Fichte and Schelling could renew our reading of Kierkegaard. I will give just two samples of such renewed reading. As is well known, Fichte opposes *Tathandlung* to *Tatsache,* act to fact. This distinction between act and fact furnishes the philosophical ground for every theory of action and for every ethics that would not be reducible to a simple theory of duty. The task of a philosophy of existence is thus to elaborate the conditions of possibility and the conditions for realizing this act of existing. I am not saying that the whole of Kierkegaard is involved in this Fichtean problematic. I am just saying that the structure of the Fichtean problematic determines the field and the ground in which and upon which the Kierkegaardian experience can be *said.* It is not the Kierkegaardian experience as such that is at issue here but the Kierkegaardian discourse that here finds the philosophical instrument for its communication.

Let us go even further with a second comment that concerns not just Fichte but also Schelling. We are too habituated to considering idealism, German idealism, as a pure game of abstractions. Yet, to the contrary, the great problem for this "idealism" was the problem of reality. Idealism signifies first of all and radically that the distinction between ideal and real is itself purely ideal. With the later philosophy of Schelling, human finitude, insofar as it has its own structure, irreducibly becomes the limitation of one object by another, and the connection between finitude, freedom, and evil receives a truly philosophical signification. The problem no longer is emotional, pathetic, or even poetic. It is the philosophical problem of finite reality.

So we have these three philosophical structures from Kant, Fichte, and Schelling that give Kierkegaardian discourse its philosophical dimension:

first, the Kantian idea of a critique of practical reason distinct from a critique of physical experience;

second, the Fichtean distinction between act and fact, as well as the definition of a practical philosophy by means of the conditions of possibility of the act of existing, along with the conditions for its realization;

finally, Schelling's problematic of finite reality, and, more precisely, the connection between finitude, freedom, and evil.

It seems to me, therefore, that to do philosophy after Kierkegaard is at the same time to return behind Kierkegaard, toward this triple problematic, to liberate him from the Hegelian yoke and to show in return that this problematic only attains its meaning—or at least one of its meanings—in Kierkegaard's lively experience.

CRITIQUE AND SYSTEM AFTER KIERKEGAARD

We are now ready for a final confrontation, the confrontation in which the dramatic, existential conflict that wholly opposes Kierkegaard to Hegel is reflected for us. This final confrontation will bring us back to our starting point. We began with a simple and naive opposition between Kierkegaard and Hegel. This opposition cannot be contested. Moreover, the question is not to attenuate it but precisely *to think* it as a *meaningful* opposition. This opposition belongs to understanding Kierkegaard. It signifies that Kierkegaard decidedly cannot be understood apart from Hegel. It is not just a biographical trait or a fortuitous encounter but a constitutive structure of Kierkegaard's thought that it is not thinkable apart from Hegel. To understand this paradoxical situation aright is the final condition for a new reading of Kierkegaard.

Let us begin with what the Hegelian thinker says—or would say—about Kierkegaard. For this thinker, Kierkegaardian discourse is just one part of Hegelian discourse. It is even possible to situate it with great precision in the system. It is the discourse of the "unhappy consciousness." Its place, its logical space, comes not at the end but at the beginning of the *Phenomenology of Spirit*. Kierkegaardian discourse itself furnishes the proof that Kierkegaard is included in the system. Since he lost the key to an authentic dialectic, which would be the very movement of its contents and the surpassing of these contents through contradiction and mediation, Kierkegaard was condemned to replace this authentic dialectic by an artificial game of paradoxes, a broken-off dialectic that remains a rhetoric of pathos covered over by a laborious didactic art. Considered in this way, Kierkegaard is just a parasite of the system, one who denies it and then invents a derisory phantom of it.

The Kierkegaardian thinker must accept this Hegelian retort as capable of having a meaning. To be philosophy's "buffoon," or its "traitor," was part of Kierkegaard's vocation. Only the person who has the courage to take up this role may call himself an existential thinker and write something like a *Concluding Unscientific Postscript*. This title indicates that derision belongs to the very structure of Kierkegaardian discourse. It is why the destiny of this discourse cannot be separated from that of Hegelian philosophy.

Yet this liaison by means of derision is itself the sign of a more intimate relation that can only be discerned by means of a second reading of Hegel himself. The Hegelian thinker's allegation that Kierkegaard is either excluded from the system because of his own discourse, understood as nonsensical, or included as a partial discourse—that, we said, of the "unhappy consciousness"— presupposes that the system exists. But we need to rediscover that the possibility of the system is both a presupposition and a question for Hegel himself. The truth of the opposition between Kierkegaard and Hegel cannot be understood unless the system is called into question by Hegel himself.

In this way, Kierkegaard and Hegel both need to be called into question and by each other. Let us consider just three critical points that result from this mutual perturbation.

First, The *Phenomenology of Spirit* has served to call into question for us the very meaning of Kierkegaard's enterprise. What, in return, is the actual situation of the *Phenomenology of Spirit* within the total system? We cannot content ourselves with saying that it is a propaedeutic to the logic. Is there not a secret discordance between an exemplary history of spirit and a logic of the absolute? Does not the prodigious richness of this history, which constitutes, so to speak, the gigantic novel of humanity, exceed any recapitulation by the system?

Favoring this mutual calling each other into question, at the level even of the "unhappy consciousness," is a curious kinship between Kierkegaard and the Hegel of the *Phenomenology.* Are they not both on the same side against all species of empty rationalism, against the *Aufklärung*? The battle between Hegel and Kierkegaard suddenly appears in a new light. Kierkegaard is neither included nor excluded by a system that remains a question for itself. The conflict between two sorts of dialectics poses a question to each of them: Is a cut-off dialectic thinkable without a philosophy of mediation? Can a philosophy of mediation be conclusive? In this way, the opposition between the Hegelian dialectic and the Kierkegaardian dialectic itself becomes a dialectical figure that needs to be understood for itself and as constituting a new structure of philosophical discourse.

If we accept this general interpretation of the relation between Hegel and Kierkegaard as an opposition that itself must become a moment of philosophical discourse, it is perhaps possible to discover a more profound signification, both of Hegel and of Kierkegaard, on two other fundamental points: that of the critique of ethics and that of the signification of religious faith.

Second, I want to begin by emphasizing the first point, which

might be omitted or misunderstood. The paradoxical situation is
that we find in both Hegel and Kierkegaard a critique of the
ethical stage of existence. Yet if Kantianism, taken as a whole,
represents the "ethical vision of the world" for Hegel,
Hegelianism, in its turn, represents the "ethical stage of existence" for Kierkegaard. This encounter and this scorn are full of
meaning. They lead to the question, What is the signification of
the ethical stage?

Hegel replies: it is the opposition of the ideal and the real, the
defaming of the real in the name of the ideal, and, in the last
analysis, any positing of transcendence as exiled from reasonable
reality. It is this transcendence that makes possible the judging
consciousness, the consciousness that discriminates and con-
demns. For Hegel, consequently, every philosophy that appeals
to the opposition between heaven and earth, between God and
the world, transcendence and immanence, is still an ethical vision
of the world and must be surpassed. In this sense, Kierkegaard's
"before God" still takes off from the ethical vision of the world
and must be surpassed. The Hegelian thinker will add an avowal
to this critique: if Kierkegaard gets beyond his ethical vision of the
world, it is because he introduces another idea, that of contemporaneity between the believer and the Christ. But this is a poetic
relation that short-circuits discourse. It may only be thought of as
an internalizing of the "before God" by which the philosophy of
transcendence is surpassed in a philosophy of love. If this can still
be said, it must also be thought. How can it be, outside of the
categories that attest to the triumph of the religion of the Spirit
over that of the Father, through the mediation of the death of the
Son? Of course, this is the very theme of the Hegelian philosophy
of religion. So runs the Hegelian reading of Kierkegaard, which
must be accepted by the Kierkegaardian thinker, just as he has to
accept his being included in the *Phenomenology of Spirit* under the
title of the "unhappy consciousness."

Yet this second critique and this second attempt to include
Kierkegaard are as little decisive as were the first ones. *We must
understand the Kierkegaardian critique of the ethical stage here in order to
understand Hegel himself.* Hegel remains in the ethical stage be-

cause he reduces the individual to the general, the subjective thinker to impersonal objective thought. The principal proposition of all Hegelian philosophy—that "the rational is the real, the real is the rational"—resounds as the prescription of every ethical thought that reduces the individual to the general. This proposition expresses the hypocritical omission of the existing individual Hegel or his delirious assumption to the rank of Spirit.

I think that this opposition between Hegel and Kierkegaard must be introduced as such into philosophical discourse. On the one side, the distance between the wholly other and man cannot be thought without the idea of an inclusive relation that puts an end to the idea of pure transcendence. As soon as we speak of transcendence, we think a totality that embraces the relation between the Other and myself. In this sense, the idea of transcendence suppresses itself, and Hegel will always be correct in resisting every pretention to think about the infinite distance between the wholly other and man. In this sense, too, every ethical vision denies itself as soon as it attempts to express itself. On the other side, this point of view without a point of view from whence one could view the profound identity of the real and the rational, the existing and the signifying, the individual and discourse, is nowhere given. With Kierkegaard, we must always return to this confession: I am not absolute discourse. Singularity is always reborn at the margin of discourse. Therefore, another discourse is required, one that takes this into account and speaks of it.

Third, a new phase of the same struggle declares itself regarding the problem of religious faith. For Hegel, religion is only an introduction to philosophy, conceived of as absolute knowledge. For Kierkegaard, there is nothing beyond faith, since it is God's gracious response to evil, for which there is no science. The opposition, therefore, seems to be a total one. But are we sure that this opposition is a disjunction? Should we not rather take these two opposed philosophies of religion as a whole? Then it is no longer at the level of the "unhappy consciousness" that one must take hold, but at the level of chapter seven of the *Phenomenology of Spirit*, which contains Hegel's true philosophy of religion and which hardly varied until the *Lectures on the Philosophy of Religion* of 1820-21. This chapter poses a problem that clarifies Kierkegaard and that Kierkegaard clarifies: the problem of religious language and, in general, of *representation*. In one sense, religion cannot be transcended—at least what Hegel calls true religion or revealed religion—because it is at one time the agony of representation and the representation of agony, at the threshold of absolute knowledge. But this absolute knowledge does not belong to us. We can barely say that there is absolute knowledge. This is why representation is both surpassed and retained. Hence, religion cannot be abolished by something external to it. It is required to live out its own agony and to understand its meaning as being that of its own suppression, that death of idols, figures, and representations, that death of God, that must be experienced and thought as its proper truth, within the religious community as well as in its worship.

In this way, we have reached the point where the opposition between the Hegelian system and the subjective, passionate thinker has become quite obviously significant. The relation between Hegel and Kierkegaard has itself become paradoxical. The reason for this paradox resides in the philosophical function of the idea "system." Perhaps we have discovered or rediscovered that the system is both philosophy's ultimate requirement and its unattainable goal. Religion is that place within philosophical discourse where the necessity to transcend images, representations, and symbols may be contemplated, at the same time as is the impossibility of dispensing with them. Here is "the place" where Hegel and Kierkegaard struggle against each other. Yet this struggle itself is henceforth a part of philosophical discourse.

I would like now to bring together the partial responses I have successively given to the question, How can we do philosophy after Kierkegaard?

First, philosophy is always related to *nonphilosophy*. In this sense, the irrational side of Kierkegaard is a source of philosophy as is all genius. If we cut the living tie between philosophy and nonphilosophy, philosophy runs the risk of being nothing other than a simple word game and, at the limit, a pure linguistic nihilism.

Second, Kierkegaard is not just the romantic genius, the individual, the passionate thinker. He inaugurates a new way of doing philosophy that we have called a *critique of existentiell possibilities.* This discourse about existence is no longer the poetic expression of an emotion. It is a genre of conceptual thought, which has its own rules for rigor, its own type of coherence, and which requires its own logic. We could say, using a Heideggerian terminology, that the problem is to pass from the existentiell to the existential, from personal decision to anthropological structures. The elaboration of this discourse requires a conjoint rereading of Kierkegaard and German idealism. Kierkegaard, in this sense, fulfills the Kantian exigence of practical philosophy, distinct from the critique of physical experience. At the same time, his existentiell analysis finds its philosophical soil: first, in the Fichtean distinction between act and fact (between the act of existing and existing facts); second, in Schelling's philosophy of reality, which was the first to tie together the problems of finitude, freedom, and evil.

Third, to finish, I returned to the initial problem of the opposition between the individual and the system. This conflict seemed to me to be something other than an alternative in the face of which we are condemned to make a choice. A new philosophical situation arises out of this conflict that invites us, on the one hand, to reread Hegel's *Phenomenology of Spirit* and *Philosophy of Religion* in light of the Kierkegaardian dialectic, and, on the other hand, to situate Kierkegaard's paradoxes within the field of the Hegelian philosophy of "representation" and absolute knowledge.

May these partial responses guard us from giving in to the disastrous alternative of either rationalism or existentialism. Science is not everything. Beyond science, there is still thinking. The question of existence does not signify the death of language and of logic. To the contrary, it requires an increase in lucidity and rigor. The question, What is existence? cannot be separated from the other question, What is thinking? Philosophy lives on the unity of these two questions and dies of their separation.

REFERENCES

Hegel, G. W. F. *Phenomenology of Spirit.* Translated by A. V. Miller. New York: Oxford University Press, 1977.

Hegel, G. W. F. *Lectures on the Philosophy of Religion, Together with a Work on the Proofs of the Existence of God.* Translated by E. B. Speirs and J. B. Sanderson. London: Routledge & Kegan Paul, 1962.

Kierkegaard, S.

Either/Or [1843]. 2 vols. Translated by D. F. Swenson and L. M. Swenson. Garden City, N.Y.: Doubleday, 1959.

Fear and Trembling and The Sickness unto Death [1843, 1849]. Translated by W. Lowrie. Garden City, N.Y.: Doubleday, Anchor, 1954.

Edifying Discourses [1843–50]. 2 vols. Translated by D. F. Swenson and L. M. Swenson. Minneapolis: Augsburg, 1943-45.

The Concept of Dread [1844]. Translated by W. Lowrie. Princeton, N.J.: Princeton University Press, 1957.

Stages on Life's Way [1845]. Translated by W. Lowrie. Princeton, N.J.: Princeton University Press, 1940. New York: Schocken Books, 1967.

Concluding Unscientific Postscript [1846]. Translated by D. F. Swenson and W. Lowrie. Princeton, N.J.: Princeton University Press, 1968.

Kroner, R. *Von Kant bis Hegel.* 2 vols. Tübingen: J. C. B. Mohr, 1921-24.

11

Aesthetic Therapy: Hegel and Kierkegaard

Few thinkers have contributed more to shaping the modern sense of self than the German philosopher G. W. F. Hegel and the Danish philosopher-theologian Søren Kierkegaard. In areas as diverse as theology, philosophy, psychology, sociology, literature, and art, the insights originally articulated by Hegel and Kierkegaard have been critically examined, imaginatively elaborated, and eagerly appropriated. Nor has their influence been restricted to that rarefied atmosphere of academic reflection and discussion removed from the confusion and vitality of everyday experience. Hegelian and Kierkegaardian categories permeate our thought and language and condition the way in which many of us understand ourselves and experience our world. Yet despite the lasting importance of the ideas of Hegel and Kierkegaard, the relationship between their contrasting points of view has only rarely been the subject of careful and thorough discussion. As a result of this oversight, many of the most important issues joining and separating Hegel and Kierkegaard continue to go unexamined. Nowhere is this more evident than in the area of psychology. Interpreters have tended to appropriate uncritically Kierkegaard's polemical caricature of Hegel as a speculative philosopher who disregards the existing individual. Consequently, the obvious differences separating Hegel and Kierkegaard frequently obscure the more subtle and significant similarities they share. In the following pages, I shall attempt to arrive at an understanding of the common purpose that informs the complex writings of these two demanding authors. My goal is to bring Hegel and Kierkegaard closer together so that their differences can emerge more clearly.

"What the Age Needs"

In the preface to his *Philosophy of Right,* Hegel remarks: "Whatever happens, every individual is a child of his time; so philosophy too is its own time apprehended in thought. It is just as absurd to fancy that a philosophy can transcend its contemporary world as it is to fancy that an individual can overleap his own age . . ." (p. 11). From Hegel's point of view, forms of reflection, be they naive or scientifically sophisticated, remain inseparably bound to the historical situation within which they arise. Although not readily apparent from his many jibes at the speculative philosopher who has forgotten what it means to be a concrete individual, Kierkegaard heartily agrees with Hegel's recognition of the situatedness of reflection. Throughout his entire authorship, Kierkegaard insists upon the conditional character of all knowing and consistently probes the multiple factors that inform the uniqueness of alternative perspectives. In keeping with their insights, Hegel and Kierkegaard regard their own work as the outgrowth of and the response to dominant intellectual and social tendencies of the day. They both begin with a diagnosis of the philosophical and existential ills of the time and proceed to offer a complex prescription for a supposed cure. More specifically, Hegel and Kierkegaard believe that their respective ages suffer spiritlessness. Each author takes as his fundamental philosophical task the articulation of the means by which the malady of spiritlessness can be overcome.

As M. H. Abrams has pointed out, "No thinker was of greater consequence than Friedrich Schiller in giving a distinctive Romantic formulation to the diagnosis of the modern malaise, to the assumptions about human good and ill which controlled this diagnosis, and to the overall view of the history and destiny of mankind of which the diagnosis was an integral part" (p. 199). For Hegel and his generation, Schiller's *On the Aesthetic Education of Man* (1795) provided a definitive interpretation of the personal

and social problems created by the industrialization and commer-
cialization characteristic of modern society. By drawing on insights garnered from Lessing's *The Education of the Human Race*
(1780), Herder's *Ideas on the Philosophy of the History of Mankind*
(1784–85), Kant's *Conjectural Origin of the History of Man* (1785),
and from the economic analyses of the Scottish philosopher and
sociologist Adam Ferguson,[1] Schiller forges a comprehensive argument in which he maintains that the essential feature of
modern experience is its fragmentation. In a world governed by
the competitive laws of an industrial economy, class divisions
emerge that create inter- and intrapersonal conflict. In a particularly penetrating passage, Schiller describes the genesis and the
consequences of the social and personal dis-integration endemic
to his age.

> That zoophyte character of the Greek States, where every
> individual enjoyed an independent life and, when need
> arose, could become a whole in himself, now gave place to an
> ingenious piece of machinery, in which out of the botching
> together of a vast number of lifeless parts a collective
> mechanical life results. State and Church, law and customs,
> were now torn asunder; enjoyment was separated from
> labor, means from ends, effort from reward. Eternally
> chained to only one single little fragment of the whole, Man
> himself grew to be only a fragment; with the monotonous
> noise of the wheel he drives everlastingly in his ears, he never
> develops the harmony of his being, and instead of imprinting
> humanity upon his nature he becomes merely the imprint of
> his occupation, of his science. But even the meagre fragmen-
> tary association which still links the individual members to
> the whole, does not depend on forms which present them-
> selves spontaneously . . . , but is assigned to them with scru-
> pulous exactness by a formula in which free intelligence is

1. The most important of Ferguson's works for Schiller was his *Essay on the History of Civil Society* (1767). For discussions of the significance of Ferguson's arguments, see Abrams, pp. 210 ff.; and Roy Pascal, "'*Bildung*' and the Division of Labor" and "Herder and the Scottish Historical School."

restricted. The lifeless letter takes the place of the living understanding, and a practised memory is a surer guide than genius and feeling. [1965, p. 40]

For the young Hegel, struggling to formulate a distinctive philosophical position, Schiller's analysis of modernity provided an important catalyst to his thinking. In his early writings on religion and politics, Hegel is preoccupied with the exploration of the nature and the origin of the fragmentation and conflict plaguing his age. Through numerous tentative and experimental writings, Hegel identifies four interrelated dimensions of disintegration that he believes to be of particular importance: political, social, religious, and personal. Hegel's deliberate probing of modern society leads him to conclude that the political integration of his native Germany had completely dissolved. "Every center of life has gone its own way and established itself on its own; the whole has fallen apart. The state exists no longer" ("The German Constitution," p. 146). Persisting language of the "German Nation" or the "Empire" reflects an actuality of a bygone age that is belied by extant political conditions of the late eighteenth century. "The old forms have remained," Hegel writes, "but the times have changed, and with them manners, religion, wealth, the situation of all political and civil estates, and the whole condition of the world and Germany. This true condition the old forms do not express; they are divorced from it, they contradict it, and there is no true correspondence between form and fact" (p. 202). With historical changes, vestigal political structures fail to address needs of the time and are experienced as strange and estranging. The forms are maintained only through "superstitious adherence to purely external formalities" (p. 197). Subjective needs and objective sociopolitical forms remain at odds with one another, creating a condition Hegel defines as "alienation."

In large measure, Hegel attributes these problems to a propensity to reify abstract individuality that he believes to be peculiar to the German people. "The German character's stubborn insistence on independence," Hegel maintains, "has reduced to a pure formality everything that might serve towards the erection of a state-power and the union of society in a state; and to this formality it has clung just as obstinately" (p. 196). Hegel's conclusion is brief and incisive: "In Europe's long oscillation between barbarism and civilization the German state has not completely made the transition to the latter; it has succumbed to the convulsions of this transition; its members have torn themselves apart to complete independence; the state has been dissolved" (p. 237).

This extraordinary distortion of political life at once grows out of and is reflected in the social existence of a people. Rather than reconciling particular interests with the common weal, individuals set themselves in opposition to one another, seeking personal benefit at the expense of others. Hegel recognizes that "once man's social instincts are distorted and he is compelled to throw himself into interests peculiarly his own, his nature becomes so deeply perverted that it now spends its strength on variance from others, and in the course of maintaining its separation it sinks into madness, for madness is simply the complete separation of the individual from his kind" (p. 242). In a different situation, one might expect the forms of a people's religious life to provide a counterbalance to the centrifugal social forces tending toward social disintegration. But Hegel contends that contemporary religious structures themselves reflect and therefore perpetuate human alienation. Instead of expressing a vital religiosity in which there is a consonance between objective forms and subjective experience, the religious life of the German people suffers from abstract formalism devoid of subjective appropriation. Consequently, faith arises only through heteronomous obedience to alien authority.

Always sensitive to the inseparability of self and world, Hegel recognizes the implications of political, social, and religious alienation for individual persons. Outward conflict manifests itself in inward disintegration;[2] political, social, and religious dissolution engender personal fragmentation. Individuals are torn between

2. To be true to the dialectics of Hegel's analysis we must, of course, stress that the converse also obtains—that is, inward conflict manifests itself in outward disintegration.

desire and duty, emotion and reason, subjective inclination and objective obligation, and long for a reconciliation of their sundered selves. From Hegel's perspective, the inward distention of the personality is reflected in the major philosophical and theological movements of the time. Be it Kant's "subjective idealism,"[3] Schleiermacher's religious feeling, or Jacobi's intuitionism, the result is the same—the reification of the bifurcation of subjectivity and objectivity that perpetuates conflict within and without. This political, social, religious, and personal fragmentation constitutes the spiritlessness that Hegel sees as the pervasive malady of his age.

In light of this interpretation of modernity, Hegel's attraction to the idealized picture of Greek life elaborated by late eighteenth-century romantics is quite understandable.[4] By contrast to the disintegration of his time, Periclean Athens appeared to represent a harmonious society in which individuals could establish personal integration through participation in political and religious structures that simultaneously embodied individual and common purpose. Hegel's infatuation with Greece, however, never leads to the longing to return to lost Arcadia expressed in the poetry of Hölderlin and Novalis. He is more sympathetic with Schiller's historical interpretation of the modern malaise.[5] Properly comprehended, the disruption of primitive Greek harmony represents a potential advance for the human spirit in which individual selfhood can become clearly differentiated and decisively defined. Hegel's question is not how to retreat to the Garden but how to advance to the Kingdom. For a while, Hegel, like so many of his contemporaries, placed great hope in the French Revolution. But when the ideals of freedom, fraternity, and equality

3. Hegel explains the significance of this term in relation to Kant's philosophy in the *Lesser Logic* (*The Logic of Hegel*, 1968). See pars. 41-45.

4. For helpful considerations of this aspect of Hegel's relation to romanticism, see Glenn Gray, *Hegel's Hellenic Ideal*, and Otto Pöggeler, *Hegel's Kritik der Romantik*. Useful related studies include Jack Forstman, *A Romantic Triangle: Schleiermacher and Early German Romanticism*, and René Wellek, *A History of Modern Criticism: 1750-1950—The Romantic Age*.

5. See, for example, Schiller's sixth letter in *On the Aesthetic Education of Man*.

gave way to the reality of the Reign of Terror, he was forced to reevaluate the means by which the dilemmas faced by his age could be resolved. Philosophical reflection comes to replace sociopolitical reform as the means of overcoming the tensions born of alienation.[6] Writing to Schelling in November of 1800, Hegel comments: "In my scientific development, which began from the more subordinate needs of men, I was bound to be driven on to science, and the ideal of my youth had to be transformed at the same time into reflective form, into a system" (*Briefe*, pp. 59–60). In his early analysis, *The Difference between Fichte's and Schelling's System of Philosophy*, Hegel explains that the "source of the need of philosophy" is "dichotomy" (p. 89), or one might add, opposition, bifurcation, fragmentation. Philosophy meets this need by attempting to mediate oppositions and to reconcile differences in a process of unification that maintains distinction while at the same time resolving conflict. Hegel's Promethean philosophical undertaking cannot be properly understood apart from the recognition of his consistent endeavor to overcome the multiple dimensions of fragmentation that he sees at the heart of alienation.

Writing in 1846, Kierkegaard describes "The Present Age" as essentially a "*sensible, reflecting age, devoid of passion, flaring up in superficial, short-lived enthusiasm and prudentially relaxing in indolence*" (*Two Ages*, p. 68). In contrast to the "essentially passionate age of revolution," in which individuals had the courage to take decisive action, contemporary man avoids decision and cultivates detachment. This "reflective indolence" is, for Kierkegaard, spiritlessness. The malady is not characterized by a fragmentation that threatens to dismember self and society through the conflict

6. Abrams notes that disappointment with the turn of events in France led many intellectuals to shift the locus of radical change from the sociopolitical arena to the domain of poetry and philosophy. His apt phrase "Apocalypse by Cognition" (pp. 348 ff.) accurately captures the high expectations for revolutionary philosophy and poetry. Left-wing critics of Hegel usually cite this change in his position as a shift to the right that ultimately leads to the reactionary conservatism of his late years in Berlin. Such a reading of Hegel's development, however, oversimplifies his understanding of the proper relation between theory and practice and obscures his view of the nature of philosophical reflection.

of contradictory forces. Quite the contrary—all-powerful reflection seeks to mediate oppositions and to abrogate the principle of contradiction. Rather than creating intolerable tensions within and among persons, bourgeois social institutions attempt "to stabilize human relationships, to establish procedures and patterns of decorum, to protect its members from unexpected contingencies and to enable them to make prudent provision for the future; to modulate the demands and perils of temporal existence so far as possible into an ordered social space" (Crites, 1972a, p. 76). The individual becomes so identified with or integrated within the social totality of which he is a member that all sense of personal uniqueness and self-responsibility is lost. Kierkegaard labels the process by which individuality evaporates in crowd-existence "levelling." "The dialectic of the present age," he argues, "is oriented to equality and its most logical implementation, albeit abortive, is levelling [*Nivellementet*], the negative unity of the negative mutual reciprocity of individuals. . . . Anyone can see that levelling has its profound importance in the ascendency of the category 'generation' over the category 'individuality' " (*Two Ages,* p. 84).

For Kierkegaard, as for Hegel, the spiritlessness that grows out of this levelling has political, social, religious, and personal dimensions. In the realm of politics, public opinion expressed in a thoughtless press holds sway. Individuals become anonymous ciphers for the viewpoints of others and personal action is transmuted into impersonal spectating. As the power of the crowd waxes, the strength of the individual wanes. In this situation, a possible revitalization of social life offers no remedy for spiritlessness. In fact, Kierkegaard holds that "The idolized principle of sociality in our age is the consuming, demoralizing principle, which in the thralldom of reflection transforms even virtues into *vitia splendida*" (p. 86). At another point, he develops this crucial insight: "In our age the principle of association . . . is not affirmative but negative; it is an evasion, a dissipation, an illusion, whose dialectic is as follows: as it strengthens individuals, it vitiates them; it strengthens by numbers, by sticking together, but from the ethical point of view this is a weakening" (p. 106). The religious faith of the nineteenth century simply exacerbates the spiritless-ness of the age by obscuring decisive distinctions between the sacred and profane and by identifying religious commitment with participation in a banal form of cultural Protestantism. When everyone is supposed to be a Christian by virtue of birth into an ostensibly Christian world, the tensions distinctively characteristic of a genuine historical career are dissipated and individuals are tranquilized into a false and a dangerous sense of security.

Kierkegaard maintains that the most important consequence of political, social, and religious developments in the modern age is the pervasive loss of authentic individual selfhood. Indeed from Kierkegaard's perspective

> the single individual . . . has not fomented enough passion in himself to tear himself out of the web of reflection and the seductive ambiguity of reflection. The environment, the con-temporary age, has neither events nor integrated passion but in a negative way creates a reflective opposition which toys for a moment with the unreal prospect and then resorts to the brilliant equivocation that the smartest thing has been done, after all, by doing nothing. [*Two Ages,* p. 69]

Through such enervating reflection, one becomes, quite literally, "nobody."

The dissipation of individual selfhood is reflected in the chief philosophical and theological movement of the time—Hegelianism. According to Kierkegaard, Hegelian reason "is the abrogation of the passionate disjunction between subjectivity and objectivity" (*Two Ages,* p. 103).[7] But, Kierkegaard adds with a note of irony, the "existential expression" of the abrogation of such decisive contradictions "is to be in contradiction" (p. 97). This

---

7. In translating this passage, Hong renders "at raisonere" as "to be loquaci-ous." He points out that although the term can be translated "to reason," Kier-kegaard's intention is better conveyed by "to be loquacious." In the present con-text, however, the use of "to reason" more accurately represents the critique of Hegel and Hegelianism implicit in Kierkegaard's remarks.

existential contradiction is the result of the individual's failure to become himself—a consequence of his self-alienation. Kierkegaard contends that what the age needs is the reintroduction of the distinctions, contrasts, and antitheses ingredient in temporal existence and requisite for the emergence of genuine individuality. Kierkegaard's literary-philosophical effort is directed to creating the possibility of overcoming the dissipation he believes to be characteristic of alienation.

It becomes apparent, then, that the complex works of Hegel and Kierkegaard are intended to serve as remedies for what they both regard as the malady of the age—spiritlessness—the sickness unto death. My analysis suggests, however, that this common diagnosis masks conflicting interpretations of the nature of the illness. Hegel insists that modern man faces the difficult task of finding his way from fragmentation and disintegration among and within individuals to a harmonious inter- and intrapersonal unification or integration. Kierkegaard concludes that the way to selfhood in nineteenth-century Europe requires the negation of the dissipation of concrete existence that results from the thoroughgoing identification of the individual with the sociocultural milieu, and that such differentiation requires a long process of distinguishing person and world. While Hegel calls for a movement from the oppositional differentiation to the reconciliation of self and other, or subject and object, Kierkegaard stresses the importance of advancing from the nondifferentiation to the differentiation of self and other, or subject and object. Nevertheless, for both the question becomes, How can spiritlessness be cured? How can the movement, development, advance, necessary for the realization of spirit be facilitated?

After considerable deliberation, Hegel and Kierkegaard arrive at the conclusion that what the age most needs is an "Aesthetic Education." Reflecting the continuing influence of Schiller, Hegel writes: "The philosopher must possess just as much aesthetic power as the poet. Men without aesthetic sense is what the philosophers-of-the-letter of our times are. The philosophy of spirit is an aesthetic philosophy. . . . Poetry gains thereby a higher dignity, she becomes at the end once more, what she was in the beginning—the *teacher of humanity.*"[8] Kierkegaard suggests his own sense of mission when he explains: "I am the last stage of the development of a poet in the direction of a small-scale reformer. I have much more imagination than a reformer as such would have, but then again less of a certain personal force required for acting as a reformer" (*Journals*, no. 6061).

In fine, both Hegel and Kierkegaard assume the role of educator—teachers of humanity whose writings are informed by a pedagogical intent.[9] Their diverse philosophical and theological works share the aim of leading individuals of their day from (*e-ducare*) spiritlessness to spirit. The alpha and the omega of this journey can be expressed in different terms. Hegel and Kierkegaard try to enable their readers to move from inauthenticity to authenticity, from immediacy to immediacy after reflection, from bondage to freedom, from abstract to concrete individuality. Moreover, the pedagogical methods employed in this aesthetic education are remarkably akin to one another. Hegel and Kierkegaard develop alternative phenomenologies of spirit that seek to lead the reader from inauthentic to authentic selfhood. While Hegel undertakes this task explicitly in his *Phenomenology of Spirit*, Kierkegaard unfolds his analysis in a series of pseudonymous writings composed over a period of years.

The methodological procedures of the authors share signifi-

8. "Earliest System-Programme of German Idealism," included in H. S. Harris, *Hegel's Development Toward the Sunlight, 1770-1801*, p. 511. Although the authorship of this fragment has been the subject of lively scholarly debate over the years, evidence now strongly supports analysts who argue that Hegel penned the work. For a convenient summary of this discussion, see Harris, pp. 249-57.

9. In his detailed reconstruction of Hegel's early years, Harris argues that "the ambition to be a *Volkserzieher*" (p. xix) provides a focus around which to organize Hegel's otherwise disparate youthful philosophical wanderings. Although Harris' study is generally quite helpful and most insightful, his effort to view all of Hegel's work prior to 1801 from the perspective of his intention to become a *Volkserzieher* distorts important aspects of his development and creates needless interpretive problems. Harris' recognition of the importance of this ideal of Hegel's is correct but need not be pursued with such relentlessness to be persuasive. For a suggestive discussion of Kierkegaard's pedagogical preoccupations, see Ronald J. Manheimer, *Kierkegaard as Educator*.

cant features. Hegel's *Phenomenology of Spirit* and Kierkegaard's pseudonymous authorship develop detailed analyses of various forms of spirit, shapes of consciousness, types of selfhood, or forms of existence. Moreover, the contrasting spiritual configurations are presented in a dialectical progression that advances from less to more complete forms of life. Since the *telos* of the journey described by Hegel and Kierkegaard is free concrete individuality, they must proceed in a way that does not violate the integrity and autonomy of the learner. Their teaching method must be subtly Socratic rather than crudely authoritarian. Most important, they must begin at the point reached by their pupils and then lead them step by step through the stages from bondage and error to freedom and truth. The works call each reader to "self-examination" and demand that he "judge for himself" the form of life he incarnates. Undertaking this educational journey exacts a price. Hegel claims that the decision to philosophize is always accompanied by "dread." Critical reflection discloses old certainties to be untenable illusions. Perplexed and bewildered, the voyager tosses and turns in a sea of doubt and despair. In fact, Hegel and Kierkegaard contend that every station along the way to the final destination remains a form of inauthentic existence that must be labeled "despair." They admit that their pedagogy leads the pupil along a painful "highway of despair" (Hegel, *Phenomenology of Spirit,* p. 49). "The life of Spirit," Hegel writes, "is not the life that shrinks from death and keeps itself untouched by devastation, but rather the life that endures it and maintains itself in it. It wins its truth only when, in utter dismemberment, it finds itself" (p. 19). The suffering of dismemberment, however, occasions the cure of the sickness unto death. Though the highway of despair constitutes a dark night of the soul, the completion of the journey holds the promise of realized selfhood.

When understood in this way, Hegel's *Phenomenology of Spirit* and Kierkegaard's pseudonymous authorship appear to be *Bildungsromanen* that chart the circuitous process of self-formation.[10] In this context, it is important to distinguish three

10. Other authors who have recognized the similarity between Hegel's *Phenomenology* and the genre of *Bildungsroman* include Abrams, pp. 225-37; Jean

different narrative strands woven together in each *Bildungsges-chichte*. In the first place, Hegel's and Kierkegaard's works are quasi-autobiographical; they summarize the phases through which they have passed in their personal development. Hegel describes the *Phenomenology of Spirit* as his "voyage of discovery," and Kierkegaard confesses, "My writing is essentially my own development . . ." (*Journals*, no. 6390). Secondly, each phenomenology of spirit recapitulates the stages of world development.[11] Finally, the different forms of spirit depicted by Hegel and Kierkegaard describe the stages that must be traversed by the reader if he is to reach the goal of genuine individuality. Hegel and Kierkegaard see this third aspect of the *Bildungsgeschichte* as essential, for it most faithfully expresses the pedagogical intention of their work. Their phenomenologies are *Bildungsromanen* that encourage the reader to educate himself—to cultivate himself, to emerge from spiritlessness and to rise to spiritual existence. The dramas unfolded never lose sight of the audience to which they are directed. If their works fail to evoke an appropriate response, Hegel and Kierkegaard are forced to regard their efforts as utter failures. It is now necessary to turn our attention to a more detailed analysis of the precise educational methods employed by Hegel and Kierkegaard.

Theoria

In his introduction, Hegel describes his *Phenomenology* as "the path of the natural consciousness which presses forward to true knowledge; or as the way of the Soul which journeys through the series of its own configurations as though they were the stations

Hyppolite, *Genesis and Structure of Hegel's Phenomenology of Spirit*, pp. 11-12; Josiah Royce, *Lectures on Modern Idealism*, pp. 147 ff. Also see W. H. Bruford, *The German Tradition of Self-Cultivation: From Humboldt to Thomas Mann*. The only author who has suggested a connection between Kierkegaard's works and the *Bildungsroman* tradition is Louis Mackey, *Kierkegaard: A Kind of Poet*, pp. 273 ff. Compare Aage Henriksen, *Kierkegaards Romaner*.

11. For support of this reading of Kierkegaard's stages, see Mark C. Taylor, *Kierkegaard's Pseudonymous Authorship: A Study of Time and the Self*, pp. 64 ff.; and Gregor Malantschuk, *Kierkegaard's Way to the Truth*, pp. 25 ff., 64 ff., and *Frihends Problem I Kierkegaards Begrebet Angest*, esp. chap. 2.

appointed for it by its own nature, so that it may purify itself for the life of the Spirit, and achieve finally, through a completed experience of itself, the awareness of what it really is in itself" (*Phenomenology*, p. 49).[12] The book attempts to provide its reader with a "ladder" (p. 17)[13] by the means of which one ascends to the scientific perspective from which spirit can grasp its own actuality. As I have suggested, Hegel believes the journey from inauthenticity to authenticity to have both universal or generic and individual or personal dimensions. "The task of leading the individual from his uneducated standpoint [*ungebildeten standpunkte*] to knowledge," Hegel maintains, "had to be seen in its universal sense, just as it was the universal individual, self-conscious Spirit whose formative education [*Bildung*] had to be studied" (ibid., p. 16). Hegel proceeds to argue that "the single individual must also pass through the formative stages [*Bildungsstufen*] of universal Spirit so far as their content is concerned, but as shapes which Spirit has already left behind, as stages on a way that has been made level with toil" (p. 16). As the analysis unfolds, it becomes apparent that the education of universal and individual spirit, in fact, forms two aspects of a single pedagogical process.

> This past experience is the already acquired property of universal Spirit which constitutes the Substance of the individual, and hence appears externally to him as his inorganic nature. In this respect formative education, regarded from the side of the individual, consists in his acquiring what thus lies at hand, devouring his inorganic nature, and taking pos-

12. Hegel's undertaking is not without historical precedent. As Werner Marx points out in *Hegel's Phenomenology of Spirit*, in both Fichte and Schelling, "we find the idea of a genetic presentation of the build-up of self-consciousness in its various capacities, conceived as a 'sequence of reflection,' in which consciousness increasingly improves in self-discernment" (p. xvii). See Fichte's *Science of Knowledge* and *Foundations of the Entire Science of Knowledge* and Schelling's *Essays to Explain the Idealism of the Wissenschaftslehre* and *System of Transcendental Idealism*. Abrams suggests similarities between Hegel's undertaking in the *Phenomenology* and Wordsworth's purpose in writing *The Prelude* (Abrams, *Natural Supernaturalism*, pp. 71 ff.).

13. The image of the ladder points to an interesting parallel with Kierkegaard's pseudonym Johannes Climacus.

session of it for himself. But, as regarded from the side of universal Spirit as substance, this is nothing but its own acquisition of self-consciousness, the bringing-about of its own becoming and reflection into itself. [pp. 16-17]

The point of departure for Hegel's educational journey is "the standpoint of consciousness which knows objects in their antithesis to itself, and itself in antithesis to them" (p. 15). Put differently, Hegel begins with a situation in which self and other are sundered; the individual subject sets himself over against an alien object that he then attempts to grasp. "Knowledge in its first phase, or *immediate Spirit*," Hegel asserts, "is spiritlessness [*das Geistlose*]" (p. 15). The arduous "initiation of the unscientific consciousness into Science" (p. 16) or the actualization of spirit involves the sublation of this opposition through the incremental reconciliation of subjectivity and objectivity. The goal of this voyage of discovery is the mediation of self and other that involves "*pure* self-recognition in absolute otherness" (p. 14). Hegel expresses the final insight toward which he leads his pupils in more technical language when he writes: "The spiritual alone is the *actual;* it is essence, or that which has *being in itself;* it is that which *relates itself to itself* and is *determinate,* it is *other-being [Anderssein]* and *being-for-self,* and in this determinateness, or in its self-externality, abides with itself; in other words, it is *in and for itself*" (p. 14). The multiple dimensions of this reconcilation of self and other, or of subject and object, eventuate in a unification that Hegel sees as overcoming the fragmentation and disintegration endemic to alienation. The dialectical integration of subjectivity and objectivity negates heteronomous determination by alien otherness and realizes authentic self-relation that is mediated by relation to other. This, for Hegel, is the freedom unique to concrete individuality.

The very nature of the end toward which his analysis is directed creates a methodological dilemma for Hegel. In order to lead the reader from inauthentic to authentic existence, it would seem necessary to employ a criterion by which to judge inadequate forms of life and through which to arrange competing structures of consciousness in a progressive sequence. And yet, if the point of the educational journey is the emergence of free autonomous selfhood, no criterion can be externally imposed in a heteronomous manner. Hegel solves this problem by arguing that every form of consciousness provides itself with a standard by which to measure itself, and hence need not be subjected to an alien criterion. Consciousness distinguishes itself from its object, which it takes to exist independent of the cognitive relationship. The self-subsistent object is the criterion by which consciousness judges itself.

> In consciousness one thing exists *for* another, i.e., consciousness regularly contains the determinateness of the moment of knowledge; at the same time, this other is to consciousness not merely *for it,* but is also outside of this relationship, or exists *in itself:* the moment of truth. Thus in what consciousness affirms from within itself as *being-in-itself* or the *True* we have the standard which consciousness itself sets up by which to measure what it knows. If we designate *knowledge* as the Notion, but the essence or the *True* as what exists, or the *object,* then the examination consists in seeing whether the Notion corresponds to the object. But if we call the *essence* or in-itself of the *object* the *Notion,* and on the other hand understand by the *object* the Notion itself as *object,* viz. as it exists *for an other,* then the examination consists in seeing whether the object corresponds to its Notion. It is evident, of course, that these two procedures are the same. [*Phenomenology,* p. 53]

Should consciousness' comparison of itself with its standard yield a negative conclusion concerning the correspondence of subjectivity and objectivity, consciousness is forced to change itself in order more adequately to grasp its object. But, Hegel argues, "in the alteration of the knowledge, the object itself alters for it [i.e., consciousness] too, for the knowledge that was present was essentially a knowlege of the object: as the knowledge changes, so too does the object, for it essentially belonged to this knowledge. Hence it comes to pass for consciousness that what it previously took to be the *in-itself* is not an *in-itself,* or that it was only an in-itself for consciousness" (p. 54). Consequently, consciousness is doubly confounded: subjective certainty becomes doubtful, and what had been seen as an objective norm now seems to have been a subjective appearance [*Schein*]. The apprehension of the illusory character of its criterion is inseparable from consciousness' recognition of a new standard of evaluation. From the viewpoint of consciousness itself, this new norm is encountered as a novel object whose origin is unknown (p. 54)[14] but that beckons consciousness to attempt to grasp it. This situation, of course, constitutes the occasion for further dialectical development.

It is necessary to stress that Hegel regards the critique of consciousness by which it progresses from less to more adequate forms as "immanent." Consciousness engages in a protracted dialogue with itself in which it subjects itself to constant questioning, revision, and reform. Hegel makes this point graphically when he writes, "Thus consciousness suffers this violence at its own hands; it spoils its own limited satisfaction" (p. 51). The conviction that consciousness engages in immanent self-criticism forms an essential presupposition of Hegel's phenomenological method. In a crucial passage, Hegel explains that "not only is a contribution by us superfluous, since Notion and object, the criterion and what is to be tested, are present in consciousness itself, but we are also spared the trouble of comparing the two and really *testing* them, so that, since what consciousness examines is its own self, all that is left for us to do is simply to look on" (p. 54). In other words, Hegel conceives his task as basically *descriptive*.[15] He attempts to represent accurately the stages through which consciousness, by its own internal dialectic, progresses. Rather than arbitrarily instructing consciousness in the errors of its ways, the

14. Hegel explains: "But it is just this necessity itself, or the *origination* of the new object, that presents itself to consciousness without its understanding how this happens, which proceeds for us, as it were, behind the back of consciousness" (p. 56).

15. This reading of Hegel's phenomenological method is developed insightfully and persuasively by Kenley Dove. See "Hegel's Phenomenological Method," and "Toward an Interpretation of Hegel's *Phänomenologie des Geistes*," esp. chaps. 2–3.

phenomenologist must sink his "freedom in the content, letting it move spontaneously of its own nature, by the self as its own self, and then contemplate this movement" (*Phenomenology*, p. 36). From this perspective, Hegel's method is radically empirical.[16] He immerses himself in the observed perspective as completely as possible in order to describe it from within in a way that simultaneously fathoms its inherent principles and discerns its latent contradictions. Interestingly enough, this empiricism is at the same time theoretical and speculative. Hegel assumes the stance of a spectator who observes and records the drama unfolding before him. Thus, the education he attempts to provide the reader is, properly speaking, "aesthetic." As Stephen Crites points out, "aesthetic" derives from the Greek verb ἀισθάγομαι, which in its most comprehensive sense means "to observe" and is the etymological root of both "theory" and "theatre."[17] Hegel offers his narrative account of the drama of human consciousness for the reader's contemplation in the hope that the observation of the spectacle will provide an aesthetic education that is cathartic.

Hegel's educational method, therefore, involves an essential distinction between observed and observing consciousness. Hegel is no mere chronicler of consciousness' own experience as it moves from standpoint to standpoint. His narrative perspective affords him an angle of vision not immediately accessible to the form of life he is describing. Having grasped the overall plot of the drama he recounts, Hegel understands the experiences of the actors better than the players themselves. He does not suffer Oedipus's tragic blindness. This comprehensive vision enables Hegel to be the educator who can serve as the reader's guide. Throughout the narrative, Hegel communicates directly with his reader in an effort to provide a map for the dangerous journey along the highway of despair. His method for offering such guidance is the employment of a device we might label "the

16. George Schrader offers an illuminating discussion of the contrast between Hegelian and British empiricism in "Hegel's Contribution to Phenomenology."

17. Stephen Crites, "Introduction," to Kierkegaard's *Crisis in the Life of an Actress and Other Essays on Drama.* Compare W. Barrett, *Irrational Man: A Study in Existential Philosophy,* p. 164.

phenomological we."[18] The repeated remarks reflecting the viewpoint of "us" or of the "we" interspersed throughout the text of the *Phenomenology* are intended to help the reader to anticipate the peripeteiae and to avoid the pitfalls to which observed consciousness inevitably succumbs.

But Hegel's direct identification with the reader through the device of the "we" should not obscure the significant difference between the points of view of instructor and pupil. As observing consciousness, both author (i.e., Hegel) and reader are distinguished from observed consciousness. Nevertheless Hegel's perspective and that of the reader are not identical; they differ as does the initiator from the initiate. The reader occupies a position suspended between the forms of life examined and the comprehensive vision of his instructor—he "hovers *between* the viewing and the viewed standpoints" (Fackenheim, p. 36). Habermas correctly points out that "the phenomenologist's perspective, from which the path of knowledge in its manifestations presents itself 'for us,' can only be adopted in anticipation until this perspective itself is produced in phenomenological experience. 'We,' too, are drawn into the process of reflection, which at each of its levels is characterized anew by a 'reversal of consciousness' " (Habermas, p. 17). Hegel's pedagogy involves a triplicity of consciousness: the consciousness of the instructor, of the instructed, and of the object of instruction.[19]

Having established the distinction between the perspectives of

18. Hegel's use of the "we" throughout the *Phenomenology* has received considerable attention in the secondary literature. See, for example, Dove (1965), chap. 2; John Findlay, *Hegel: A Reinterpretation*, pp. 87 ff.; Martin Heidegger, *Holzwege*, pp. 173 ff.; Hyppolite, *Genesis and Structure*, pp. 3 ff.; R. Kroner, *Von Kant bis Hegel*, 2: 369 ff.; G. Lukacs, *Der junge Hegel: Uber die Beziehungen von Dialektik und Okonomie*, pp. 602 ff.; Herbert Marcuse, *Reason and Revolution: Hegel and the Rise of Social Theory*, p. 94. None of these authors, however, adequately distinguishes the "we" of the author from the "we" of the reader.

19. The emphasis on the triplicity of consciousness in the *Phenomenology* distinguishes this line of analysis from an interpretation such as that of Abrams (pp. 225 ff.), in which consciousness is seen as merely double. If the threefold distinction is allowed to slip into simple duality, Hegel's pedagogical purpose becomes overshadowed by autobiographical preoccupations.

teacher and student *within* observing consciousness, we are in a position to analyze the precise way in which Hegel distinguishes viewing and viewed consciousness. The basis of the difference between these two forms of awareness lies in the nature of their respective objects. We have seen that observed consciousness sees itself involved in an effort to establish knowledge by relating to an object that it takes to be both independent of consciousness and true in itself. Since this very knowledge is the object of observing consciousness, observed consciousness' contrast between subject and object, being-for-consciousness and being-in-itself, now is seen as a distinction that falls *within* consciousness. The criterion that consciousness encounters as external and imposed upon itself is, for the phenomenologist, immanent in consciousness itself. In other words, "consciousness provides its own criterion within itself, so that the investigation becomes a comparison of consciousness itself" (*Phenomenology*, p. 53). Hegel stresses that "the essential point to bear in mind throughout the whole investigation is that these two moments, 'Notion' and 'object,' 'being-for-another' and 'being-in-itself,' both fall *within* that knowledge which we are investigating" (p. 53). This insight proves to be central to Hegel's argument.

We have noted that consciousness apprehends the progressive experience it undergoes as resulting from a series of contingent encounters with different external objects. Hegel contends that the reflective description of the experience of consciousness sublates both the externality of subject and object and the contingency of the stages of development from error to truth. The empathetic identification with other forms of consciousness discloses the inherent contradictions that lead to the self-negation of every particular viewpoint. Each perspective is internally related to its opposite in such a way that it bears within itself the seeds of its own destruction. Hegel argues, however, that dissolution is at the same time resolution. The new object encountered by consciousness is not a creation *de novo*, but is the result of consciousness' own negation of its prior object.

> Consciousness knows *something*; this object is the essence of the *in-itself*; but it is also for consciousness the in-itself. . . .

We see that consciousness now has two objects: one is the first *in-itself*, the second is the *being-for-consciousness of this in-itself*. The latter appears at first sight to be merely the reflection of consciousness into itself, i.e., what consciousness has in mind is not an object, but only its knowledge of that first object. But . . . the first object, in being known, is altered for consciousness; it ceases to be the in-itself, and becomes something that is the *in-itself* only *for consciousness*. And this then is the True: the being-for-consciousness of this in-itself. Or, in other words, this is the *essence*, or the *object* of consciousness. This new object contains the nothingness of the first, it is what experience has made of it. [ibid., p. 55]

The sequence of experiences undergone by consciousness is generated by a continual process that Hegel calls "determinate negation." The distinguishing characteristic of any particular object is mediated by the specificity of the object through whose negation it arises. Since each object harbors a necessary relation to its antithesis, the progressive unfolding of the experience of consciousness is not arbitrary and inflicted in an external manner but grows out of a necessary process of immanent dialectical development. The stages through which spirit passes in moving toward its full realization form a necessary progression in which beginning and end are implicitly identical.[20] In itself, spiritlessness is spirit; of itself, inauthentic selfhood advances to authentic individuality. The apprehension of the necessity of this dialectical progression is the lesson taught by the reader's phenomenological guide. Hegel summarizes:

Our account implied that our knowledge of the first object, or the being-*for*-consciousness of the first in-itself, itself becomes the second object. It usually seems to be the case, on the contrary, that our experience of the untruth of our first

20. Hegel points out: "Because of this necessity, the way to Science, is itself already *Science*, and hence, in virtue of its content, is the Science of the *experience of consciousness*" (*Phenomenology*, p. 56). In recent years, the question of relationship between the *Phenomenology* and Hegel's mature system has provoked heated debate among German commentators. The best discussion of the problem is Friedrich Fulda's *Das Problem einer Einleitung in Hegels Wissenschaft der Logik*.

notion comes by way of a second object which we come upon by chance and externally, so that our part in all this is simply the pure *apprehension* of what is in and for itself. From the present viewpoint, however, the new object shows itself to have come about through a *reversal of consciousness itself*. This way of looking at the matter is something contributed by *us*, by means of which the succession of experiences through which consciousness passes is raised into a scientific progression—but it is not known to the consciousness that we are observing. [*Phenomenology*, pp. 55–56]

Despite his persistent pedagogical purpose, Hegel, in one sense, has nothing to teach his pupil. His method of educating is Socratic to the extent that it seeks to render the implicit explicit. As Hyppolite observes, "The rise of empirical consciousness to absolute knowledge is possible only if the necessary stages of its ascent are discovered within it. These stages are still within it; all that is needed is that it descend into the interiority of memory by an action comparable to Platonic recollection" (1974, p. 39). Through the process of recollection (*Er-innerung*), the individual who follows Hegel's guidance internalizes or appropriates as his own the stages necessary for full self-realization. Prior to this inwardization, the phases of spirit's cultivation remain external to one another in outward temporal dispersion (*Entäusserung*). Recollection renders spirit transparent to itself and brings a fulfillment that "consists in perfectly *knowing* what *it is*, in knowing its substance" (*Phenomenology*, p. 492).[21] The journey Hegel invites his reader to undertake turns out to be a voyage of *self*-discovery whose destination is spirit's adequate comprehension of the actuality it has become.

Poiesis

Our consideration of Kierkegaard's analysis of his age has disclosed that he holds spiritlessness to arise from the dissipation of

---

21. For the twentieth-century reader, Hegel's recognition of the therapeutic value of recollection suggests interesting parallels with Freud's psychoanalytic method. Consider Paul Ricoeur, *Freud and Philosophy*, and Hyppolite, "Hegel's Phenomenology and Psychoanalysis."

individual selfhood created by abstract reflection. When reflection obscures vital distinctions and "dispels the urge to decision," the individual becomes absent to himself—a mere "spectator" of his own life, devoid of the passionate "inwardness" constitutive of genuine individuality (*Two Ages,* pp. 76, 81, 80). Kierkegaard is not suggesting a thoroughgoing condemnation of all reflection. To the contrary, responsible deliberation is a presupposition of free selfhood. But when carried to extremes, reflection can paralyze decisive action. "Reflection is not the evil," Kierkegaard insists, "but a standing state of reflection and a standstill in reflection are the fraud and the corruption, which by transforming the conditions for action into means of escape lead to dissipation" (p. 96). Although he acknowledges that "beyond a doubt there is no task and effort more difficult than to extricate oneself from the temptations of reflection" (p. 77), Kierkegaard believes that precisely such an undertaking is required to overcome the spiritless dissipation of his day. The purpose of Kierkegaard's diverse writings is to engender inwardness by making people aware of the depths to which they have fallen and by creating the possibility for them to begin the journey from despair to realized selfhood. Since he is convinced that "rescue comes only through the essentiality of the religious in the single individual" (p. 88), Kierkegaard's works have from the outset a religious orientation. More specifically, Kierkegaard's belief that concrete individuality can be fully actualized only through Christian existence leads him to conclude in *The Point of View for My Work as an Author* (posthumous) that the sole antidote to spiritlessness is the clarification of "how to become a Christian" (p. 13). He explains: "The contents of this little book affirm, then, what I truly am as an author, that I am and was a religious author, that the whole of my work as an author is related to Christianity, to the problem 'of becoming a Christian,' with a direct or indirect polemic against the monstrous illusion that in such a land as ours all are Christians of a sort" (pp. 5–6).

Paradoxically, however, Kierkegaard could combat the pathological reflection of his age only reflectively. "My task," he writes, "was to cast Christianity into reflection, not poetically to idealize it (for the essentially Christian, after all, is itself the ideal) but with poetic fervor to present the total ideality at its most ideal—always ending with: I am not that, but I strive" (*Journals,* no. 6511). An aesthetic age calls for an aesthetic education. Kierkegaard, like Hegel, could not accomplish his end by attempting to force his viewpoint on others. His understanding of the nature of free selfhood requires him to employ a method that constantly respects the integrity of the individual. Consequently, in a manner similar to Hegel, Kierkegaard decides that spiritlessness can be overcome most effectively by the depiction of alternative forms of life that provide the reader the occasion for self-examination and self-judgment. The various personae of Kierkegaard's pseudonymous authorship comprise the cast of characters through which the dramatic struggle toward authentic selfhood is acted out.

Each pseudonym represents a particular shape of consciousness, form of life, type of selfhood. In order to present every standpoint as completely and as accurately as possible, Kierkegaard, like Hegel, withdraws and allows each persona to speak for itself. In the course of the ensuing dialogue, the characters uncover the unique contours, nagging tensions, and destructive contradictions of their different perspectives. Taken together, the pseudonyms present a coherent account of what amounts to a phenomenology of spirit analogous, though alternative, to the course plotted by Hegel. The Kierkegaardian forms of life are arranged as dialectical stages in a progressive movement toward genuine individuality. As educator, Kierkegaard hopes to enable the reader to achieve more adequate self-knowledge and to provide the occasion for the reader's movement from spiritlessness to spirit. In intention and execution, therefore, there are significant parallels between the philosophical and theological projects of Hegel and Kierkegaard.

Despite these noteworthy similarities, equally essential differences distinguish their works. Most important in this context, Kierkegaard's pseudonyms do not represent descriptions of the stages through which consciousness *has passed* in the process of its actualization. The various personae are imaginative projections of existential possibilities that *might be realized* in the course of becoming an authentic individual. In place of Hegel's theoretical description of spirit's actuality, Kierkegaard creates poeticized possibilities that confront the sojourner along life's way. *Poiesis,* not *theoria,* is Kierkegaard's element. To understand more adequately the distinctive features of Kierkegaard's aesthetic education, we must consider his interpretation of the person of the poet and the nature of the poetic work of art.[22]

We have already noted that Kierkegaard regards himself as "essentially a poet" (*Journals,* no. 6383). In the following *Journal* entry, he identifies the distinguishing characteristic of a poet: "What is it to be a poet? It is to have one's own personal life, one's actuality in categories completely different from those of one's poetic production, to be related to the ideal only in imagination, so that one's personal life is more or less a satire on the poetry and on oneself" (no. 6300). Put differently, the poet's thought and being, word and deed, ideality and reality, do not coincide, but contradict one another. Since he sees his "purely ideal task" as involving "casting Christianity completely and wholly into reflection" (no. 6237), Kierkegaard ever insists that he is not a Christian. The denial of the poet masks a definite pedagogical strategy.

> [If] it is an illusion that all are Christians—and if there is anything to be done about it, it must be done indirectly, not by one who vociferously proclaims himself an extraordinary Christian, but by one who, better instructed, is ready to declare that he is not a Christian at all. That is, one must approach from behind the person who is under an illusion. Instead of wishing to have an advantage of being oneself that rare thing, a Christian, one must let the prospective captive enjoy the advantage of being the Christian, and for one's own part have resignation enough to be the one who is far behind—otherwise one will certainly not get the man out of his illusion, a thing which is difficult enough in any case. [*Point of View,* pp. 24–25]

22. In his excellent study *Kierkegaard: A Kind of Poet,* Mackey also stresses the importance of Kierkegaard's understanding of poetry and the poet. See esp. chap. 6.

Kierkegaard's interpretation of the poet represents his version of the principle of Socratic ignorance. In fact, Kierkegaard's educational technique is thoroughly informed by his appropriation of the central features of Socratic method. While Kierkegaard's understanding of Socrates is profoundly influenced by Hegel's consideration of Socrates' viewpoint, his criticisms of Hegel's analysis point to crucial differences between their methodological commitments. Kierkegaard's interpretation of Socrates consists of a radicalization of Hegel's insights. Here as elsewhere, Kierkegaard assumes Hegel's perspective in order to negate it.[23] Kierkegaard admits that Hegel correctly identifies the essence of the Socratic position as irony. Moreover, he agrees with Hegel's definition of irony as "infinite absolute negativity" (*Concept of Irony,* p. 287). Hegel's error lay in his failure to carry through his insight with sufficient rigor. Rather than allowing Socrates to remain "infinitely negative," Hegel urges him toward a positive resolution of the dilemmas he discovers. Consequently, irony becomes a "mastered moment"; negativity ceases to be a perduring perspective and is itself negated by the "higher" positivity it is supposed to generate.

In an important passage in his magister dissertation, Kierkegaard distinguishes his reading of Socrates from that of Hegel.[24]

> It is towards this point of exhibiting Socrates as the founder of morality that Hegel unilaterally allows his conception of Socrates to gravitate. It is the Idea of the good that he seeks to claim for Socrates, but this causes him some embarrassment when he attempts to show how Socrates has conceived the good. It is essentially here that the difficulty with Hegel's

23. This line of analysis opposes those authors who maintain that in *The Concept of Irony* Kierkegaard is fundamentally a Hegelian. See, for example, Vilhelm Andersen, *Tider og Typer af Dansk Aands,* part 2, 2:65–108; and Harold Høffding, *Søren Kierkegaard som Filosof.*

24. For helpful discussions of the differences between Hegel's and Kierkegaard's views of Socrates, see Robert L. Perkins, "Hegel and Kierkegaard: Two Critics of Romantic Irony" and "Two Nineteenth-Century Interpretations of Socrates: Hegel and Kierkegaard."

conception of Socrates lies, namely the attempt is constantly made to show how Socrates has conceived the good. But what is even worse, so it seems to me, is that the direction of the current in Socrates' life is not faithfully maintained. The movement in Socrates is to come to the good. His significance for the development of the world is to arrive at this (not at one point to have arrived at this). His significance for his contemporaries is that they arrived at this. Now this does not mean that he arrived at this toward the end of his life, as it were, but that his life was constantly to come to this and to cause others to do the same. . . . He did not do this once and for all, but he did this with every individual. He began wherever the individual might find himself, and soon he was thoroughly involved in issuing clearance papers for each one of them. But as soon as he had ferried one of them over he immediately turned back for another. No actuality could withstand him, yet that which became visible was ideality in the most fleeting suggestion of its faintest configuration, that is, as infinitely abstract. . . . Socrates ferried the individual from reality over to ideality, and ideal infinity, as infinite negativity, became the nothingness into which he made the whole manifold of reality disappear. . . . Actuality, by means of the absolute, became nothingness, but the absolute was in turn nothingness. In order to be able to maintain Socrates at this point, in order never to forget that the content of his life was to undertake this movement at every moment, one must bear in mind his significance as a divine missionary. Yet this has been ignored by Hegel, although Socrates himself places much emphasis upon it. [*Irony,* pp. 254–55]

According to Kierkegaard, Hegel does not adequately distinguish Socrates' existential and Plato's speculative dialectic. Therefore, at Hegel's hands, Socratic questioning and irresolution become speculative answering and resolution. "One may ask a question," Kierkegaard points out, "for the purpose of obtaining an answer containing the desired content, so that the more one questions, the deeper and more meaningful becomes the answer; or one may ask a question not in the interest of obtaining an answer, but to suck out the apparent content with a question and leave only an emptiness remaining. The first method naturally presupposes a content, the second an emptiness; the first is the speculative, the second the ironic. Now it was the latter method which was especially practised by Socrates" (ibid., p. 73).

To correct the errors into which Hegel's interpretation falls, one need simply return to the Hegelian notion of "infinite absolute negativity" and apply it consistently to the person and position of Socrates. For Kierkegaard, Socrates' standpoint is "exclusively ironic" (ibid., p. 232). He never allows negativity to give way to a "higher" positivity; the disquiet of ignorance always fails to win the peace of knowledge. "The reason Socrates could content himself with this ignorance was because he had no deeper speculative need. Instead of pacifying this negativity speculatively, he pacified it far more through the eternal unrest wherein he repeated the same process with each particular individual" (p. 201). Unlike the systematic philosopher, the Socratic educator offers no results. Question marks and not periods punctuate his dialogue.

The attraction Socrates exercises over Kierkegaard becomes more understandable when we recall that he sees the spiritlessness of modernity as arising from the complete identification of the individual with his sociocultural milieu. Kierkegaard maintains that the entire point of Socratic questioning is to raise "the individual out of immediate existence" (p. 85), or to precipitate the differentiation between self and social totality. "By means of his questions," Socrates "sawed through the virgin forest of substantial consciousness in all quietude, and when everything was ready, all these formations suddenly disappeared and his mind's eye enjoyed a prospect such as it had never before seen" (p. 215). This prospect is nothing less than the free individual that Socrates' "art of midwifery" seeks to bring to birth. Such a birth is possible, however, only if "the umbilical cord of substantiality" (p. 215) is severed. Kierkegaard contends that Socratic midwifery involves a justified deception intended to dispel the interlocutor's illusions. The ignorance resulting from this dis-illusionment forms "the nothingness from which a beginning must be made" (p. 222). Poetic and ironic dissimulation is never without pedagogical purpose, for it attempts "to mystify the surrounding world not so much in order to conceal itself as to induce others to reveal themselves" (p. 268). To understand the nature of this evoked self-revelation, we must turn our attention from the person of the poet to the nature of the poem. As Mackey points out:

> The speech of a poet does not utter his inner states, but rather builds meanings into a free-standing structure of language. Paradox, self-concealment, plural connotations, distentions of metaphor and the like are the shears by which he clips the umbilical of his fancy's child and sends it out on its own. His art is not the externalizing of himself, but the objectifying of a work of words: *poiesis*. What the poet produces is a verbal object (*poiema*) in which meanings, released from any personal interest he may vest in them, are neither affirmed nor denied, but simply placed. A poem in this sense does not *mean*—it does not urge the feelings and opinions of the poet on the reader. It *is*—as a thing made it is self-sufficient (*perfectum*) and bears no message not indigenous to its perfection. But the poetic object, however much it dispatches the poet's words from the poet, is nevertheless an object (*objectum, Gegenstand*) and as such commands a response. [Mackey, pp. 284–85]

To command such a response, Kierkegaard composes his pseudonymous authorship. He explains that "a pseudonym is excellent for accentuating a point, a stance, a position. It creates a poetic person."[25] The "poeticized personalities" who act out the Kierkegaardian drama of existence are "personified possibilities,"[26] imaginative projections of fantastic, fictitious forms

25. *Papirer*, X^1 510, in *Armed Neutrality and an Open Letter*, p. 88. For an elaboration of the points being made here, see Taylor, *Kierkegaard's Pseudonymous Authorship*, chap. 2.

26. Paul Holmer, "Kierkegaard and Ethical Theory." Holmer has analyzed this aspect of Kierkegaard's thought with unusual insight. Compare "Kierkegaard and Religious Propositions" and "On Understanding Kierkegaard."

of life that can serve as models for the despairing person's self-interpretation and self-judgment. The ideality of these imagined possibilities is essential to their function in Kierkegaard's aesthetic education.

Drawing on his understanding of Hegelian aesthetics, Kierkegaard maintains that the genuine work of art embodies an ideal form in the medium singularly appropriate to the idea it seeks to express. As Crites indicates, "the idea comes to consciousness only in the process of artistic creation itself, and only in the appropriate medium. The problem in art, as Hegel had shown, is to shape the material or medium in such a way that it will become as transparent as possible to its proper idea, so that the idea can, as it were, shine through the medium employed."[27] This artistic transparency is achieved only through abstraction from the tensions of finitude. The timeless ideality of the work of art articulates pure possibilities that stand in marked contrast to the confusing options faced in temporal experience. This atemporal ideality provides the occasion for aesthetic education. Borrowing a term from Hegel and the Platonic tradition, Kierkegaard argues that a person apprehends the aesthetic object by a process of "recollection." In recollection, one grasps ideal forms that are antecedent to and the presupposition of temporal existence. Aesthetic education affords the opportunity for self-clarification by transporting the individual from the conflicts and confusions of actual life to the momentary repose and clarity of the ideal realm of pure possibility. To attempt to remain in such aesthetic repose is, however, to fall victim to spiritlessness. Kierkegaard indicates that "art and poetry have been called anticipations of the eternal. If one desires to speak in this fashion, one must nevertheless note that art and poetry are not essentially related to an existing individual; for their contemplative enjoyment, the joy over what is beautiful, is disinterested, and the spectator of the work of art is contempla-

27. Stephen Crites, "Introduction," *Crisis in the Life of an Actress,* p. 29. Crites gives an excellent account of Kierkegaard's aesthetic theory and of its relation to Hegel's position. Compare "Pseudonymous Authorship as Art and as Act." I have benefited greatly from these two essays.

tively outside himself *qua* existing individual" (*Concluding Unscientific Postscript*, p. 277 n.).

In contrast to Hegel, Kierkegaard's aesthetic education is not an end in itself but has an unaesthetic, ethical purpose. On the one hand, "The aesthetic and intellectual principle is that no reality is thought or understood until its *esse* has been resolved into its *posse.*" On the other, "The ethical principle is that no possibility is understood until each *posse* has really become an *esse*" (p. 288). Reflection becomes doubly reflected as recollection gives way to repetition. Explaining his poetic productions, Kierkegaard, under the guise of Johannes Climacus, writes: "A communication in the form of a possibility compels the recipient to face the problem of existing in it, so far as this is possible between man and man" (p. 320). Through his pseudonymous authorship, Kierkegaard attempts to extricate his reader from "the temptations of reflection" by occasioning a crisis of decision. His poeticized personalities force the reader to confront difficult choices; they lay a claim upon the will as well as upon the imagination. Pure possibilities, of course, must initially be grasped reflectively. But this reflective apprehension of imagined ideality is the propaedeutic to the existential act of "double reflection" in which possibility becomes actual and ideality is reflected in reality by means of the individual's free decision. A person does not achieve transparency (*Gjennemsigtighed*) simply by the appreciation of an ideality already implicit in his reality, but by volitional activity in which he struggles to become a living expression of the ideal he has conceived. In striving to "reduplicate" concept in being, one attempts to "'exist' in what one understands."[28] To the extent that this

---

28. *Training in Christianity*, p. 133. Elsewhere Kierkegaard explains more fully: "However, coming into existence may present a reduplication, i.e., the possibility of a second coming into existence within the first coming into existence. Here we have the historical in the stricter sense, subject to a dialectic with respect to time. The coming into existence which in this sphere is identical with the coming into existence of nature is a possibility, a possibility which for nature is its whole reality. But this historical coming into existence in the stricter sense is a coming into existence within a coming into existence." *Philosophical Fragments*, p. 94.

endeavor is successful, truth develops or the individual becomes truthful.

With respect to human existence, the identity of thought and being definitive of truth is not primordial but is historically emergent, born of the individual's free activity. Kierkegaard contends that in ethical and religious matters, "truth is subjectivity," or, as he explains, "*An objective uncertainty held fast in an appropriation-process of the most passionate inwardness is truth,* the highest truth attainable for an *existing* individual" (*Postscript,* p. 182). The important phrase in this definition for our purpose is "an appropriation-process" (*Tilegnelse*). Because the existing individual is in a state of becoming, his life is a constant approximation of the ideals he conceives. "Subjectivity" indicates the process by which an individual appropriates what he thinks, or constitutes his actuality by realizing his possibilities. Kierkegaard proceeds to identify subjectivity with truth for the existing individual: "The truth consists in nothing else than the self-activity of personal appropriation" (p. 217). As should be clear, this argument is not intended to deny the notion of truth as the conformity of thought and being. However, because the existing individual is in a process of becoming, Kierkegaard holds that such conformity is never reached as long as existence continues but remains an ideal that is asymptotically approximated. "Not for a single moment is it forgotten that the subject is an existing individual, and that existence is a process of becoming, and that therefore the notion of the truth as identity of thought and being is a chimera of abstraction, in its truth only an expectation of the creature; not because truth is not such an identity, but because the knower is an existing individual for whom the truth cannot be such an identity as long as he lives in time" (p. 176).

This understanding of the nature of religious truth further illuminates Kierkegaard's pedagogical strategy. Since true selfhood presupposes an individual's free actualization of possibility, the teacher must communicate with the pupil in an indirect manner. Instead of constantly identifying with and offering direct guidance to the reader,[29] the author must withdraw himself from

29. As Hegel does through the "phenomenological we."

the dialogic relation and leave the reader alone with imagined possibilities expressed in the poetic work. By insisting on the disparity between his ideas and his life, the poet directs the reader away from his person and toward his poetic creation. Kierkegaard's pseudonymity is the curtain separating him from the drama he stages. His multiple literary devices seek to focus the reader's attention on the play his personae enact rather than on the complex behind-the-scenes maneuvers necessary to mount the production.

For Kierkegaard, however, observation of the drama is not itself cathartic. The purification of spirit that cures the sickness unto death lies not in passive speculation but in practical action. Theoretical reflection is a necessary but not sufficient condition of the development of the inwardness necessary for authentic selfhood. To recollection must be added repetition, a movement Hegel never makes.

> The dialectic of repetition is easy; for what is repeated has been, or it could not be repeated, but precisely the fact that it has been makes the repetition something new. When the Greeks said that all knowledge is recollection, they were saying that everything that comes into existence has been. When one says that life is a repetition, one is saying that the existence that has been now becomes. If one has neither the category of recollection nor that of repetition, the whole of life is dissolved into a vain and empty noise. Recollection is the pagan life-outlook, repetition is the modern. Repetition is the *interest* of metaphysics, and also the interest on which metaphysics is stranded; repetition is the solution of every ethical outlook; repetition is the *conditio sine qua non* for every dogmatic problem. [*Repetition*, p. 149]

From Kierkegaard's perspective, inwardness is not the result of a retrospective dialectic of recollection that grasps reality as the necessary outworking of ideality. To the contrary, inwardness presupposes a prospective dialectic of repetition that posits an abyss between ideality and actuality which can be bridged only by the contingent leap of the free individual. The stages of Kierkegaard's journey to selfhood are not internally related and do not constitute a *necessary* progression. They represent distinct forms of life that can be realized only if they are willed by the individual. In a sense, Kierkegaard, too, has nothing to teach his pupil. He questions, but does not answer—his aesthetic education ends without result. He confesses that the "result is not in my power; it depends upon so many things, and above all it depends upon whether he [i.e., the reader] will or not. In all eternity it is impossible for me to compel a person to accept an opinion, a conviction, a belief. But one thing I can do: I can compel him to take notice. In one sense this is the first thing, for it is the condition antecedent to the next thing, i.e., the acceptance of an opinion, a conviction, a belief. In another sense it is the last—if that is, he will not take the next step" (*Point of View*, p. 35). The journey to which Kierkegaard calls his reader is unending. *Omega* ever recedes, for the concluding chapter of the drama of selfhood can only be written after the final curtain falls.

Spiritlessness

Though our course has been long, our conclusion can be brief. The intricate philosophical and theological works of Hegel and Kierkegaard share a common purpose: they seek to meet the need of the age by providing an aesthetic education that leads the individual from spiritlessness to spirit, from bondage to freedom, from inauthentic to authentic selfhood. And yet their educational journeys lead in opposite directions. What Hegel regards as self-realization Kierkegaard sees as self-alienation, and what Hegel interprets as self-estrangement is for Kierkegaard self-fulfillment. Conversely, what Kierkegaard views as authentic selfhood, Hegel believes to be inauthentic selfhood, and what Kierkegaard sees as inauthenticity is for Hegel authenticity. Hegel's *Phenomenology of Spirit* leads the reader to the contemplative re-cognition of the ideality of actuality through cognitive recollection. Kierkegaard's pseudonymous authorship leads the reader to the brink of decision by presenting idealities yet to be actualized through volitional repetition.

In light of such significant differences, the question of the basis of the many ostensible similarities between the undertakings of Hegel and Kierkegaard inevitably arises. We can solve this final puzzle by recalling that both Hegel and Kierkegaard believe their respective pedagogies must begin with the standpoint of the pupil. For Kierkegaard, this means that the educational process has to commence with the spiritlessness of Christendom and its philosophy, Hegelianism. Kierkegaard's appropriation of Hegel's insights is consistently ironic. He assumes Hegel's perspective in order to negate it from within. Like Socrates before him, the poet Kierkegaard "allows the existent to exist though it has no validity for him, yet he pretends that it has and under this guise leads it on towards its certain dissolution. Insofar as the ironic subject is world historically justified, there is in this a unity of what is genial with artistic sobriety and discretion" (*Irony*, p. 281).

REFERENCES

Abrams, M. H. *Natural Supernaturalism: Tradition and Revolution in Romantic Literature.* New York: Norton, 1973.

Andersen, V. *Tider og Typer af Dansk Aands.* Copenhagen, 1916.

Barrett, W. *Irrational Man: A Study in Existential Philosophy.* New York: Doubleday, 1962.

Bruford, W. H. *The German Tradition of Self-Cultivation: From Humboldt to Thomas Mann.* New York: Cambridge University Press, 1975.

Crites, S. "Introduction." In S. Kierkegaard, *Crisis in the Life of an Actress and Other Essays on Drama.* New York: Harper & Row, 1967.

————. *In the Twilight of Christendom: Hegel vs. Kierkegaard on Faith and History.* Missoula, Mont.: Scholars Press, 1972a.

————. "Pseudonymous Authorship as Art and as Act." In J. Thompson, ed., *Kierkegaard: A Collection of Critical Essays.* New York: Doubleday, 1972b.

Dove, K. "Toward an Interpretation of Hegel's *Phänomenologie des Geistes.*" Ph.D. dissertation, Yale University, 1965.

————. "Hegel's Phenomenological Method." In W. E. Steinkraus, ed., *New Studies in Hegel's Philosophy.* New York: Holt, Rinehart and Winston, 1971.

Fackenheim, E. L. *The Religious Dimension of Hegel's Thought.* Bloomington: Indiana University Press, 1967.

Findlay, J. *Hegel: A Reinterpretation.* New York: Collier Books, 1962.

Forstman, J. *A Romantic Triangle: Schleiermacher and Early German Romanticism.* Missoula, Mont.: Scholars Press, 1977.

Fulda, F. *Das Problem einer Einleitung in Hegel's Wissenschaft der Logik.* Frankfurt: V. Kostermann, 1965.

Gray, G. *Hegel's Hellenic Ideal.* New York: King's Crown Press, 1941.

Habermas, J. *Knowledge and Human Interests.* Translated by J. Shapiro. Boston: Beacon Press, 1971.

Harris, H. S. *Hegel's Development Toward the Sunlight, 1770–1801.* New York: Oxford University Press, 1972.

Hegel, G. W. F. *Briefe von und an Hegel.* Vol. 1. Edited by J. Hoffmeister and R. Flechsig. Hamburg: F. Meiner, 1961.

———. *The Difference between Fichte's and Schelling's System of Philosophy.* Translated by H. S. Harris and W. Cerf. Albany: State University of New York Press, 1977.

———. "Earliest System-Programme of German Idealism." Included in Harris, 1972.

———. "The German Constitution." *Hegel's Political Writings.* Translated by T. M. Knox. New York: Oxford University Press, 1964.

———. *The Logic of Hegel.* Translated by W. Wallace. New York: Oxford University Press, 1968.

———. *Phenomenology of Spirit.* Translated by A. V. Miller. New York: Oxford University Press, 1977.

———. *Philosophy of Right.* Translated by T. M. Knox. New York: Oxford University Press, 1969.

Heidegger, M. *Holzwege.* Frankfurt: V. Kostermann, 1957.

Henriksen, A. *Kierkegaards Romaner.* Copenhagen: Gyldendal, 1969.

Høffding, H. *Søren Kierkegaard som Filosof.* Copenhagen, 1892.

Holmer, P. "Kierkegaard and Ethical Theory." *Ethics* 63 (1953): 157–70.

———. "Kierkegaard and Religious Propositions." *Journal of Religion* 35 (1955): 135–46.

———. "On Understanding Kierkegaard." In H. A. Johnson and N. Thulstrup, eds., *A Kierkegaard Critique.* Chicago: Henry Regnery, 1962.

Hyppolite, J. "Hegel's Phenomenology and Psychoanalysis." In W. E. Steinkraus, ed., *New Studies in Hegel's Philosophy.* New York: Holt, Rinehart and Winston, 1971.

———. *Genesis and Structure of Hegel's Phenomenology of Spirit.* Translated by S. Cherniak and J. Heckman. Evanston, Ill.: Northwestern University Press, 1974.

Kierkegaard, S.
   Journals and Papers [1834–55]. Translated and edited by H. and E.
      Hong. Bloomington: Indiana University Press, 1967.
   The Concept of Irony with Constant Reference to Socrates [1841]. Translated
      by L. M. Capel. Bloomington: Indiana University Press, 1968.
   Repetition: An Essay in Experimental Psychology [1843]. Translated by W.
      Lowrie. Princeton, N.J.: Princeton University Press, 1946.
   Philosophical Fragments [1844]. Translated by D. Swenson and revised
      by H. Hong. Princeton, N.J.: Princeton University Press, 1967.
   Concluding Unscientific Postscript [1846]. Translated by D. F. Swenson
      and W. Lowrie. Princeton, N.J.: Princeton University Press, 1968.
   Two Ages: The Age of Revolution and the Present Age: A Literary Review
      [1846]. Translated by H. and E. Hong. Princeton, N.J.: Princeton
      University Press, 1978.
   Armed Neutrality and an Open Letter [1849]. Translated and edited by H.
      and E. Hong. New York: Simon & Schuster, 1969.
   Training in Christianity [1850]. Translated by W. Lowrie. Princeton,
      N.J.: Princeton University Press, 1967.
   The Point of View for My Work as an Author: A Report to History [1859;
      posthumous]. Translated by W. Lowrie. New York: Harper & Row,
      1962.
Kroner, R. *Von Kant bis Hegel. Naturphilosophie zur Philosophie des Geistes*,
   vol. 2. Tübingen: J. C. B. Mohr, 1924.
Lukacs, G. *Der junge Hegel: Uber die Beziehungen von Dialektik und
   Okonomie*. Zurich: Europa, 1948.
Mackey, L. *Kierkegaard: A Kind of Poet*. Philadelphia: University of
   Pennsylvania Press, 1972.
Malantschuk, G. *Kierkegaard's Way to the Truth*. Minneapolis, Minn.:
   Augsburg, 1968.
————. *Frihends Problem I Kierkegaards Begrebet Angest*. Copenhagen:
   Roskenkilde og Bagger, 1971.
Manheimer, R. J. *Kierkegaard as Educator*. Berkeley: University of
   California Press, 1977.
Marcuse, H. *Reason and Revolution: Hegel and the Rise of Social Theory*.
   Boston: Beacon Press, 1960.
Marx, W. *Hegel's Phenomenology of Spirit: Its Point and Purpose—A Com-
   mentary on the Preface and Introduction*. Translated by P. Health. New
   York: Harper & Row, 1975.
Pascal, R. "Herder and the Scottish Historical School." *Publications of the
   English Goethe Society*, n.s. 14 (1938–39): 23–42.

———. "'*Bildung*' and the Division of Labor." In *German Studies Presented to Walter Horace Bruford*. London, 1962.

Perkins, R. L. "Two Nineteenth-Century Interpretations of Socrates: Hegel and Kierkegaard." *Kierkegaard-Studiet,* international edition 4 (1967): 9–14.

———. "Hegel and Kierkegaard: Two Critics of Romantic Irony." In *Hegel in Comparative Literature*. Baltimore: St. John's University Press, 1970.

Pöggeler, O. *Hegel's Kritik der Romantik*. Bonn: H. Bouvier, 1956.

Ricoeur, P. *Freud and Philosophy*. New Haven: Yale University Press, 1970.

Royce, J. *Lectures on Modern Idealism*. New Haven: Yale University Press, 1964.

Schiller, J. C. F. von. *On the Aesthetic Education of Man: In a Series of Letters*. Translated by R. Snell. New York: Frederick Ungar, 1965.

Schrader, G. "Hegel's Contribution to Phenomenology." *The Monist* 48, no. 1 (1964): 18–33.

Taylor, M. C. *Kierkegaard's Pseudonymous Authorship: A Study of Time and the Self*. Princeton, N.J.: Princeton University Press, 1975.

Wellek, R. *A History of Modern Criticism: 1750–1950—The Romantic Age*. New Haven: Yale University Press, 1955.

12

Kierkegaard's Negativistic Method

MICHAEL THEUNISSEN

I. Introduction

1. ON THE PSYCHOLOGICAL AND
PSYCHIATRIC RECEPTION OF KIERKEGAARD

As Jaspers' *Allgemeine Psychopathologie (General Psychopathology)*[1] shows, Kierkegaard exercised, from an early time on, a certain influence on the sciences of the disturbed psyche. In the last decades, however, several developments have started to take place in psychology, psychiatry, and psychoanalysis which have either awakened a new interest in Kierkegaard or made him potentially interesting for these sciences. I should like to comment on only two tendencies here. The first is the reconsideration of the "self." We can observe this particularly well in the history of psychoanalytical theory.[2] Although Kierkegaard never worked out a concept of the unconscious and thus does not conceive becoming self as becoming conscious of the unconscious,[3] he has

---

This essay was translated by Charlotte Baumann under the supervision of the author.

1. K. Jaspers, *Allgemeine Psychopathologie* (Berlin/Heidelberg: Julius Springer, 1913) [*General Psychopathology*, trans. J. Hoenig and M. W. Hamilton (Chicago: University of Chicago Press, 1963)]. Jaspers refers to Kierkegaard only in the later editions of the book.

2. Cf. H. J. S. Guntrip, *Psychoanalytic Theory, Therapy, and the Self* (New York: Basic Books, 1971), and H. Kohut, *The Analysis of the Self* (New York: International Universities Press, 1971).

3. Cf. B. Wilshire, "Kierkegaard's Theory of Knowledge and New Directions in Psychology and Psychoanalysis," *Review of Existential Psychology and Psychiatry* 3 (1963): 249–61.

in the light of these developments actually been seen as a
forerunner of Freud,[4] who himself at the most presupposed the
wholeness of person so important for Fairbairn and Sullivan and
who also on the way to the ego only had "a substructure of personality" as his goal.[5] Other psychological systems as well have
arisen under Kierkegaard's influence, some of which—such as
"existential psychology"[6]—even declare the self their whole object; and ideas of psychologies have been proposed which at least
build on the concept of self, such as "the psychology of the fully
evolved and authentic self."[7] In addition, psychotherapeutic
practice, both within and without the psychoanalytical schools,
found itself confronted with the task posed by Kierkegaard—
namely, helping patients discover their real self.[8]

The other change that made the new relevance of Kierkegaard
evident is the revolutionizing of our ideas on psychic normality
and anomaly. These opposites seem to have lost their sharpness
of contrast. On the one hand, what was previously considered
"normal" is now suspected of being a "psychopathology of the
average."[9] On the other hand, people are seeing even in serious
psychoses a corrective for our usual understanding of our self
and our world: for Foucault madness is merely the price the
modern age has to pay for its reason,[10] and Laing hears such

4. Rollo May, *The Meaning of Anxiety* (New York: Ronald Press, 1950), p. 17; O.
H. Mowrer, *Learning Theory and Personality Dynamics* (New York: Ronald Press,
1950), pp. 534, 541.

5. H. Hartmann, "Psychoanalysis as a Scientific Theory," in S. Hook, ed.,
Psychoanalysis, Scientific Method, and Philosophy (New York: New York University
Press, 1959), p. 14.

6. Cf. Rollo May, E. Angel, and H. F. Ellenberger, eds., *Existence: A New Dimension in Psychiatry and Psychology* (New York: Basic Books, 1958); Rollo May, ed.,
Existential Psychology (New York: Random House, 1961).

7. A. H. Maslow, "Existential Psychology—What's in It for Us?," in R. May, ed.,
Existential Psychology, 2d ed. (New York: Random House, 1969), p. 57.

8. Cf. particularly C. F. Rogers, *On Becoming a Person: A Therapist's View of
Psychotherapy* (Boston: Houghton Mifflin, 1961), pp. 108, 110, 166. Rogers calls
Kierkegaard "a sensitive and highly perceptive friend" and thanks him for "deep
insights and convictions which beautifully express views I have held but never
been able to formulate."

9. Maslow, "Existential Psychology," p. 57.

10. M. Foucault, *Histoire de la Folie* (Paris: Librairie Plon, 1961).

"truth" from the lips of a schizophrenic as would ordinarily be doomed to silence.[11] In any event the opinion has been severely shaken that normal social behavior is a sure guide for "a certain standard way of being human to which the psychotic cannot measure up."[12] The practice of stereotyping neurosis as a mere deviation from normality has become particularly dubious.[13] Even those who adhere in principle to nosological differentiation have as a rule a propensity for comparative studies that take "normal" behavior into consideration in critical testing.[14] In such a situation Kierkegaard must necessarily attract the attention of the experts. For in the first place he is greatly concerned with the "sickness" of man; second, he ascribes a "universality" to this sickness, under the conditions of which "health" is a rare exception;[15] and third, he is thus in a position to locate clinical illnesses in the context of a preclinical deficiency in human life.[16] Thus an effort has been made to bring Kierkegaard to fruition for the discussion of this problem area. The wish to bring him up to date has even induced some to read into his work the concepts *neurosis* and *psychosis*, which he, of course, did not know.[17]

11. R. D. Laing, *The Divided Self* (New York: Pantheon Books, 1969), p. 28.

12. Ibid., p. 27.

13. Cf., for example, R. May, "Existential Bases of Psychotherapy," in May, *Existential Psychology* (1961), p. 75: "Neurosis is not to be seen as a deviation from our particular theories of what a person should be."

14. I should particularly like to point out E. Jacobson, *Depression: Comparative Studies of Normal, Neurotic, and Psychotic Conditions* (New York: International Universities Press, 1971).

15. S. Kierkegaard, *The Sickness unto Death*, Samlede Vaerker, 2d. ed., ed. A. B. Crachmann, J. L. Heiberg, and H. O. Lange (Copenhagen: Gyldendal, 1920 ff.), 11: 153-59. The page numbers given in the body of the text of the essay refer to this edition. Vol. 4 refers to *The Concept of Dread* and vol. 7 to *Concluding Unscientific Postscript*.

16. Cf. especially the section, "The somatic-psychic loss of freedom" in *The Concept of Dread* (4: 445-47); and on this point May, *The Meaning of Anxiety*, p. 42.

17. Cf. May, *The Meaning of Anxiety*, pp. 33, 38, 40. Whether a condition is to be designated normal or neurotic in the Kierkegaardian sense depends, according to May, upon the individual's ability to master his conflicts. May orients himself thus on the neurosis concept of Karen Horney, who herself defines the difference in degree between normal and neurotic conflicts by means of a Kierkegaardian distinction (i.e., conscious and unconscious despair). K. Horney, *Our Inner Conflicts: A Constructive Theory of Neurosis* (London: Routledge & Kegan Paul, 1946),

In accordance with both these concentrations of interest, those works of Kierkegaard that develop the concept of "self" (or "spirit") and simultaneously investigate deficient forms of human life have received the greatest attention from psychology, psychiatry, and psychoanalysis: primarily *The Concept of Dread* (1844), *The Sickness unto Death* (1849), and the second volume of *Either/Or* (1843). Attention thus centers on the phenomena of melancholy[18] (described particularly in the 1844 work), anxiety,[19] and despair—which Kierkegaard, in allusion to John 11:4, interprets as "sickness unto death." In the following I should like to illustrate my thesis in respect to the relation between despair and self in the work of 1849.[20] In these introductory remarks I shall therefore more extensively go into only such attempts as have been made to relate Kierkegaard's concept of despair to psychic illnesses.

Before Kierkegaard begins his presentation in *The Sickness unto Death* he sums up his whole theory in a kind of heading: "Despair is a Sickness in the Spirit, in the Self, and So It May Assume a Triple Form: in Despair at Not Being Conscious of Having a Self (Despair Improperly So Called); in Despair at Not Willing to be Oneself; in Despair at Willing to be Oneself." This titlelike sen-

---

pp. 31–32. At the same time, nevertheless, Horney refers to the sentence in *The Sickness unto Death*, "Real life is far too multifarious to be portrayed by merely exhibiting such abstract contrasts as that between a despair which is completely unconscious, and one which is completely conscious" (p. 181). Mowrer's assertion that according to Kierkegaard a leap leads "from normality to neurosis" is completely ungrounded (*Learning Theory and Personality Dynamics*, p. 539). This assertion is based on the unjustified identification of these concepts with the concepts of "objective dread" and "subjective dread."

18. H. Tellenbach, *Melancholie*, 2d ed. (Berlin/Heidelberg/New York: Springer, 1974), pp. 128–29.

19. Mowrer, *Learning Theory and Personality Dynamics*, pp. 531–61, particularly pp. 540–46; May, *The Meaning of Anxiety*, pp. 32–45, and further, May's contributions to the anthology edited by himself and others, *Existence:* "The Origins and Significance of the Existential Movement in Psychology" and "Contributions of Existential Psychotherapy."

20. Kierkegaard transferred this book to his pseudonym Anti-Climacus. Since it belongs to the so-called "ungenuinely pseudonymical works" (E. Hirsch, *Die Krankheit zum Tode* [Dusseldorf: 1954], p. x), it is permissible to speak of Kierkegaard as being the author. I shall do so here for reasons of clarity.

tence in its entirety can be taken as a starting point for the understanding of psychic illnesses if one chooses Kierkegaard's concept
of despair as a basis for such understanding; one accepts his translation of "despair" into "not being oneself" and endows the latter
with a structure according to the above scheme. F. A. Weiss reproduces this scheme with the greatest precision: he explicates
"self-alienation" as "self-anaesthesia," "self-elimination," and
"self-idealization," respectively.[21] The scheme is wholly or partially applied to all psychic illnesses, wherever they are understood in terms of despair in a Kierkegaardian sense.

Karen Horney has attempted this for neurosis. Here the kind
of despair that Kierkegaard described as desperately wanting to
be oneself—that is, as striving for a merely "hypothetical" or
"abstract" self, plays a prominent role. It appears in Horney's
theory as the despair of the person who creates "an idealized
image of himself" by compounding parts of his real self with
fictitious elements.[22] However, under the heading "hopelessness"[23] she actually treats all three types of despair discerned by
Kierkegaard, laying particular emphasis on unconscious and
half-conscious despair, whose subject does not know he despairs
over himself because he is distracted by something external. Finally, she applies the Kierkegaardian scheme in a somewhat different form when she derives the various types of neurosis also
from the failure of the "synthesis," with which Kierkegaard, as we
shall see, identifies being human: namely, either from claiming
"possibility" as absolutely real, which we may refer to Kierkegaard's "desperately wanting to be oneself," or from laying
similar claim to "necessity," which corresponds to Kierkegaard's
"desperately not wanting to be oneself."[24]

21. F. A. Weiss, "Self-Alienation: Dynamics and Therapy," in J. L. Rubins, ed.,
Developments in Horney Psychoanalysis (Huntington, N.Y.: Robert E. Krieger, 1972),
p. 214.

22. Horney, *Our Inner Conflicts*, pp. 16–17, 110–12.

23. Ibid., pp. 179–90; cf. K. Horney, *The Neurotic Personality of Our Time* (London: Routledge & Kegan Paul, 1937), p. 227: "I do not believe that one can
understand any severe neurosis without recognizing the paralyzing hopelessness
which it contains."

24. Cf. thereto particularly K. Horney, *Neurosis and Human Growth: The Struggle
Toward Self-Realization* (London: Routledge & Kegan Paul, 1951), p. 35.

In the field of the psychoses, depression or melancholia as well as schizophrenia have been examined from the perspective of despair as analyzed by Kierkegaard. Tellenbach describes the "melancholic-psychotic initial situation" as despair—that is, the beginning of the clinical melancholic phase, into which the pre-melancholic may lead.[25] Tellenbach treats not being oneself, which Kierkegaard conceives as despair, under "remanence" (*Remanenz*), with which he means a lagging behind oneself, and "includence" (*Inkludenz*), being shut up within oneself, respectively.

Laing declares with the same conviction, "Schizophrenia cannot be understood without understanding despair."[26] It is precisely the despair investigated in *The Sickness unto Death* that Laing brings in to enhance understanding first of the schizoid and then of the schizophrenic—"a disruption of his relation with himself."[27] On the basis of this "disrelationship," as Kierkegaard would say, Laing works out primarily his "false-self system," which, like Kierkegaard's "abstract self," is merely "an amalgam of various part-selves."[28] Shirley Sugerman, who traces this and other common elements back to Laing's making explicit the meaning of Kierkegaard's concept of sin through his own concept of madness, applies both of their analyses on her part to narcissism, which is certainly fertile ground for schizophrenic illness, by interpreting narcissism as desperate "self-destruction."[29]

Another concept that can be mentioned in connection with research into schizophrenia is Leslie H. Farber's "therapeutic despair," a despair that, in his personal experience, overtakes the therapist himself during psychotherapy with schizophrenics.

25. Tellenbach, *Melancholie*, pp. 143–47.

26. Laing, *The Divided Self*, p. 39.

27. Ibid., p. 15. Cf. also L. Binswanger, "The Case of Ellen West," in May et al., *Existence: A New Dimension in Psychiatry and Psychology*. On this: H. M. Ruitenbeek, "Some Aspects of the Encounter of Psychoanalysis and Existential Philosophy," in H. M. Ruitenbeek, ed., *Psychoanalysis and Existential Philosophy* (New York: E. P. Dutton, 1962), pp. xxii–iii.

28. Laing, *The Divided Self*, p. 76.

29. S. Sugerman, *Sin and Madness: Studies in Narcissism* (Philadelphia: Westminister Press, 1976).

This despair is "therapeutic" not only in referring to the therapy but in itself as well: if it evokes sympathy and thus a healthy impulse in the patient, it also becomes a "remedy," which Kierkegaard, too, saw in despair.[30]

2. THE THESIS

The adoption by some psychiatric and psychoanalytic literature of the equation of despair with not being oneself gives us ample cause to investigate the relationship between self and despair in *The Sickness unto Death*. The result of the investigation I should like to conduct in the following will show that Kierkegaard does not make his idea of the self the presupposition of his theory of despair, but rather uses despair, in a certain sense, as his point of departure and allows it to dictate what self is. Obviously, the verification of this thesis would not be without relevance to both of the problem areas sketched at the beginning, through the discussion of which the sciences of the psyche, particularly of the sick psyche, have today become so receptive to Kierkegaard, or ought indeed to have become so. On the one hand we may assume that in a situation where the antithesis between normality and anomaly has lost its self-evidence Kierkegaard is not only significant for the three aforementioned reasons but also because he above all principally avoids raising any preconceived idea of health to a norm in order to judge sickness as an anomaly but rather develops from the idea of being sick an idea of being healthy. On the other hand, for this very reason it would no longer be legitimate to demand from Kierkegaard a philosophy and psychology of the self without any reservations. At any rate it would no longer be possible to consider his thinking an example and a model of a

---

30. L. H. Farber, "The Therapeutic Despair," in *The Ways of the Will: Essays Toward a Psychology and Psychopathology of Will* (New York: Basic Books, 1966). Farber admits in the preface of his book to having "an affection for the writings of Sören Kierkegaard." See in the same volume, "Despair and the Life of Suicide," where Farber shows in "a brief account of the landscape of despair" that despair is both "destroying and renewing" (p. 83); and the beginning of the essay, "Schizophrenia and the Mad Psychotherapist" (p. 184). Concerning "suicidal tendencies" of despair and hopelessness, cf. also Horney, *Our Inner Conflicts*, p. 188.

theory that builds on the self as if it were an empirically evident fact. While he would indeed remain a powerful aid to orientation in the reflection on the self, he could nevertheless at the same time be called to account by those who warn against careless use of the concept of *self* and doubt the suitability of basing a philosophical and psychological doctrine of man upon it.[31]

Before endeavoring to support my thesis, I should like to clarify it somewhat and also to formulate more explicitly the principles upon which it is based. Kierkegaard terms the sickness of despair a "negativity" (p. 176). Not in the same sense but nevertheless in an analogous one, anxiety and melancholy are also considered to be such negativities, for each of these phenomena points to conditions under which the person is not yet or no longer that which he should be. To the extent that they occupy the foreground in Kierkegaard's thought, we may characterize it as "negativism." It is of no matter that this word designates in the vocabulary of psychiatry an illness or a symptom. For Kierkegaard, standing "beside the sickbed," as he writes in the preface to the work of 1849, and thus speaking *about* a sick person *to* a sick person, also knows he is diagnosing sickness *as* a sick person. Seen more closely, his negativism has both a contentual or material aspect and a methodical or formal aspect. Contentual negativism refers simply to the fact that despair is ordinarily understood as a

31. For philosophy cf., for example, B. Mayo, *The Logic of Personality* (London: Jonathan Cape, 1952); H. W. Johnstone, Jr., *The Problem of the Self* (University Park: Pennsylvania State University Press, 1970). Johnstone subscribes essentially to Mayo's linguistically supported critique of the concept *self,* but nevertheless advisedly chooses as a motto for the chapter in which he discusses this critique the first sentences of *The Sickness unto Death.* In psychology, Allport draws constructive conclusions from his somewhat skeptical view of the tendencies that have led to "a revival of the self-concept." G. W. Allport, *Becoming: Basic Considerations for a Psychology of Personality* (New Haven: Yale University Press, 1955), pp. 38–39. In addition, some of the psychiatrists and psychotherapists oriented toward Kierkegaard retain a critical distance from the self concept (cf. Laing, *The Divided Self,* p. 17; May, "The Emergence of Existential Psychology," in *Existential Psychology,* pp. 34–35). See also R. Schafer, *Aspects of Internalization* (New York: International Universities Press, 1968), p. 27; H. Loewald, review of *The Analysis of the Self, Psychoanalytic Quarterly* 42 (1973): 441–51.

negative. Methodological negativism refers to Kierkegaard's method of learning from the sick self what a healthy self is. We shall soon see that on still closer analysis we must distinguish two different aspects of his contentual negativism.

For the present I am limiting myself to Kierkegaard's orientation on phenomena in which this "negativity," in the sense of a deficiency in human life, manifests itself. My thesis focuses on the methodical as opposed to the contentual aspect of negativism; it maintains that Kierkegaard also begins with the "negative" phenomena, on which he orients himself in order to reveal successful human existence through them. According to *The Sickness unto Death,* successful human existence, being oneself, is health, which can be achieved only through "faith." Anti-Climacus, the pseudonymous author of this work, "merely describes the sickness, defining at the same time little by little what *faith* is" (*Papirer* X 5 B 23).[32] He describes *merely* the sickness and *at the same time* defines faith. Instead of beginning with faith and then proceeding to its opposite—to despair conceived as sin—he confronts himself *directly* with despair alone in such a way as to define faith only *through* the analysis of its negation.

The quotation demonstrates that at least the author of *The Sickness unto Death* consciously adheres to his negativistic method. The question must remain open here to what extent Kierkegaard is also reflecting in his other writings what he actually does. One may be sure only that this negativism objectively ensues from his appraisal of man's historical situation. Kierkegaard, one of the greatest critics of his time, came to the conclusion that genuinely being human has practically disappeared in "Christendom" and that we today hardly know what it is to be human, let alone Christian. It is this real distortion of modern man that forces Kierkegaard to part company with a naive normative psychology. Because the so-called anomalies themselves have practically become the norm, he finds it necessary to begin with them and from them

32. I quote the *Papirer* of Kierkegaard according to the edition of P. A. Heiberg and V. Kuhr (Copenhagen: Gyldenal, 1909 ff.). The roman numeral (and occasionally the first arabic number as well) refers to the volume number, the letter to the section, and the arabic number at the end to the number of the entry.

to gain access to that which once was the sure standard against which they were judged.

II. Corroboration of the Thesis by the Beginning of The Sickness unto Death

Nothing would seem to disprove this thesis more drastically than the fact that *The Sickness unto Death* begins with statements concerning man and his self. Yet there is no other text in all of Kierkegaard's writing that is more important for our subject than the exposition of this work on despair. For here his view of human existence and thus basically his whole thought attains to its conclusive and consummate expression. What he says here may be considered as valid for his other works, too—that is, for the pseudonymous writings as well as for the "edifying" discourses. Kierkegaard himself was of the opinion that he had developed "a splendid scheme" at the beginning of *The Sickness unto Death*, which he could apply in spite of its high level of abstraction in "discourses" as well (*Papirer* VIII A 651). Therefore, we shall in the following put the anticipated thesis to the test on this text. Whereas the numerous extant interpretations devote themselves exclusively to questions of content, completely neglecting the methodic structure of the text, I should like to restrict myself in the framework of this essay to the methodical aspect of negativism.[33]

33. Among the interpretations given up to now, the following are particularly noteworthy: R. Guardini, "Der Ausgangspunkt der Denkbewegung Sören Kierkegaards," *Hochland* 24 (1927): 12–33; H. Fahrenbach, *Kierkegaards existenzdialektische Ethik* (Frankfurt: Vittorio Klostermann, 1968); J. Holl, *Kierkegaards Konzeption des Selbst. Eine Untersuchung über die Voraussetzungen und Formen seines Denkens* (Meisenheim: Anton Hain, 1972). I, too, have already analyzed the text several times, albeit also nearly always from contentual viewpoints: "Sören Kierkegaard," in M. Landmann, ed., *De Homine* (Freiburg/Munich: Karl Alber, 1962); "῍Ο αἰτῶν λαμβάνει," in *Jesus—Ort der Erfahrung Gottes* (Freiburg: Herder, 1976); M. Theunissen and W. Greve, eds., *Materialien zur Philosophie Søren Kierkegaards* (Frankfurt: Suhrkamp, 1979), pp. 67 ff. This anthology also contains a reprint of my aforementioned essay of 1962, under the title "Das Menschenbild in der 'Krankheit zum Tode.'" In the following I refer to various theses contained in these writings.

I shall first reproduce here in its entirety the text relevant to our purposes, dividing it into sections from whose connection, according to my thesis, it is possible to read the methodic structure of the whole.

[I] Man is spirit. But what is spirit? Spirit is the self. But what is the self? The self is a relation which relates itself to its own self, or it is that in the relation [which accounts for it] that the relation relates itself to its own self; the self is not the relation but [consists in the fact] that the relation relates itself to its own self. [2] Man is a synthesis of the infinite and the finite, of the temporal and the eternal, of freedom and necessity, in short it is a synthesis. A synthesis is a relation between two factors. So regarded, man is not yet a self. [1]

In the relation between two, the relation is the third term as a negative unity, and the two relate themselves to the relation, and in the relation to the relation; such a relation is that between soul and body, when man is regarded as soul. If on the contrary the relation relates itself to its own self, the relation is then the positive third term, and this is the self.

Such a relation which relates itself to its own self (that is to say, a self) must either have constituted itself or have been constituted by another.

If this relation which relates itself to its own self is constituted by another, the relation doubtless is the third term, but this relation (the third term) is in turn a relation relating itself to that which constituted the whole relation.

Such a derived, constituted, relation is the human self, a relation which relates itself to its own self, and in relating itself to its own self relates itself to another. [3]

[II] Hence it is that there can be two forms of despair properly so called. If the human self had constituted itself, there could be a question only of one form, that of not willing to be one's own self, of willing to get rid of oneself, but there would be no question of despairingly willing to be oneself. This formula is the expression for the total dependence of the relation (the self namely), the expression for the fact that the self cannot of itself attain and remain in equilibrium and rest by itself, but only by relating itself to that Power which constituted the whole relation. [1] Indeed, so far is it from being true that this second form of despair (despair at willing to be one's own self) denotes only a particular kind of despair, that on the contrary all despair can in the last analysis be reduced to this. [2] [Translation: Walter Lowrie]

In this text two parts contrast sharply with one another. The first part—I have marked it [I]—outlines a particular anthropology,[34] the second [II] a concept of despair. The first contains essentially three points[35]: (1) Man is a synthetic relation of the infinite and the finite, of the temporal and the eternal, of freedom and necessity, but as such relation not yet a self. (2) Man only becomes a self when that relation relates to its own self. (3) His self is constituted by another, so that he can only be that which he is when he relates himself simultaneously to the Power that constituted the relation. Section II expresses primarily the following thoughts: (1) Despair "properly so called"—conscious despair—takes two and only two forms, namely, either the person wants desperately to be himself, or he wants desperately not to be himself. (2) The despair of not wanting to be oneself can be traced back to his desperately wanting to be himself. Kierkegaard supplements the second point in what follows (p. 151) by saying that desperately wanting to be oneself may conversely be reduced to desperately not wanting to be oneself. We ultimately have here the assertion that either form may be reduced to the other.

1. THE GENERAL CONNECTION BETWEEN SELF AND DESPAIR

1.1 Two possible interpretations. Clarifying the methodical structure of the text means rendering the connection between I and II

34. I use the concept *anthropology* here in the sense in which one speaks in Germany of "philosophical anthropology," but with this use I do not intend any prejudicial judgment in favor of the view that Kierkegaard pursues philosophy entirely "from the standpoint of anthropology" (L. Feuerbach). L. H. Farber (*The Ways of the Will*, pp. 156, 161) borrows this term from Martin Buber.

35. I reverse the sequence of 1 and 2 used in the text because the train of thought thus comes out better. This reversal has no essential significance.

evident. Two possibilities, which seem alternative, are available for the explication of this connection. One possibility is to regard it as a deductive connection.[36] In this case one would have to assume that Kierkegaard claims to derive both forms of despair and their mutual reducibility from the constitution of man and his self. One would then, however, be forced to conclude that Kierkegaard can in no way substantiate such a claim. Above all, one would have to reproach him for the dogmatic character of his three initial assertions (I.1-3). As they stand they are without any support whatsoever. Were they in themselves entirely evident, surely they would require no support; but they obviously are not. On the contrary: they appear to be fraught with metaphysical assumptions that carry no conviction.

If we are to take Kierkegaard seriously as a thinker, we have therefore no choice but to seize the other possibility. We must then proceed from the assumption that assertions I. 1-3, in keeping with a distinction made by Marx,[37] represent only the beginning in the *presentation*, not in the *investigation*—that is, the foregoing revelation of the material; primary in order of knowledge would be rather the idea of despair outlined by assertions II. 1-2, reached through immersion in the phenomenon itself.

Were this the case, the three statements at the beginning about man and his self would assume the function of indicating the conditions under which despair is possible. To actually assign such a function to them would be quite desirable, since under this presupposition one would no longer need to take offense at their apodictic form. Their form may confidently be regarded as external as soon as one presupposes that the assertions answer the question, how must man be constituted and how is his self to be conceived for the despair he experiences as his actuality to be

36. Thus B. Meerpohl, *Die Verzweiflung als metaphysisches Phänomen in der Philosophie Sören Kierkegaards* (Wurzburg: C. J. Becker, 1934), p. 44.

37. K. Marx, *Das Kapital.* Karl Marx/Friedrich Engels, *Werke* (Berlin: Dietz, 1971), vol. 23, p. 27: "Of course, the mode of presentation must differ formally from the mode of investigation. One's research must adopt its subject matter in detail, analyze its various forms of development and discover the relations entertained among them. Only when this work has been done can the true movement of the subject matter be appropriately presented."

possible? For, seen as answers to these questions, the initial assertions are conclusions anticipated in the presentation, gained re-
gressively by returning from the actuality of despair to the conditions themselves that render it possible.

1.2 An objection to the alternative chosen.   I should like to avert a
misunderstanding that might easily arise from this suggestion. In
no way do I intend to create the impression that Kierkegaard
considers what he describes as despair an empirical fact that he
need only record. While despair is indeed the material with which
he commences, it has nevertheless already been examined and
hence also interpreted; he does allow himself to be led by the
phenomenon, but he gleans from it an idea that already contains
the germ of his whole theory. If this were not so, his contentual
and methodical negativism would at the same time be positivism
in the usual sense. Such positivism, however, does not in the least
apply to the author of *The Sickness unto Death.* Anti-Climacus lays
no claim to uninterpreted description but only to "a fundamental
apprehension consistently carried through" (p. 153), whose consequences alone can be the validity of a theory.

Of course, the defense itself against the positivistic misunderstanding provokes an objection to my suggestion. Kierkegaard not only begins with a *theory* of despair but also introduces a theory that interprets despair in the context of *self.* He
obviously believes he can divide despair "properly so called" into
desperately wanting to be oneself and desperately not wanting to
be oneself only because he presupposes the self as the standard of
judgment here. In the same way the self provides him with the
criteria according to which he measures despair "improperly so
called." In the passage preceding sections I. 1–3 and II. 1–2,
which summarizes the germ of the theory in a kind of heading,
Kierkegaard more closely defines all despair, that properly so
called as well as that improperly so called, through *negation* of the
self. Only this negation holds together "proper" and "improper"
despair, which are otherwise separated by an abyss; and it similarly provides the link between the two forms of the former: even
as desperately wanting to be oneself is also desperately not want-

ing to be oneself, inasmuch as the self, which the person desperately wants to be, "is a self, which he is not" (p. 151). In view of this, however, the idea that Kierkegaard derives the self from despair seems untenable. He rather appears to have proceeded the other way round, as all philosophy before his had done, and inferred despair from the self. Indeed, in light of his procedure of so determining despair from the self that he determines it by the self's negation, the "negativity" as ascribed to the self appears to be the merely formal negativity common to all that is known *ex negativo* in the order of knowledge. It would therefore seem as if his point of departure were not merely the self but even an in itself positive self whose positivity precedes all negativity.

So much of the objection based on Kierkegaard's interpretation of despair with help of the concept *self* is correct that the second possible interpretation, for whose choice I plead, does not entirely exclude the first. I was aiming at this when I said the two possibilities only seem to be alternatives. Just as Kierkegaard views the self from the vantage point of despair, so he surely also conversely view despair from the perspective of the self. Not only does he do this, but he knows full well that he does so. Just as a doctor must be conversant with the health of the body and the soul in order to diagnose a somatic or a psychic illness as such, so despair can only be understood as a "sickness in the spirit" if one has a notion of "what spirit is," as Kierkegaard expressly remarks (p. 154).

Notwithstanding, we must come to a decision here, and that is the decision for negativism. Although one must concede that despair and the self are interdependent in Kierkegaard's epistemological thought, the choice we have made remains essentially unaffected by the objection. Above all, there are two arguments that speak in favor of upholding the choice. One rests on the specific structure of the interdependence relation, the other on the status Kierkegaard accords to the self. The first substantiates our negativism thesis at least within the bounds to which it is confined following our admission of interdependence; the second makes it clear that the thesis retains its full validity within its limitations and must be even more forcefully asserted.

The first indispensable step is the recognition that the path leading from the self to despair and from despair back to the self is not the usual circle, unless, if one likes, perhaps the "hermeneutic" (as articulated by Heidegger and by Ricoeur). For the self at the point of departure lacks the determination of the self in which the movement culminates. At the outset Kierkegaard propounds but a preliminary concept, which must yet be proved with respect to the material of despair and reaches its final form only through this material. Such a method is indebted to the Hegelian dialectic. It was, however, the antidialectician Heidegger who endowed this method with the form in which it has attained its widest dissemination. In *Sein und Zeit* (*Being and Time*) (1927) Heidegger takes three steps, both on the large and the small scale in his work, namely: the sketch of a preliminary concept, the "phenomenal diagnosis," and the concluding ontological interpretation, which by virtue of the meanings acquired through the phenomenon relieves the preliminary concept of its tentative nature. This procedure, however, is closely related to that chosen by Marx and, according to our thesis here, is also applied by Kierkegaard—namely, making the result of one's investigation the beginning of the presentation. Because of their common origin in Hegel,[38] both of their methods belong together. Of course, the reminder of the method taken over from Heidegger would be useless if the unity did not also entail a difference. Both their methods are essentially one and for that reason actually unifiable, insofar as the sketching of a preliminary concept can be the still vague anticipation of the investigation's result in the presentation. If one reconstructs the first step of existential ontology with respect to the dialectic of presentation, one only draws particular attention to the fact that the preliminary concept, even before its examination, has already been gleaned from that very material against which it is supposed to be tested. Compared with this, the new element added to the dialectic method of presentation by that

38. My thesis can be further articulated with the help of a distinction drawn by Hegel: whereas the definition of man and his self given in I is "first [*das Erste*] in the course of thought," yet it is not "the earlier [*das Prius*] for thinking." G. W. F. Hegel, *Wissenschaft der Logik*, ed. G. Lasson (Leipzig: Felix Meiner, 1951), 1: 52.

inherited from existential ontology lies in taking into consideration that the material used to verify the preliminary concept is no independent authority but instead one that itself has been structured by the former. If we wish to salvage our negativism thesis, we must demonstrate that for Kierkegaard the preliminary concept is indebted to the material evidence in a more elementary way than is this material to the preliminary concept.

The demonstration will be completely successful only in recourse to the status Kierkegaard ascribes to the self. At this point we can but pave the way for it. We need first to establish that Kierkegaard applies the procedure I have described in referring to *Sein und Zeit* both in his dialectic of presentation and in itself. The titlelike heading does not belong to the presentation. Accordingly, Kierkegaard here outlines a preliminary concept not yet conceived in terms of the presentation's dialectic, the phenomenological demonstration of which occupies the whole following inquiry. As opposed to the heading—and this is at any rate my position—section I outlines a preliminary concept that anticipates the result of the investigation in the presentation. The text in its entirety, which I have subdivided into I and II, relates in such a way to the heading that it expresses verbally what happens, as gleanings from the material, even prior to the preliminary concept's sketch.

Now there is a striking difference in the proof of the preliminary concept between the nondialectical and the dialectical procedure. The former represents in Kierkegaard and in Heidegger, too, a mere filling in of the structure introduced at the beginning, no restructuring; the latter, however, as we shall observe, changes the structure of the preliminary concept. Here we see the predominance of the material element. The methodical difference, however, is associated with one of content. In the first case the material element is despair and the preliminary concept is the sickness in the self, the latter being the meaning Kierkegaard assigns to despair. The phenomenological check of the preliminary concept here consists in Kierkegaard's detailed description of how the self becomes ill in despair. The description is only a concretizing, since the examination nowhere breaks through the bounds set it by the preliminary concept of despair as sickness in the self. In the second case, Kierkegaard sketches a preliminary concept of the healthy self, while its sickness is the material. The predominance of the material, to which the qualitative change of the preliminary concept seems to point, shows, therefore, that within the dialectical circuit to which *The Sickness unto Death* solders the healthy self and its sickness together, the sickness or the material negativity possesses a gnoseological preponderance. That Kierkegaard conceives the self from the aspect of despair, as I said, means more precisely this: he conceives the healthy self from its sickness. The interpretation implied therein of despair as sickness in the self implies in turn a prior understanding of the self and its health—that is, of its proper realization. Yet Kierkegaard must find out from the sick self what a healthy one is, because the latter in his view results only through being cured from the sickness. The whole inquiry rests on the premise, "There is no immediate health of the spirit" (p. 156).[39] Thus its method is predetermined: if spiritual health is not immediately given as a condition preceding the sickness, then it cannot be immediately apprehended but only ascertained from its opposite. While Kierkegaard indeed conceives the healthy self from sickness, he does not explain the sick self in the same way by *starting* with health, but rather by *aiming* at health.

The status of the self anticipated in the presentation confers complete conviction to these reflections. In retrospect Kierkegaard limits the scope of the presentation's beginning by emphasizing that the self anticipated here is only the "negative form of the self" (p. 204). This negative form does not in his view attach to any in itself positive self; it is rather negative because it is the form of an in itself "negative self" (p. 203). As we shall see, Kierkegaard describes the self at the beginning as reflection or, more precisely, as infinite reflection, in keeping with the fact that he also characterizes the aforementioned form as "infinite"

39. This concept of health is diametrically opposed to that which Maslow has taken as the basis of his empirical investigations. A. H. Maslow, "Self-actualizing People: A Study of Psychological Health," in C. E. Moustakas, ed., *The Self: Explorations in Personal Growth* (New York: Harper, 1956).

(p. 203). He calls this reflection "the reflection of nothing" (p. 157), that is, a reflection that itself is nothing. Hence from the fact that he defines despair through negation of the self, its positivity in no way follows for him. The status he ascribes to the self even allows us to strengthen our negativism thesis, for there thus accrues a further aspect to the negativistic approach we have already observed. We have certainly already contrasted the contentual from the methodical side of this negativism in the preceding. However, it seemed up to now as if only Kierkegaard's orientation on the "negativity" that characterizes such phenomena as anxiety, melancholy, and despair fell on the contentual side. Now we are discovering that in *The Sickness unto Death* we are dealing with a negativism of content insofar as Kierkegaard invests the self, too, with negativity. The self's negativity pertains to the content as the determination of the form in which alone it can be anticipated in the presentation.

To be sure, in all of this, "negative" is as yet an empty word. It could only be filled with meaning if we were, first, to set forth Hegel's negation theory and, secondly, to show how Kierkegaard appropriates the theory and transforms it at the same time. For *The Sickness unto Death,* by its expression of the negativity of the self, picks up the thread of Hegel's *Wissenschaft der Logik (Science of Logic).* The assurance that the reflection identical with the self is that of nothing reproduces the definition given there: reflection is "the movement from nothing to nothing and from there back to itself."[40] We should also have to turn to Hegel's logic to answer the question why, according to section I, the two terms of the synthetic relation are joined together in a "negative unity," and in what sense the self, on the other hand, represents "the positive third term," and how this positivity is compatible with the negativity also maintained. A merely doxographical answer is easy: the positivity of the positive third term is but Hegel's "absolute negativity," which arises from the reflection of the negative (of the "negative unity"). It would, however, be difficult to render these matters more tangible. And it would cause yet greater diffi-

---

40. Hegel, *Wissenschaft der Logik*, 2: 13.

culties to present Hegel's thought in such a way that one could follow through on how Kierkegaard uses speculative negation theory to grasp the healthy self by means of a diagnosis of its illness. Such a reconstruction of the path leading from Hegel to Kierkegaard would burst the confines of this essay. For this reason suffice it to show here with respect to the issue raised by Kierkegaard that by employing the means made available by speculative negation theory he serves his purpose—namely, to establish his negativistic method on a stable foundation. In order to do this, however, one must anticipate the interpretation of the text.

In Hegel, "absolute negativity" means an activity that through reflection becomes pure activity—that is, a process that rests without substratum within itself. We also shall encounter the self at the beginning of *The Sickness unto Death* as such a process. However, we shall also note that Kierkegaard perceives this process from the point of view of despair; he interprets the self as pure process, as constant annihilation of the possibility of despair. How Hegel arrives at his interpretation of all activity as negation does not admit of completely rational explanation. However, Kierkegaard's designating the particular activity of the self as negation appears completely reasonable. For this is the activity we commonly understand as negation: a no-saying, ordinarily tacit. It consists in a person's saying "no" at every moment to the despair mounting within him. This thought presupposes that the self not be considered as any different from the act of being oneself. Yet this presupposition itself follows conclusively from the negativity of the self. As negative in the sense described, the self cannot be a substance underlying its own realization. The necessity of resolving self into being oneself, which Kierkegaard further resolves into an incessant becoming oneself, is also the reason he does not first describe the self per se and then separately the healthy self. Where he speaks of self at the beginning he already has in truth the healthy self in mind, for only when realized is the self what it is. If, however, the self is only healthy in resisting the danger of despair, then it must be understood in terms of the sickness, through combating which it attains health.

2. THE SPECIAL CONNECTION BETWEEN THE
STATEMENTS MADE AT THE BEGINNING ABOUT THE
SELF (I.1–3) AND THOSE CONCERNING DESPAIR (II.1–2)

2.1 Provisional determination of the relation of I.3 to II: the constitution of the human self by God. In order to disarm the objection that may be made against the interpretation proposed here, I have jumped ahead considerably. To the extent that the arguments brought forward against the objection make use of conclusions the reader cannot yet evaluate, they do not justify the acceptance of the proposal. The proposal is actually to be tested against the text I have chosen as a paradigm. Still open to discussion is the methodical relationship between the two main segments into which the text is divided. I have rejected the possibility that Kierkegaard would like to have the relation understood as a deductive one and instead have chosen the other possibility—that he presents in I what must be accepted to clarify II.

In examining more closely the individual statements contained in I and II, it is appropriate to approach first those statements that Kierkegaard himself brings into connection. He obviously associates the statement that the human self has been constituted by another (I.3) with the assertion that (conscious) despair is either desperately not willing to be oneself or desperately willing to be oneself (II.1). Yet he connects I.3 with II.1 in a way that allows interpretation in a sense congenial to our thesis concerning his negativistic method. The first sentence of II ("Hence it is that there can be two forms of despair properly so called") seems to express the conviction that the constitution of the self by another formulated in I.3 is a hypothesis necessary to understanding the duality in the forms of conscious despair. This supposition is confirmed by the form of presentation of I.3. It is consistent with the apparently purely assertive style of the text that Kierkegaard in I.3, as has often been observed,[41] while mentioning the alternative of the self's having constituted itself or having been constituted by another, tacitly ignores the former in what follows. The

---

41. Guardini, loc. cit.; Meerpohl, op. cit., pp. 51–52; H. Fahrenbach, *Kierkegaard's existenzdialektische Ethik*, p. 31.

simplest explanation for this is offered by the proposed reading: of the two forms of despair, at least desperately willing to be oneself would be incomprehensible in the event the self had constituted itself.

What appears plausible in view of the form of I.3 can be made conclusive by looking at the content of this thesis. Section A in *The Sickness unto Death*, from which the text to be explicated here has been taken,[42] closes with "the formula which describes the condition of the self when despair is completely eradicated: by relating itself to its own self and by willing to be itself the self is grounded transparently in the Power which constituted it" (p. 145). Originally "in God" stood behind this text (*Papirer* VIII B 170, 2). If Kierkegaard decided to eliminate the reference to God and to rest content with the characterization of the constituting through the neutral terms "another" and "the power," then it was not because he wished to deny any of his theological premises. He by no means qualifies the final version of the beginning as anthropology prefixed to the theological result, in itself free of Christian elements. The thoroughly dialectical character of *The Sickness unto Death* prohibits us from understanding the exposition of the book as basic anthropology free from theology. What we can observe in the introductory passage shows in the general outline as well: in accordance with the presentational principle of dialectical thought, the beginning is the anticipated end and already contains in germ what its continuation renders explicit. It therefore presupposes even the second part of the book, according to which "the Qualification 'Before God'" makes despair sin. But why does Kierkegaard suppress this qualification at the beginning? Why did he ultimately find it right *not* to address the self's constitution from the outset as constitution through God? I believe because he wanted to stress the difference between that which can already be known and that which must be merely accepted at first.

In light of this general account, the methodical relation between I.3 and II.1 becomes readily apparent. The point in II.1 is

42. Since my reflections refer exclusively to the first part of *The Sickness unto Death,* here and in the following I shall not expressly identify as parts thereof the sections marked by Kierkegaard with capital letters.

that despair also assumes the form of desperately willing to be oneself. In the further development of his thought Kierkegaard pursues this form of despair to the concept of defiance. In defiance he sees a revolt against God. The fact of such revolt, however, indicates in his view that the human self has not been merely constituted in general, but actually went forth from the hand of a god. Accordingly, the necessity of introducing the assumption of the self's constitution through God as a hypothesis that alone can adequately explain the circumstances of despair previously glimpsed also emanates from this view.

Thus, of course, Kierkegaard does not make the significance of this assumption *totally* dependent upon the analysis that follows. The self's having been constituted should already make sense per se at the beginning. However, its having been constituted *through God* can only be demonstrated with respect to the phenomenon of defiance, as required by the methodical precept. Here it is for Kierkegaard the personal quality of defiance that points to a personal God as constituting agent. The personal dimension, in which the passion of defiance calls attention to the living nature of Him against whom he rebels, does not appear in this conception as a third level, beneath that of having been constituted per se and that of such a constitution as in itself is clearly comprehensible as constitution through another in general. Accordingly, a person discovers that his self has been constituted by another only when he defiantly experiences himself as having been constituted by God. Kierkegaard's speaking of "another," a Power, is thus part of his anticipation of the not yet really knowable. Only having been constituted per se is a priori intelligible. In order to see in what way this nevertheless can be known at the beginning and not merely acknowledged, we must also bring out the relation between the first two theses of part I and the theses of part II. Only at the end can we return to the thesis in I.3

2.2 *The relation of I.1 to II: man as a synthesis of opposites.* The assertion that all three anthropological statements formulate the conditions that render despair possible should have been verified first on the basis of the proposition I.3, because this last determination of man and his self is the only one that the text expressly correlates with the exposition of the concept of despair. That this is the case reveals something significant about its relative importance. Of the three anthropological statements, this one is primary in respect to the matter at hand. As a result, the overlapping relation of I and II is repeated in its relation to I.1 and I.2. These earlier statements already presuppose the proposition that the self has been constituted and, indeed, in its full significance as the proposition that the human self has been constituted by God. It was thus not only meaningful to commence with I.3, but necessary.

   2.2.1 The opposites.   According to I.1, man is a relation of the temporal and the eternal (I.1.1), of the infinite and the finite (I.1.2), and of freedom and necessity (I.1.3), a relation that is to be understood as a synthesis. Later we shall have to ask in what sense man "is" such a synthesis. For the present, however, let us concentrate on the factors involved. If we do not take the theologically determined proposition of the self's having been constituted into account, the three respective pairs of factors in the synthesis are neither in themselves nor in their relation to one another adequately intelligible. With respect to their relation, we can observe a gradient as measured against the criterion of phenomenological demonstrability between the respective syntheses of freedom and necessity, of infinitude and finitude, and of the temporal and eternal. The assurance that man is a time-eternity synthesis is the least obvious. It appears to be a purely metaphysical doctrine that admits of no phenomenological demonstration. However, Kierkegaard takes the liberty of posing the concept of the eternal only because he is presupposing the concept of God, that is, the concept of the God Whom man in his despair experiences as absent.

   2.2.1.1   THE TEMPORAL AND THE ETERNAL.   I should first like to show how Kierkegaard in this way ultimately conceives I.1.1 from the standpoint of despair. The dependence of the whole statement in I.1 upon I.3 is but the beginning of its dependence upon II. For the former dependence means that the criterion by which I.1 becomes comprehensible is the full theological content of I.3. Consequently, it points beyond I.3 to the analysis of despair expounded in II. Only this analysis thus clarifies the meaning of speaking of a synthesis of the temporal and the eternal at the very beginning. It may at first look as if Kierkegaard neglected this version of the synthesis in the further development of the book. For in his analysis of the forms of despair according to the aspects of the synthesis he fails to dedicate a particular section to the relation of the eternal and the temporal, as opposed to "the aspects finitude/infinitude" and "the aspects possibility/necessity." However, he is able to proceed in precisely this manner because he *always* bears in mind man's belonging on the one hand to the temporal or "earthly" and on the other to the eternal. Evidence for this is that the time-eternity synthesis exercises a leading function from beginning to end in the analysis according to the degree of consciousness, which in *The Sickness unto Death* reveals first of all the truth about despair dissected according to the aspects of the synthesis. Kierkegaard conceives despair ultimately with respect to the eternal. This means, however, that he conversely conceives the eternal from the standpoint of despair. Support for this is the assertion, "We can demonstrate the eternal in man from the fact that despair cannot consume his self" (p. 151). That the despairer, as *The Sickness unto Death* teaches us, basically always despairs about the eternal means, however, that he no longer finds solace therein nor hopes for his salvation therefrom. To despair over the earthly means "to despair about the eternal, that is, not to let oneself be comforted and saved by the eternal, to ascribe such value to the earthly that the eternal can offer no comfort" (p. 205). *That* eternal, then, which Kierkegaard perceives from the standpoint of despair, is imbued with meaning through the Christian experience of God. We encounter it in the double viewpoint of salvation and reconciliation as the place of healing and the spring of consolation.

In spite of this I by no means wish to imply that Kierkegaard's interpretation of the eternal through despair succeeds completely without metaphysics. It cannot be denied that the eternal in his sense is *also* the *aei on* of Plato, the everlasting being through which the *kosmos noētos* is different from the *kosmos aisthētos*. As a matter of fact, I am of the opinion implied above that the idea of

man's being a synthesis of the temporal and eternal *at the beginning* can *only* have metaphysical import and thus removes itself
from the realm of phenomenological examination. Furthermore,
one will have to admit that the eternal also retains a Platonic sense.
Without it Kierkegaard would certainly have found no reason for
hoping to "prove" the indestructibility of the self through despair. The statement that man's despair cannot "consume his self"
is a sophisticated way of stating the simple fact that no despairer
who wants to get rid of himself can actually do so. He cannot
because he is and stays what and who he is. His not being able to
do so is, therefore, based on the impossibility of cancelling his
factual existence. Wanting to "prove" the eternal element in man
on the basis of his factual existence can only occur to the admirer
of Plato, because he has already hypostasized this existence under
the heading of self to an enduring substance. He thus presupposes the goal of his proof, in the form of everlasting being, which
provides the basis for Plato's reckoning the soul to the realm of
ideas.

Still, the Platonic concept of eternity agrees quite well with
Christian religious experience. Kierkegaard the Christian adjusts
the Platonic concept to this experience by considering it from the
standpoint of consolation, which can also be maintained from a
metaphysical perspective. An underground movement in Kierkegaard's thought comes to our attention here, which emerges
most clearly from the *Philosophical Fragments:* the evident opposition of Platonism and Christianity on the surface is itself made
possible by mediation on a deeper level, which is accomplished in
the *Fragments* by Climacus' developing exactly the alternative to
Plato (or, as he says, to Socrates)—namely, the paradoxical unity
of time and eternity, from the Platonic concept of eternity. Nevertheless, as in the *Fragments,* so likewise in *The Sickness unto Death,*
the Platonic beginning—continued here, too, like a *basso ostinato*
throughout—is counterbalanced by the context as a whole, which,
conceived through an interest in reconciliation and ultimately in
redemption, reduces it to a single aspect.

2.2.1.2 INFINITUDE AND FINITUDE, FREEDOM AND NECESSITY
We must distinguish between the confirmation of the passage at

the beginning, which occurs throughout the work, and its immanent logic. The certainty rooted in the latter gives the complementary propositions I.1.2 and I.1.3 precedence over the assertion
of man's affinity to the eternal. The two other syntheses, or
more appropriately, the two other modes of one and the same
synthesis, do not belong together for this reason alone. Kierkegaard makes their correlation clear by subsuming them under
the antithesis of *apeiron* and *peras*, the boundary and the bound-
lessness (p. 167). Of course, only in the case of freedom and
necessity is it at once clear what Kierkegaard has in mind. Let
us, therefore, turn first to this version of the synthesis. We will
notice immediately that there is also a great difference in the
degree of evidence possessed by I.1.2 and I.1.3, respectively.

Restricting the concept of freedom for good reasons to the self
that the person per se as yet is not, subsequent to having made I.1
more specific, Kierkegaard replaces it with the concept of possibility when he later returns to the aspects of the synthesis. This
operation discloses the structure of the relation described in I.1.3.
The necessity Kierkegaard means here characterizes man's being
with respect to his past; possibility marks it in the direction of his
individual future. Kierkegaard thinks thus what Heidegger's and
Sartre's existential ontology, as a result of his influence, conceives
as *Geworfenheit* and *Entwurf*, factual existence and transcendence.
As necessity and possibility, *peras* and *apeiron* must therefore be
construed as essentially temporal: man encounters his limit especially when his given existence and his life's history hem him in,
and he experiences himself as limitless chiefly in respect to his still
open future.

That man in this way leads a twofold existence is phenomenologically evident. Compared to this it may seem less compelling to concede to him an infinity beyond his finitude. Above
all, the infinitude ascribed to man in I.1.2. has no unequivocal
meaning. Kierkegaard speaks of it in two different senses. On
the one hand, both the concepts used in I.1.2. have merely the
status of predicates of necessity and possibility. The predicate of
finitude belongs to my actual existence, in and as which I always
find myself; correspondingly, to my still-open not-yet-being

infinitude is predicated—namely, the infinitude of possibilities that Kierkegaard, like Heidegger after him, unites in the single possibility of my own self-determination. On the other hand, he understands the synthesis of finitude and infinitude in such a way that a person by means of fantasy reflects himself out of the complete determination of his existence; here we encounter infinitude as an attribute of reflection and fantasy. Doubtless only in this meaning does it do justice to its concept. For it is understatement to call infinitude a predicate of possibility. Here infinitude is merely endlessness and as such does not even possess reality for the existing human being, for possibility is finitized by its bond with necessity. The "reflection of the process of infinitizing" ("*den uendeliggjørende Reflexion*") and fantasy as "the medium of the process of infinitizing" ("*det uendeliggjørendes Medium*") (p. 162) possess compared with this an infinitude that is not merely endlessness but indeed the character of the absolute ascribed by Hegel to reflection. Yet this reflection that fantasy renders productive is, strictly speaking, inappropriate to the person described here, who as a relation of finitude and infinitude "is not yet a self." Reflection *is* the self, or more precisely, the self in its "infinite form" (pp. 202 ff.).

Thus, we are confronted with a dilemma: to the extent that Kierkegaard is really talking about what he is ostensibly talking about, he is not really talking about infinity; and where he really means infinity, he does not stick to the subject of being oneself, in contradistinction to being a human being. Yet it is precisely his intention to draw this distinction, and in accordance with it we must assume that the synthesis of possibility and necessity provides the phenomenological foundation upon which the synthesis of infinitude and finitude rests, even if it does not allow for an authentic concept of the infinite. That means it is the first and most fundamental of all the syntheses involved. Indeed, Anti-Climacus presents it as such when he defines reality itself—and that means for him as well as for Climacus the reality of the human individual—as the "unity of possibility and necessity" (p. 168). That this unity provides the basis not only for the unity of finitude and infinitude but also for that of the temporal and the eternal, at least according to Kierkegaard's anthropological premises, results from its own temporal character. For Kierkegaard is of the opinion that time, if defined by one of its modes, is "past time" (IV, 393), while "the future is the incognito in which the eternal, although incommensurable with time, still wants to maintain its relations with time" (IV, 396).

We have established the priority of the unity of opposites represented by possibility and necessity before that represented by infinitude and finitude only in order to locate precisely the point at which the dependence of the *apeiron-peras* complex from the proposition that the self has been constituted becomes clear. This dependency strikes us first in connection with the concept of necessity, insofar as the use of this concept within the framework of I.1 cannot fully be justified. For it is indeed not in the least obvious that the factuality of existence, the state in which I always find myself as myself already existent, should be termed necessity. This could be obvious least of all for Kierkegaard, since in the Interlude to the *Fragments* he had torn open a gap between possibility and reality as the modalities of being on the one hand and necessity as expression of essence on the other, renewing the Platonic *chorismos,* so that he came to the conclusion that the future (the possible) in becoming the past (the real) in no way assumes the character of necessity. What Anti-Climacus calls "necessity" has in common with this quite different concept only that it, too, means immutability. The situation into which I was born, the decisions already made during the course of my life, are necessary to the extent that I can no longer change them.

However, they are only relatively immutable. Kierkegaard was profoundly convinced that repentance can transform at least the past history of an individual's life. The fact that he nevertheless calls this factual existence necessity has already been traced by Johannes Sløk to Kierkegaard's proposition that the self has been constituted.[43] Notable in the interpretation Sløk proposes is his thesis that theologically substantiated necessity includes that very

43. J. Sløk, *Die Anthropologie Kierkegaards* (Copenhagen: Rosenkilde & Bagger, 1954), pp. 61–62.

element of mutability. According to this interpretation, the concept is supposed to indicate that I relate correctly to the hardly bearable circumstances I am expected to assume with my factual existence and being-as-I-am only when I accept that they cannot be altered by me and at the same time I also believe that they can be cancelled by God. Thus, factuality attains its sense of necessity by being accepted, yet not, however, accepted as unalterable because accepted from God's hand.[44] It seems even more likely that the Kierkegaardian concept actually possesses such a motivation when one understands its dialectical version—which declares necessity to be nonnecessity—as an answer to the Greek concept *anankē*—which interprets the constraints of nature and the toils ensuing therefrom as fate, which not even the gods can alter.

Such use implies that Kierkegaard also realigns the meaning of the word "possibility," used in place of freedom, from the aspect of the proposition that the self has been constituted. Its realignment makes anticipatory use of the concept with which Kierkegaard identifies the concept of God—by no mere coincidence only later in the course of his concrete analysis of despair: "God is that all things are possible, and that all things are possible is God" (p. 172). The necessary can only be also not necessary because for and with God it is the possible. The conclusion Kierkegaard drew from Luke 1:37, identifying God with universal possibility, must in turn, however, have consequences for the possibility belonging to man's being. If we understand this from the bottom up, it reveals itself to be the sum of all that is possible for man because God has rendered it possible.

2.2.2 *Man "is" a synthesis.*   From our explication of the concept of possibility it may already be inferred that I.1 with respect to the synthesis of necessity and possibility, together with I.3, presupposes the theory of despair sketched in II. This dependency upon II, which is of dominant interest to us, finally becomes evident when we call to mind the sense in which man as he is portrayed at

44. For the psychoanalytical reception of Kierkegaard's concept of acceptance, see A. Wenkart, "Self-Acceptance," in Rubins, ed., *Developments in Horney Psychoanalysis,* particularly p. 170.

the beginning of *The Sickness unto Death* "is" the synthetic relation between the aspects described above.

He "is" a synthesis, in Kierkegaardian terms, not in the sense that without any further ado on his part he is simply given as such. For only the self synthesizes necessity and possibility, the finite and the infinite, the temporal and the eternal. By pointing to the self Kierkegaard answers the question of what spirit is. Yet in respect of the spirit, it is written in the treatise on anxiety: "In that moment when the spirit constitutes itself, it constitutes the synthesis"; before then the spirit is 'not real' (IV,353). Of course, before the spirit constitutes the synthesis, in a certain sense the person also is not real. Kierkegaard indicates this lack of reality by dissolving the person into a relation, thereby expressing that a person who is not yet a self also has no substantial being; he is by no means ready-made substance. One cannot even say that he exists substantially in the aspects of the relation, for they only become what they are in relation to each other (i.e., aspects) when they are being synthesized. Only thus do they become human. Temporal-finite necessity is in itself an inhuman reality, the brutality of a *factum brutum* or the bare actuality of the given; eternal-infinite possibility is in itself an inhuman ideality, the abstractness of a *fictum* or of the merely possible that for me is no real possibility.

Thus, there is really nothing from which one could deduce what the self is. The self of the human being is the human being himself. But if before becoming himself man has no specific reality, then one can also not specify what comes to itself when he comes to himself. To be sure, contrary to one's first impression Kierkegaard defines the self in I.1, where he takes for his immediate subject what "is not yet a self." Man's being a self may not be complete, but it is already essentially determined when determined as synthesizing. It consists for Anti-Climacus, as well as for Climacus (cf. VII, 289), in "holding together" the contrary factors whose relation man is. Anti-Climacus is thinking of such holding together when he formulates this sentence, "But to become oneself is to become concrete" (p. 161). For he conceives becoming concrete, trusting in Hegel's etymology of the word *concrescere,* as the growing together of elements that separately would be abstract. Later he even expressly analyzes the two contrasting nuances of meaning contained in the concept of holding together. According to this view, "the opposites are held together in a double sense: they are held together (continentur), not allowed to separate from one another; but by being thus held together the differences display themselves all the more strikingly, as when one speaks of holding colors together: opposite juxta se posita magis illucescunt" (p. 261). In realizing himself man holds together the limbs of the relation that constitutes him, first in the sense of uniting them, secondly in being aware of them as extremities.

Of course, all these explanations already presuppose that becoming oneself is indeed an act of synthesizing. However, this presupposition seems to be rendered legitimate only by the definition of man as a relation. Surely, it is somewhat plausible to say that from the relationship character of man the challenge follows of holding the limbs of the relation together. However, the definition of man as a relation rests in truth on a previous understanding of becoming oneself as synthesizing. The whole, in itself obscure, complex of assertions—which characterizes man as a relation, introduces the relation as a synthesis, and names its factors by falling back on more or less conventional dualisms— finally gains in intelligibility only in light of the statement that becoming oneself fulfills the function of holding together. Yet whence does this statement claim its justification?

It is justified solely by Kierkegaard's looking ahead at despair. In the section where Kierkegaard views despair "in such a way that one reflects only on the factors of the synthesis," he distinguishes between the two basic forms that Karen Horney and others[45] have proposed for understanding psychic illnesses, relegating two of the four *expressis verbis* dissected types to each of them. The two types that he designates "despair of necessity" and "despair of finitude" have in common that the person gets stuck in his factuality and leads a life adapted to prescribed norms. This is the state of affairs that Kierkegaard somewhat

45. Cf. also, for example, Sugerman, *Sin and Madness*, p. 31.

too subtly expresses when he says that in the despair of necessity man lacks possibility, and in the despair of finitude, infinity escapes him. Correspondingly, too, the difference between "despair of possibility" and "despair of infinitude" is based on a deeper unity, for in both forms man evaporates into his transcendence; in the former he loses himself in fantastic abstractions from his concrete personality, and in the latter he dissolves into innumerable projects for life in which a continuous shift of possibilities substitutes for their realization. Thus the *apeiron* and *peras* forms of despair are contrary deformations of being a person insofar as the individual in the former never reaches out *beyond* himself as factually given and in the latter never *returns* to himself—that is, to his existence in its present condition. The self's inability to reach out beyond itself and its failure to return to itself are, so to speak, the premises from which Kierkegaard draws the conclusion that the act of becoming oneself failed in both forms is identical with the "double movement" that, according to Johannes de Silentio in *Fear and Trembling* (1843), characterizes faith. Becoming oneself, says Anti-Climacus, "consists in moving away from oneself infinitely by the process of infinitizing oneself, and in returning to oneself infinitely by the process of finitizing" (p. 161). However, he reads this definition off precisely those contrary modes of existence in which the double movement is not working.

2.3 The relation of I.2 to II: the self as process without substratum. The differentiation of despair into the two basic forms of not reaching out beyond oneself and of not returning to oneself can be correlated with the distinction subsequently developed between the despair of weakness and that of defiance, as my introductory remarks on the psychologic, psychoanalytic, and psychiatric reception of Kierkegaard imply.[46] With this distinction Kierkegaard merely repeats the division of his subject matter made in the exposition of his theory of despair into desperately not willing to be oneself and desperately willing to be oneself. Thus, the methodical correlation between the distinction as elucidated and

46. Problems that cannot be discussed here are involved in the kind of coordination which should not be considered an identification.

the initial statement of man's being a synthesis is already conceived in the beginning itself. Like I.3—according to the above
division of the introductory passage—I.1 depends gnoseologi-
cally upon II. Finally, the same dependence pertains between II
and I.2.

We shall now turn to this second anthropological assertion and
its foundation at the root of the theory of despair. In doing so we
must depart from the fact that assertions I.1 and I.2 alternately
presuppose one another. We have seen that Kierkegaard in I.1, at
the same time that he is dealing with his direct subject matter, man
who is "not yet a self," concomitantly defines the self as well.
Conversely, in I.2, where the self is the subject, he makes use of
the definition of man as a relation, which is only later made
explicit in the text. The main point now is how to evaluate what is
added in I.2 to the description of man that is peculiar to the self.

According to the description of the self Kierkegaard gives, the
specific difference between it and man as a "selfless" being seems
to lie in the self's reflectivity. Yet if one were to assume that Kierkegaard actually defines the self by reflexivity, one would be im-
puting to him first of all a violation of the logic of defining. Seen as
a definition, the second anthropological statement is defective
because it breaks the rule that the definiendum may not be repeated in the definiens. Furthermore, one would have to concede
that Kierkegaard does not yet know what he later expressly
says: *being* oneself is more than self-*consciousness,* namely, will (cf.
p. 160)—and that, moreover, he has a dubious notion of self-
consciousness. The latter would imply that he falls back behind
Fichte, of whom his choice of words and train of thought in the
text remind us. For Fichte himself had already penetrated the
notion that self-consciousness is reflexive consciousness and
found it dubious.[47] From the assumption that Kierkegaard
equates being a self with self-consciousness would follow that in
taking the step in which he goes beyond Fichte he was utterly
blind to its relevance. For what is new with Kierkegaard over and

47. Cf. D. Henrich, *Fichtes ursprüngliche Einsicht* (Frankfurt: Vittorio Klostermann, 1967).

against idealism is precisely the existential character of being a self, which as such cannot be reduced to a phenomenon of consciousness.

If one follows the inner logic of the beginning of *The Sickness unto Death* and not its external appearance, then one also comes to a different conclusion: Kierkegaard can at the most ascribe reflexivity to the self as one of two predicates. The other predicate is pure processuality. For this, too, is left over, according to the text, when one throws the self into relief against everything human that "is not yet self." The train of thought in I.2 fulfills even the sole purpose of bringing this out: the assertion that the self is a relation which relates to its own self must be corrected, because the self is nothing but the occurrence *that* the relation relates to itself. In fact, Kierkegaard makes the notion of pure processuality so fundamental that reflexivity by contrast is diminished to a secondary characteristic. He creates the impression that both predicates are equally fundamental only because he is still under the spell of the Hegelian thought that any process without a substratum must *eo ipso* be self-referent. Kierkegaard was hardly moved to escape from this influence, as he sought to find the absoluteness that he, together with Hegel, ascribed to the process without substratum, in reflexivity as well. For, again with Hegel and the whole Aristotelian tradition, the absoluteness of infinite reflection seemed to him certain.

To make use of the connection established between the concept of the self developed in I.2 and the exposition of the concept of despair, we must therefore take a closer view of this pure processuality. In doing so we must not forget that it, too, is merely a property of holding together, as we know being oneself from I.1. Being oneself is in its concrete connotation a holding together, both uniting and extremitizing at once, of factors of a relation that man, in being himself, reveals himself to be, a holding together having the form of a process without substratum. The application to the self, however, of the idea of the pure act (*Tathandlung*), which was Fichte's characterization of the absolute ego, is in *The Sickness unto Death* a hypothetical procedure compelled by the need to formulate the conditions that render possible the despair already sighted in reality. We gain insight into this procedure in the section, early in the work, on the "possibility and actuality of despair."

Aside from the actuality of despair named by the title of this section, yet another actuality is the theme here, namely, that of successfully being oneself, a state in which—as the end of the very first section declares—"despair is completely eradicated." This actuality has an unusual status in respect to possibility, according to Kierkegaard. For actually being oneself is no "fulfilled" possibility like ordinary actuality; it is merely "the annihilated possibility" of despair. The latter can only be prevented from becoming a competing reality when its possibility is annihilated *incessantly:* "if it is to be true that a man is not in despair, he must annihilate the possibility every instant" (pp. 145 ff.). Therefore, being oneself— and therein lies its negativity—succeeds exclusively *in constant carrying out* of the annihilation of the possibility of despair. Only this insight enables Kierkegaard to realize his program of pure processuality. His apparently traditionalistic interpretation of the self as *Tathandlung* is based in truth on the experience that despair can break through at any moment. It formulates only a necessary condition man must fulfill if he does not want to fall prey to despair.

It is easy enough to put this to the test. The observation on the actuality of being oneself made in "Possibility and Actuality of Despair" returns at the end to characterize the actuality of despair. Here Kierkegaard illuminates factual despairing under the aspect of its duration and compares it in this light with natural illness. While a natural illness arises at a certain point in time and continues from there until another time, without one's continually contracting it, man can only find himself in his despairing "state," which precisely for this reason is not really a state, because he is continually casting himself into despair. Therefrom Kierkegaard derives his instructions to "trace" the actuality of despair "back to possibility." If we follow these instructions, we reach the conclusion: the actuality of despair is one and the same with not annihilating its possibility. Being oneself is accordingly such an unremitting process that it turns promptly into its opposite if the annihilation of the possibility of despair ceases for a single moment.

One may well object that for the explanation of despair, which incessantly threatens to overwhelm man, the restlessness of the process to which Kierkegaard reduces the self appears indeed to be a reasonable hypothesis but that the absoluteness he claims for the process because it has no substratum does not. One would have to concede to such an objection that his making the self absolute certainly has no adequate support in the preliminary concept of despair. Yet it is another question whether Kierkegaard bases his assertion of the self's absoluteness on a trait gleaned from despair that, even if it is per se nothing absolute, can be interpreted metaphysically in the sense of the assertion. And that is really the case. We realize this as soon as we confirm the overlapping connection of "Possibility and Actuality of Despair" with "Despair is 'The Sickness unto Death'" and "The Universality of This Sickness." Kierkegaard makes this connection by continuing the comparison begun at the end of "Possibility . . ." between the "sickness in the spirit" and natural illness in the two following sections. Just as he distinguishes between the duration of natural illness and *creatio continua,* on the strength of which despair has no continuity separable from its origin, so he also contrasts against the same background the impossibility of despair's willing to put an end to itself (in "Despair is 'The Sickness . . .'") and the lack of a beginning of despair (in "The Universality . . ."). According to the former, despair is "self-consuming, but it is an impotent self-consumption which is not able to do what it wills" (p. 149). The following section culminates in the sentence: "As soon as despair manifests itself in a person, it is manifest that the person was in despair" (p. 155). The theme here is that despair does not have the beginning in which its subject first believes, and the thesis of the preceding section emphasizes that it does not have the end for which its subject strives. Such an, as it were, negative eternity, however, points to the endlessness and beginninglessness to which the circle movement—which the self according to the first section executes—owes the predicate of the absolute inherited from metaphysics.

2.4 Final determination of the relation between I.3 and II: having been constituted per se.

   2.4.1 Possibility and actuality of the self.   Our task was to demonstrate that the concept of the self, which in *The Sickness unto Death* makes the beginning of the presentation, itself is the result of an investigative process whose point of departure is despair. To that end it was necessary to go beyond the first section and draw on further sections, particularly "Possibility and Actuality of Despair." Here we must once again look ahead to something that appears later in order to prepare, by means of a concluding clarification of the concept of self introduced in I.2, the still-missing answer to the question of the self's being constituted per se, maintained in I.3.

   Later material must be considered in the concluding clarification of the self because the determination of the self essential to the strategy of presentation is not merely explained and rendered concrete in the course of the book but itself undergoes a fundamental change. This shift, as well, has to do with Kierkegaard's treating the self with continuous regard to despair. We encounter here the situation already introduced in defense of the proposed interpretation against the objection nearest at hand; we find, namely, that the preliminary concept of the self, whose form is that of the dialectical presentation, transforms itself qualitatively in passing through the matter of despair. Kierkegaard is evidently only partially capable of apprehending the self from the outset as it ought to be grasped from the perspective of despair. Not in spite of but rather because of its being his most individual subject, in the formulation of the statement with which he introduces it he remains obedient for the most part to a terminology in which the philosophical tradition expressed precisely what is not the self. Despair must instruct him on the self to such an extent that this concept itself only becomes clear, or at least somewhat clearer, through its progressive description. It is no coincidence that he resorts here to the same categories that he employs when trying to elucidate the process of despairing and nondespairing existence—"possibility and actuality of despair." Possibility and actuality are just as much the modal qualifications that predominate in his revision of the concept of self drawn up initially.

Wherever Kierkegaard really conceives possibility and actuality as characteristics of the self, he places them in a relation to each other constructed inversely to the synthetic relation between possibility and necessity. In the synthesis that defines man per se, not in that which constitutes his being a self, possibility is dependent upon necessity as that which is given. In the self possibility is the absolutely primordial, which can neither itself be called actual nor rest on any prior actuality. The self assigned man as possibility bears in *The Sickness unto Death* the title of "the self κατὰ δύναμιν." But "the self κατὰ δύναμιν does not actually exist; it is only something that must come into being" (p. 161). This conception adopts the initial view of the self as a process without substratum in a form modified by modal theory.

Now in the compass of his attempt to render the initial determination of the self more specific by means of the concepts "possibility" and "actuality," Kierkegaard certainly also makes use of the modal difference through which he had defined the synthesis, the difference between possibility and necessity. "The self κατὰ δύναμιν is just as possible as it is necessary; for though it is itself, it has to become itself. Inasmuch as it is itself, it is necessary, and inasmuch as it has to become itself, it is a possibility" (p. 167). It is nonetheless to be noted that Kierkegaard here implants the difference "possible"-"necessary" into the context of the self conceived according to possibility. The concept of a possibility that embraces the difference "possible"-"necessary" is modeled after the figure of the whole that contains itself and its opposite developed in the Hegelian dialectic.[48] The following sentence aims at this kind of overlapping possibility: "The self is reflection, and imagination is reflection, it is the counterfeit presentment of

48. Concerning the dialectical concept of the whole, see M. Theunissen, "Krise der Macht. Thesen zur Theorie des dialektischen Widerspruchs," in *Hegel-Jahrbuch 1974* (Cologne: Pahl-Rugenstein, 1975), pp. 318-29; *Sein und Schein. Die kritische Funktion der Hegelschen Logik* (Frankfurt: Suhrkamp, 1978), particularly p. 28.

the self, which is the possibility of the self" (p. 162). The self's possibility, equivalent to the self *kata dynamin* treated above, is that which appears in the appearance that Kierkegaard, following Hegel, construes reflection to be, or it is that which is imagined in the productive imagination, which via inspiration from Kant and Fichte provides the meaning of Kierkegaard's own concept of fantasy; yet the self's possibility is this in such a way that it itself remains in original unity with reflection or fantasy. Thus Kierkegaard handles it, too, in an idealistic fashion that is with reference to the theory of intellectual intuition developed by Schelling in which the intuited object has no autonomy outside the act of intuition. The self as possibility *is* imagining itself, and it is nothing else because only thereby does a self-image come into being. The self in its determination of actuality must be understood as just such processuality, for actuality here means a self-actualizing that makes the image created by imagining oneself actual. As this process of self-actualization, actuality can by no means occupy the position held by necessity in the synthesis. And also the necessity implied by possibility must be related to this possibility in a way quite different from the synthetic relation of necessity to possibility. The question of what it is, positively expressed—if no pattern for the possibility of self—can be answered with a view to the identification of this possibility with creative imagination thus: it is *having* to imagine oneself. The possibility to be actualized contains the necessary as the necessity of itself.

2.4.2 The necessity of the self's possibility. We have now arrived at the point at which we can resume the work on I.3 left incomplete above. It remained to be seen with respect to I.3 how in contradistinction to the self's having been constituted *by God*, which in its entirety at the beginning must be merely acknowledged, the self's having been constituted per se, initially knowable, can be conceived. The expectation was expressed that the clarification previously made for I.3 of the methodical connection also existing between the two initial theses and the theory of despair expounded in II can be of assistance here. The wording Kierkegaard later gives to the concept of self formulated in I.2 confronts us precisely with the problem that the state of having been constituted per se already became visible with it. This reconfirms the assertion that the backward reasoning by which II guarantees I is continued in the relation of the theses of I among themselves. The proposition of the self's having been constituted substantiates the characterization of the self earlier in the presentation, merely making the conditions explicit, without which the characterization cannot be adequately appreciated.

In this connection we must bear in mind that the web of substantiating relationships within I also here points beyond I.3 to the theory of despair propounded in II. For, indeed, Kierkegaard can clearly visualize the constellation within which the state of the self's having been constituted per se already emerges from the general concept of the self, the constellation into which in the case of the self possibility and actuality enter, only in the course of the explication of his thought on despair. Thus, we must still futher differentiate the distinction made in interpreting I.3 between that which must be simply acknowledged at the beginning and that which can be known from the outset. At the beginning, strictly speaking, there is no such thing as being absolutely evident in Husserl's sense of perfect intelligibility in and of itself. The proposition of the self's having been constituted—provided that the entire doctrine of the possibility and actuality of the self is in fact concealed in it—is understandable on the spot, at least in the concrete sense Kierkegaard demands, only via the insight into the idea of despair this doctrine articulates.

We glimpse that which in its thus restricted meaning is immediately knowable in I.3 when we begin by asking why Kierkegaard felt it imperative to replace the concept of freedom, which he had at first used as a title for one aspect of the synthesis, with the concept of possibility. He was undoubtedly moved to this step by his striving for maximal differentiation between merely being human and being a self. This motive, however, rests on the idea that the concept of freedom must be reserved to the self per se because it coincides absolutely with freedom. The copula of the lapidary sentence, "The self is freedom" (p. 160) functions as a sign of identity. The self is, as Kierkegaard wrote just preceding this, "a relationship which, though it is derived, relates itself to itself, which means freedom." According to this, "freedom" does not accrue to the self as a predicate merely inherent in it. Kierkegaard's identification of freedom with relating itself to its own self indicates rather its identification with the self, which itself should indeed be identical with relating itself to its own self.

Now it is the totality of the possibility and actuality of the self that Kierkegaard reduces to the concept of freedom. The self is freedom, according to his view, as the pure process of self-imagining and of self-realization (cf. II, p. 231). Therefrom follows how the self's having been constituted per se should be determined: it amounts to the necessity that is contained in the possibility of the self as a factor. In the dimension of immediate phenomenological demonstrability the self's having been constituted means the necessity even of its possibility. We may therefore translate this formula obtained by the analysis of the self concept directly into the concept of freedom. If we do so, a situation results that I have on a previous occasion with respect to freedom characterized thus: "It is free in respect to everything allowed to possibility by prescribed necessity, but it is not free to be or not to be the freedom that it is. For itself it is unqualified necessity."[49]

It is quite obvious that freedom is not free for itself. This fact and only this fact supports the self's having been constituted, which I call its having been constituted "per se" because no arguments are required to justify its assertion beyond the phenomenological *hic et nunc* verifiable experience of man with himself. Of course, we encounter here, too, the previously established fact that Kierkegaard's negativistic method subjects even the apparently evasive vestiges of a priori intelligibility to the conditions it dictates. For in such concreteness as that in which Kierkegaard would like to demonstrate the necessity of freedom indicated here we come to know even this necessity only if we have already traced the way back with him from later in the presentation. For in a concrete manner Kierkegaard derives the self's having been constituted per se from the fact that the despairer wants to get rid of himself but cannot do so. In his view, only

49. Theunissen, "Sören Kierkegaard," p. 506.

through this impotent attempt do I experience existentially that I could only escape from the necessity of being free if I were to sacrifice myself along with it and choose death.

The fundamental significance of this procedure for Kierkegaard's methodical negativism becomes obvious through the systematic relevance of the phenomenon, from which Kierkegaard demonstrates the necessity of freedom as experienced reality. Wanting to get rid of oneself is in his view not merely coincidental despair, let alone a reaction to it. The reducibility of all despair to desperately not willing to be oneself means for him that all human despairing boils down to wanting to get rid of oneself. That "the second form of despair (in despair at willing to be oneself) can be followed back to the first (in despair at not willing to be oneself)" can also be formulated: "To despair over oneself, in despair to will to be rid of oneself, is the formula for all despair" (p. 151). Yet desperately wanting to get rid of oneself would not be what it is—namely, desperate—if not being able to get rid of oneself did not belong so inexorably to it as wanting to get rid of oneself does to despair. By making the self's having been constituted per se understandable, without prejudice to the evidence it bears in and of itself, from the fact that the despairing subject wants to get rid of himself and cannot do so, he presents it to the reader principally in the same way as the self's having been constituted by God, namely by referring back to it from the midst of despair.

Index